W9-CBW-021

Fourth Edition

Patient Practitioner Interaction

An Experiential Manual for Developing the Art of Health Care

CAROL M. DAVIS, PT, EdD, MS, FAPTA

PROFESSOR AND ASSISTANT CHAIR
DEPARTMENT OF PHYSICAL THERAPY
UNIVERSITY OF MIAMI MILLER SCHOOL OF MEDICINE
CORAL GABLES, FLORIDA

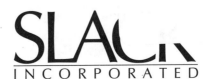

SLACK
INCORPORATED

Delivering the best in health care information and education worldwide

ISBN 10: 1-55642-720-4
ISBN 13: 978-1-55642-720-6

Patient Practitioner Interaction, Fourth Edition Instructor's Manual is also available from SLACK Incorporated. Don't miss this important companion to *Patient Practitioner Interaction: An Experiential Manual for Developing the Art of Health Care, Fourth Edition*. To obtain the instructor's manual, please visit http://www.efacultylounge.com.

The procedures and practices described in this book should be implemented in a manner consistent with the professional standards set for the circumstances that apply in each specific situation. Every effort has been made to confirm the accuracy of the information presented and to correctly relate generally accepted practices. The author, editor, and publisher cannot accept responsibility for errors or exclusions or for the outcome of the application of the material presented herein. There is no expressed or implied warranty of this book or information imparted by it.

The work SLACK publishes is peer reviewed. Prior to publication, recognized leaders in the field, educators, and clinicians provide important feedback on the concepts and content that we publish. We welcome feedback on this work.

Davis, Carol M.
 Patient practitioner interaction : an experiential manual for developing the art of health care / Carol M. Davis.-- 4th ed.
       p. ; cm.
Includes bibliographical references and index.
ISBN-13: 978-1-55642-720-6 (softcover)
ISBN-10: 1-55642-720-4 (softcover)
1. Physical therapist and patient. 2. Allied health personnel and patient 3. Professional socialization.
 [DNLM: 1. Physical Therapy Techniques. 2. Burnout, Professional--prevention & control. 3. Helping Behavior. 4. rofessional-Patient Relations. WB 460 D261p 2006] I. Title.
RM705.D38 2006
610.69'6--dc22

                                          2005022063

Printed in the United States of America

Published by: SLACK Incorporated
                  6900 Grove Road
                  Thorofare, NJ 08086 USA
                  Telephone: 856-848-1000
                  Fax: 856-853-5991
                  www.slackbooks.com

Last digit is print number: 10   9   8   7   6   5   4   3   2   1

DEDICATION

This edition of *Patient Practitioner Interaction* is dedicated to:

Geneva R. Johnson, PhD, PT, FAPTA—collegue, mentor, and dear friend.

My students and graduates who embody therapeutic presence.

My family and friends who help nurture my soul and keep my quadrants balanced and my lenses straight.

and to Jamie, for the fourth time, for supporting the original work, and the subsequent editions.

Thank you, each of you, from the bottom of my heart.

Carol M. Davis
Miami Beach, Florida
2005

CONTENTS

Dedication .... *iii*

Acknowledgments .... *vi*

About the Author .... *vii*

Contributing Authors .... *viii*

Preface .... *ix*

Preface to the First Edition .... *x*

Foreword .... *xii*

SECTION I: AWARENESS OF SELF **1**

   Chapter 1:   Basic Awareness of Self 3

   Chapter 2:   Family History 17

   Chapter 3:   Values as Determinants of Behavior 33

   Chapter 4:   Identifying and Resolving Moral Dilemmas 55

SECTION II: INTERACTING WITH OTHERS **79**

   Chapter 5:   The Nature of Effective Helping: Empathy and Sympathy vs Pity 81

   Chapter 6:   Effective Communication: Problem Identification and Helpful Responses 95

   Chapter 7:   Assertiveness Skills and Conflict Resolution 109

   Chapter 8:   Communicating to Establish Rapport and Reduce Negativity 131
                 Using Neurolinguistic Psychology
                 Helen L. Masin, PT, PhD

   Chapter 9:   Communicating With Cultural Sensitivity 149
                 Helen L. Masin, PT, PhD

   Chapter 10: The Helping Interview 167

   Chapter 11: Health Behavior and Effective Patient Education 189
                 Kathleen A. Curtis, PT, PhD

   Chapter 12: Communicating With Persons Who Have Disabilities 205
                 Kathleen A. Curtis, PT, PhD

   Chapter 13: Sexuality and Disability: Effective Communication 221
                 Sherrill H. Hayes, PT, PhD

   Chapter 14: Communicating With the Dying and Their Families 243

   Chapter 15: Stress Management 261

Afterword 277

Index 281

ACKNOWLEDGMENTS

Special thanks to my patients and students who continue to keep this work fresh right in front of me. I get to practice what I write about each day as I interact with them.

Special thanks to my boss, Sherill H. Hayes, PhD, PT, Professor and Chair of the Department fo Physical Therapy, who supports my writing and the infusion of affective domain competencies throughout the curriculum as we constantly work together with our faculty to develop mature healing professional physical therapists at the University of Miami.

Thanks to my collegues, coauthors, and friends—Dr. Helen Masin and Dr. Kathy Curtis—who both serve as marvelous role models of professional compassion for our students, and content experts for me.

Thanks to my good friends who enrich my life, both within and outside physical therapy, and thanks to my my sister Susan and brother Bill who are always there for me with love and a home to come in to Maine.

ABOUT THE AUTHOR

Carol M. Davis, PT, EdD, MS, FAPTA received her undergraduate degree in biology from Lycoming College, an MS in physical therapy from Case Western Reserve University, and a Doctorate in Humanistic Studies (psychology and philosophy) in the School of Education at Boston University.

As a faculty member at the University of Miami School of Medicine, Dr. Davis has served as Clinical Assistant Professor with Family and Internal Medicine from 1983 to 1985, where she coordinated the Fellowship in Clinical Geriatrics, and from 1987 to present, serves as Professor and Assistant Chair of Physical Therapy. Additionally, she has held the positions of clinical staff and clinical instructor at Massachusetts General Hospital, Assistant Professor and Co-Chair *ad Interim* of Physical Therapy at Sargent College of Boston University.

She is an internationally recognized speaker and consultant in teaching and developing curriculum in attitudes and values, ethics, geriatrics, and complementary therapies in rehabilitation. Dr. Davis authored this book, *Patient Practitioner Interaction: An Experiential Manual for Developing the Art of Health Care*, now in its fourth edition. She is the editor of *Complementary Therapies in Rehabilitation: Holistic Approaches for Prevention and Wellness*, now in its second edition, and with Dr. Christine Williams, she coauthored the text, *Therapeutic Interaction in Nursing*.

Today, Dr. Davis is an active researcher, teacher, and practicing physical therapist in Miami, Florida. She conducts research in complementary therapies, clinical geriatrics, and ethics; teaches entry-level doctoral studies and PhD students in physical therapy; and treats patients. She has studied Myofascial Release since 1989 and uses it regularly as a complement to her physical therapy treatments. In 2003, she was awarded the Catherine Worthingham Fellow award for a lifetime of outstanding service to the profession by the American Physical Therapy Association.

CONTRIBUTING AUTHORS

Kathleen A. Curtis, PT, PhD, is Associate Dean *ad Interim* in the College of Health and Human Services and former chairperson of the Department of Physical Therapy at California State University, Fresno. Dr. Curtis received her Bachelor of Science degree in Physical Therapy at Northeastern University, Boston, Massachusetts. She received her master's degree in Health Science from San Jose State University and received her PhD in Education at University of California, Los Angeles.

In addition to cofounding the interdisciplinary Disability Studies Institute and the Central Valley Health Policy Institute at California State University, Fresno, she is a well-known speaker and author. She has published extensively in the rehabilitation literature and serves as a manuscript reviewer for several journals. She is a recipient of the California Physical Therapist Faculty Research Award and the prestigious President's Award of Excellence at California State University, Fresno. Her books, *The Physical Therapist's Guide to Health Care, Physical Therapy Professional Foundations,* and *The PTA Handbook* (coauthored with Peggy DeCelle Newman) have been used as texts in a majority of college and university physical therapy and physical therapist assistant professional education programs.

Sherrill H. Hayes, PT, PhD, is Professor and Chair, Department of Physical Therapy, and Assistant Dean for Women's Health at the University of Miami, Miller School of Medicine. She has a bachelor's degree in physical therapy and an advanced master's degree in allied health/neuroscience education from the University of Connecticut, and a PhD in higher education/administration from the University of Miami. She is a former President of the Education Section of the American Physical Therapy Association, and an international consultant in physical therapy education. Her clinical specialties are in neuropathology, neurological dysfunction, and women's health, and she has been teaching sexuality and rehabilitation for over 20 years. She teaches in both the entry-level doctorate (DPT) and PhD programs at the University of Miami.

Helen L. Masin, PhD, PT, is currently a clinical associate professor in the Graduate Programs in Physical Therapy in the Department of Physical Therapy at the Miller School of Medicine at the University of Miami. She also holds joint appointments in the Department of Psychiatry and Behavioral Sciences in the University of Miami School of Medicine and the Department of Pediatrics. She received her Bachelor of Science in Physical Therapy from New York University, her Master of Medical Science in Pediatric Physical Therapy and Education from Emory University, and her PhD in Educational Leadership from the University of Miami.

Her clinical experience in physical therapy has included hospitals, public schools, private practice, and child development centers. She served as Director of Physical Therapy at the University of Miami Mailman Center for Child Development for 14 years. Currently, she teaches in both the entry-level DPT and the PhD programs in physical therapy.

Dr. Masin's professional interests include pediatric assessment and treatment, clinical education, professional socialization, communications, and intercultural aspects of health care. She is a consultant in physical therapy for the Debbie School Program for children who are Deaf and Hard of Hearing. Dr. Masin is certified in Neurodevelopmental Treatment in Pediatrics (NDT) and Sensory Integration and Praxis Testing (SIPT). She is a certified practitioner in Neurolinguistic Psychology (NLP) and assists in teaching NLP for Health Professionals, as well as for Self Development at the University of Miami School of Medicine. She is a certified instructor for the Rape Aggression Defense Systems (RAD) and teaches the course for students, faculty, and staff at the University of Miami.

Dr. Masin has consulted with a wide variety of organizations in the utilization of NLP to enhance rapport, facilitate team building, promote cultural competency, and resolve conflict. She has taught the principles of NLP for a wide variety of organizations. She has published articles on incorporating NLP principles in clinical settings, and has been a contributing author in two physical therapy textbooks.

PREFACE

"One of the nicest things that happens to you when you write a textbook," I wrote in the Preface to the Second Edition of this text, "is that people who know you only from your written work feel free to come up to you in a crowd and begin talking to you about what you've written, as if you were picking up a conversation you'd started long ago. What a pleasure it has been for me to receive feedback from many over the past 4 years in this and other ways." Well, it is now 2005 and this is the Fourth Edition; the years have now grown to 15, and I feel even more strongly about this. As with all previous editions, the nature of my approach has been to use many examples from my life, from my students, and from my patients, so that the material in the text really does give readers information with which to converse with me on a more personal basis. I have enjoyed this tremendously, and I thank all of you who have given me helpful suggestions about what worked for you from previous editions, and what didn't.

The changes—the improvements—that are here in the Fourth Edition are nicely summarized in the Foreword, graciously written by my close friend, colleague, and most valued mentor, Geneva R. Johnson, PhD, PT, FAPTA. This book includes the entire Preface to the First Edition, in which I tell a story that it was she who sat me down in 1986 and instructed me to get my ideas about values and ethics, professionalism, and communication skills down in a textbook that could be used in health professional education. I am eternally grateful to her for her support in my work and in my life.

Again from the Preface of the Second Edition, "I've been teaching since 1971, and more than ever I feel grateful for each of my students who helped me to refine this material for maximum usefulness and relevance to them in their professional careers. Every once in a while, I hear from them in serendipitous ways. They share important news with me about their growth and their professional and personal lives. I feel humble to have walked the path with each of them for awhile, and am grateful when something I say or have written makes their way easier or more effective.

"One of the intentions of this book is to assist the reader in deciding the best thing to do for the patient when the system would insist otherwise. Since the publication of *PPI*, First Edition, my mother died. Her death was an important moment for me in many ways, for, along with my twin sister Susan, I was able to be with her and hold her hand as we kept the 17-hour vigil. We were both tested by a series of events, and by people who would have allowed her dying to be more traumatic and painful than it was. Because we persisted in fighting assertively for what we knew she wanted, and what we knew was right and humane to do, she died peacefully and with dignity.

"I have come to see that writing this text has helped me to clarify and integrate principles that have resulted in a richer life for me as a health professional. I am grateful for my boss, Sherri Hayes, who encourages me to do the things that I most love to do. I am grateful to my colleagues at the University of Miami and in Physical Therapy for their collegial support, and for encouraging me to research and write about matters that are not circumscribed by pure thought or theory alone. Most of all, I am grateful to my kindred spirits around the world who are ready in a heartbeat to be present to me in all my incompleteness. They are the ones who assist me with keeping my quadrants balanced. In their hearts, they know who they are, and I am there with them in that knowing. Thank you."

And again, from my perspective in 2005, thank you from the bottom of my heart.

PREFACE TO THE FIRST EDITION

This book is a workbook designed for students and professionals who are willing to embark on a path of growth, specifically, the path of professional socialization. The professional socialization process is an induction into a professional role. When novices become health professionals, they are expected to learn how to act as professionals. Historically, it was assumed that this learning how to act would take place automatically along with the incorporation of new knowledge and skills. Students were expected to develop a kind of sixth sense and, with careful observation, grasp the right things to say and do, and discern the right values and attitudes to embody as a professional. If one failed this process of osmosis, he or she stood out from the rest and became suspect.

We now understand the process of professional socialization more adequately, and realize that novices and young professionals can be assisted in learning the professional role. This text is designed to help this process.

How can a text/workbook assist you to grow, to change, to mature, to develop as a mature healing professional? This book represents one aspect of the socialization process that will offer you material to read, reflect upon, respond to, and, in general, experience. The goal is to help you, the reader, to think about various carefully chosen topics in such a way as to raise your consciousness about your "self," about your self interacting with the goal of promoting healing, and about your self working with groups with a professional purpose. Using an interactive format, learning is designed to be personally meaningful and as intense as the reader allows. Hopefully, changes will occur in how well you know yourself, your attitudes will be invited to conform to those believed to promote healing, and your perceptions will become clearer and more global, less idiosyncratic and more in line with the norms and values of healing professions.

The text/workbook format is designed for individual interaction. Section I is devoted to helping you increase awareness of your "self." One's basic attitudes, beliefs and values are rarely examined and less often discussed. But those basic constructs are the framework upon which judgments are made and comprise the fundamental operating principles out of which our perceptions of ourselves and the world emerge. Each of us carries around a kind of voice which tells us things about the world, even when the opinion of that voice isn't asked. What are your basic beliefs about yourself, about people in general, about men versus women, about old people and children, about rapists and murderers? What are your feelings about your body? What perceptions do you have about your communication skills, your ability to be helpful? What right do people have to health care? What is stressful to you? How do you handle stress? What are your personal values of compassionate and effective health care?

These beliefs and attitudes lead to a basic philosophy of life which may, in most instances, be quite in harmony with the healing process. But sometimes we find ourselves feeling anxious. Anxiety emerges both when we're not sure about the right thing to do, and when we know the right thing to do, but we don't want to do it. Section I concludes with a chapter that teaches you how to identify and resolve moral or ethical dilemmas.

Section II deals with interaction. The nature of effective helping is explored; a process of assertive therapeutic communication is taught and then expanded to instruction in patient interviewing. A closer look at caring for patients who are dying will assist you in clarifying your ideas about life and death and will give you useful ideas with which to interact in an emotion-laden circumstance. The workbook concludes with a close look at professional stress, or burnout.

These topics represent material I have been using for the last 20 years in my teaching of health professionals. They are offered with the hope that they will assist students and professionals alike in the important growth process on the path to becoming a mature healing professional. Each exercise is followed by an opportunity for you to journal, to write out specific reflections you have about the material just considered. I encourage you to take full opportunity to record your growth as it unfolds.

It is well established that the journaling process is an invaluable aid in the identification of one's feelings as well as one's thoughts. Until you are fully aware of what you feel, as well as think, you unwittingly will act in ways that sometimes don't make sense. A health professional not in full awareness of feeling invites disaster. An invaluable lesson in maturing is to realize that the work that we do will

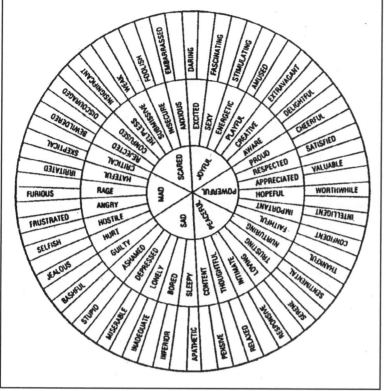

Figure 1. The Feeling Wheel. Reprinted with permission from *Transactional Analysis Journal.* 12(4):276.

inevitably arouse strong feelings. Feelings happen. We can't block them except at great emotional cost. Alternatively, we can identify them and choose how and when to act on them. And assisting you to know how and when to act appropriately is one of the main goals of this text/workbook.

To assist you in the identification of your feelings, the Feeling Wheel (Figure 1) offers a framework that delineates the six basic feelings. The middle circle further refines the basic feelings, and the outer circle describes how one might appear to others while experiencing this emotion. As you journal, if you experience yourself struggling to identify a feeling, this figure might help. College students are overdeveloped in their abilities to intellectualize. Resist the urge to talk about your thought and the facts of the situation, and force yourself to journal about what feelings are aroused by the experience. And remember, feelings are one word. "I feel that" is the introduction to a thoughts, not a feeling. I feel ____ is the expression most useful to discover your emotions around a topic.

This book was first envisioned in Chicago in June of 1986 over lunch with Geneva Johnson, my mentor and friend. Through her encouragement and support, I was linked with Harry Benson from SLACK Incorporated, and the book was conceptualized over lunch in Boston later that year. Harry, Lynn Borders and Cheryl Willoughby at SLACK have been key supporters in the effort, and I thank them for all of their help.

I would like to acknowledge the contributions of all those who have helped me on my path, but the number is great. I would be remiss, however, not to mention the feedback and new learning over the years that I have gleaned from my students, as well as the profound contributions made by Ruth Purtilo, Jane Mathews, Elsa Ramsden, Margaret Moore, Geneva Johnson, Dorothy Pinkston, Don Lehmkuhl, Marjorie Ionta, Dorothy Voss, Marilyn Gossman, Judy Cantey, Brenda Munsey, Helen Hickey, Patricia Yarbrough, Ruth Ouimette, Susan Doughty, Mary Ann Douglas, Victor Kestenbaum, and James Sebert, not only to my professional life, but to my growth as a person as well. And you see, this is what it is all about. One day you realize that who you are as a person and who you are as a professional have merged, gently, delightfully into a comfortable whole. At that point you feel yourself traveling the road to self-actualization. It is my belief that the work you will do with this text will assist you in that vitally important process. So, welcome to a set of experiences designed just for you. Most of all, have fun!

Foreword

The fourth edition of *Patient Practitioner Interaction* remains true to the first one authored by Dr. Carol M. Davis in 1988. That First Edition opened a new era in literature published by physical therapists. In that early, unique work, Dr. Davis shared her knowledge of and experiences in the Art of Healing as an essential complement to the Science of Physical Therapy.

Why does this text merit a Fourth Edition? One answer is that Dr. Davis gave voice to a critical process that lacked prominence in physical therapy curricula in 1988 and that lack continues in some curricula today. With this Fourth Edition, *Patient Practitioner Interaction* has achieved status as a classic in health professional literature.

In later editions of her book, Dr. Davis chose to enhance the content of the original by inviting presentations by other experts in communications. However, none of the superb content of the first edition has been lost in subsequent editions. In this edition, each of the 15 chapters is followed by new and varied exercises that can be used by learners preparing for practice in a health care profession, by new graduates, and by practitioners who have years of experience. The new exercises are designed to reflect the substantial growth of evidence in the past several decades that has changed the practice of all professional health care practitioners. The exercises also reflect the challenge of the changes that will continue to occur as new evidence is uncovered and as health care practices evolve in the years ahead.

With the inclusion in later editions of chapters by three outstanding physical therapists, Helen L. Masin, PT, PhD (Chapters 8 and 9), Kathleen A. Curtis, PT, PhD (Chapters 11 and 12), and Sherrill H. Hayes, PT, PhD (Chapter 13), *Patient Practitioner Interaction* expanded the wealth of knowledge available to learners at any level. Like Dr. Davis, each of these authors has shared a wealth of knowledge and experience in a personal and engaging written format.

Developing knowledge and skills in communicating with therapeutic presence with patients, clients, caregivers, peers, colleagues, supportive personnel and the public requires a commitment to acquiring needed behaviors, such as observation, active listening, careful interpretation of oral and body language, and patience with self and others. The significance of those essential behaviors, and others, is addressed in this text. Beginning with the first chapter, Dr. Davis provides the foundation for the adoption and refinement of communication behaviors by learners who are preparing for practice as health care providers, for novice practitioners, and for experienced practitioners.

The first chapter focuses on enabling learners to gain a perception of themselves as individuals and the impact self-awareness has on their roles in society and on their effectiveness as health care practitioners. Chapter 2 continues to lead learners to a deeper understanding of themselves as individuals who are influenced by many factors in their life history, especially their involvement with parents and siblings. When families live in a loving, supportive atmosphere, children may learn to be responsible, assertive, generous individuals. Conversely, the effect of negative behaviors and attitudes in a family environment that failed to nurture the growth of the individual as a person of worth, may interfere with the development of behaviors expected of health care practitioners. Exercises following this chapter assist learners in identifying both positive and negative influences that have shaped their behaviors as children and adults.

Learners and health care practitioners continually must confront and resolve ethical and moral dilemmas. In Chapters 3 and 4, Dr. Davis discusses the importance of a strong, positive, personal value system as a basis for dealing with and solving those dilemmas. The exercises following Chapters 3 and 4 are designed to encourage learners to identify their value systems and to appreciate the personal experiences that have influenced their value systems and style of making decisions.

In Chapters 5, 6, and 7, emphasis is placed on the communication skills required to interact in a therapeutic and productive manner with others: patients, families, peers, colleagues, supportive personnel, and the public. The exercises following these chapters invite learners to examine the meaning and importance of effective helping, developing the knowledge, skills, and values needed to be an effective helper and an effective communicator, and creating a helping environment.

Chapters 1 through 7 by Dr. Davis are foundational and set the tone for the remainder of this text. The impressive result is the coordination of content to create unity. Comments on the chapters that follow verifies that unity. In the Chapters 8 and 9, Dr. Masin encourages learners to deepen skills in observing the actions of patients and others as they interact in treatment skills, in confronting issues important to the learner and others and skills in establishing rapport with patients and others. Dr. Masin also stresses the importance of understanding the impact of culture on the response of patients and their families to proposed treatments; how to adapt or eliminate some treatment procedures to avoid refusal of treatment on the grounds of invasion of a family's cultural norms; and how to eliminate threats to health care practices dictated by cultural norms. By being sensitive to embedded health care cultures of groups, Dr. Masin believes that, in time, opposition to some scientific treatment measures may be reduced or eliminated. The six universal aspects of health care that exist in all cultures is a sparkling gem that Dr. Masin has added to this book.

In the Chapter 10, Dr. Davis provides the learner with a blueprint for conducting a helpful interview. The principles are applicable to the practitioner as evaluator, diagnostician, planner, and intervener in any environment or situation. Dr. Davis also cautions the learner about those behaviors that can produce an unproductive, even harmful, interview.

In Chapters 11 and 12, Dr. Curtis moves into the application of principles of interaction to the patient or client who needs the unique knowledge, skills, and values of the health care practitioner. She adds to the unity of this text by addressing the factors that influence acceptance of responsibility for prevention of health problems; the significance of how individuals view control of their health care; and the importance of gathering much more than surface data from a patient or client prior to initiating evaluation, establishing a diagnosis, creating a plan of care, and initiating the plan. A discussion of patient education is followed by excellent comments on the planning and presentation of patient education materials and activities.

Chapter 12 is designed to help learners rid themselves of false notions about the person who has a disability. Dr. Curtis presses the learner to accept the person with a disability as an individual who has intelligence, talent, abilities, emotions, needs, and goals—in other words, a person of value who is not seeking pity, but acceptance.

In Chapter 13, Dr. Hayes brings different parts together to make a whole. She writes of sexuality and disability in a direct, sensible manner in a discussion that is under-girded by the basic sciences, the humanities, the social sciences, and the science and art of physical therapy. She has a depth of knowledge that is not common to many health care practitioners. That makes this outstanding chapter one of prime importance for learners in all stages of development. As the population of older individuals grows in number, and more of them have disabling conditions from disease or injury, information in this chapter is vital to health care practitioners, especially those who are in close contact with elders. Frequently, the health care practitioner who sees a person with a disability on a regular schedule becomes the confidant and advisor of individuals who are patients or clients in an out-patient or home environment. This chapter adds another sparkling gem to the treasure trove to be discovered in *Patient Practitioner Interaction*.

In Chapter 14, Dr. Davis presents yet another subject that makes many health care practitioners uncomfortable. Like all of the chapters in this book, linked as they are to the theme of interaction, this one is another gem. From her own experience of being with and preparing patients and others for death, she writes movingly of the opportunity to share that special time with a person who is coming to terms with the end of an earthly life. She cites the effects of death on caregivers because they grieve for the loss of a patient, sometimes long before the actual death. Recovery for those who care for dying persons comes in predictable, but variable stages, described also in Chapter 14.

The relationship of the content in Chapter 15 on stress to the preceding 14 chapters is undeniable. Practice in a busy treatment environment may be stressful, especially for a practitioner who has not developed sufficient coping skills to deal with professional and moral issues that arise daily. Interaction with others—patients, clients, peers, colleagues, the public—may cause extreme stress for some health care practitioners. Dr. Davis describes how stress can threaten the physical, psychological, and emotional well being of health care practitioners. In this chapter, the discussion includes ways to avoid or reduce stress. One practical means available to all is the establishment of behaviors that lead to making timely and effective decisions, especially those that affect the care of patients and clients.

What makes *Patient Practitioner Interaction* so special is the way all chapters are linked to form a sequential, comprehensive, cohesive text that can serve learners at many levels of professional development. Another aspect is that each presenter draws the learner into a thought provoking dialogue as the learning process advances, chapter by chapter. The extensive, pertinent references included with each chapter add to the quality of the text.

Dr. Davis is acknowledged for her ability as a teacher who can engage learners in discussion, no matter how large or small her audience, nor where in the world her audience is addressed. In this exceptional text, her collaborators share that unique ability with her.

Faculty searching for a text designed to foster positive interactive behaviors in their learners will find that *Patient Practitioner Interaction* is the one to adopt.

Geneva Richard Johnson, PhD, PT, FAPTA

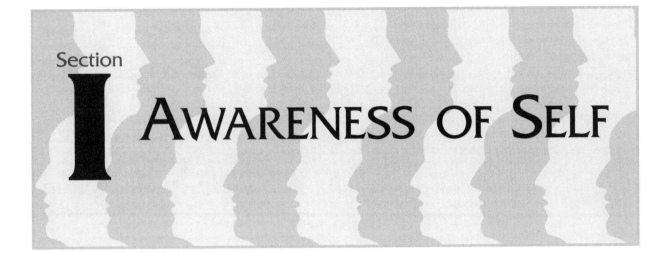

Section I

AWARENESS OF SELF

This first section is composed of 4 chapters: Basic Awareness of Self, Family History, Values as Determinants of Behavior, and Identifying and Resolving Moral Dilemmas. The process of professional maturation requires an in-depth look at who we are at any given time. Who we are includes awareness of our basic ideas, beliefs and feelings about the physical, intellectual, emotional, and spiritual aspects of ourselves. These ideas, beliefs and feelings grow out of the sum total of all our experiences, some say even before birth. **Chapter 1** examines some of our basic ideas about ourselves and the perceptions we hold at this particular time of who we are as individuals. **Chapter 2** takes us back to our growing up years and to the memories we have of the influence our family members had on our current beliefs about the world and about ourselves. **Chapter 3** brings us back to the current day, with an invitation to look at our current values, many of which will directly influence the behaviors we manifest in the therapeutic process. **Chapter 4** examines how we develop our ideas about right and wrong behavior, based on personal values, and how those values can be compared to the values of a profession.

Each chapter begins with a set of objectives which is designed to point out the goals for learning. In order to really learn about your self and your current values, ideas, and communication patterns, it is necessary for you to interact with the content in these pages. Learning implies action, a change in behavior. The more senses involved in the learning process and the more reflection and consideration of thought that the learner expends, the more likely that change will take place in a deep and integrated way. Thus, at the conclusion of each chapter, experiential exercises are offered which are designed to help you achieve the goals for that chapter.

The aim of this book is to teach you how to learn about yourself, about others, and about the world in which you interact with others. And so, in essence, this is a beginning for some, and for others a continuation of lifelong learning that many assert is necessary for effective and compassionate health care. Let's begin!

Basic Awareness of Self

Carol M. Davis, PT, EdD, MS, FAPTA

Objectives

1. To introduce the concept of the "self."
2. To emphasize the importance of self-knowledge in relation to the quality of one's life and the choices one makes.
3. To facilitate self-awareness through reading, completing exercises, and journaling about oneself.

What is the "Self?"

How well do you know yourself? Why would anyone ever ask that question? Some would say that the better you know yourself, the more aware you are of your thoughts and feelings, your strengths and weaknesses, the more you feel in control of your life, then the less stressed and helpless you feel, the less surprised you are by your responses to life. Thus, it might be said that the quality of one's life is, in part, measured by the amount of personal control one feels over day-to-day happenings and choices.

People who are forced to live in institutions to be cared for by others especially feel the negative effect of powerlessness in being forced to succumb to the rules of the larger order, the system. For example, few personal choices are preserved in nursing homes and hospitals.

What is the "self?" How is the self different from the body? What are people asking when they ask, "Who am I, really?" "Why am I here?" These are timeless questions that curiously seem to become more the focus of concern as we live the second half of life than the first. It has been said that the first half of life for many of us is the "doing" half, and the second half of life becomes the "being" half. When we are very busy achieving and working for security and happiness, questions like, "Who am I?" seem distracting. Once we grow beyond our mid 30s, these questions take on greater importance as we reflect on the meaning of life.

Young children are unable to be truly self-aware. But you may remember that delicious moment when you first discovered, all by yourself, that you were uniquely different from anyone in all the world. You were probably 6 or 7. Richard Zaner, in his text, *The Context of Self*,[1] describes a colleague's recounting of this moment:

> *As far as I can tell, I must have been younger than 8 years old when I began having what I now call I-am-me experiences. On such occasions I would tell myself insistently, "This is me, me..." (or rather in my native German: "Das bin ich, ich..."). The inner pronouncing of these words and especially the repetition of the personal pronoun were accompanied with the feeling of a cave-in, a dropping down from a surface level of self-awareness to a more and more personal me-myself. Along with it went a feeling of being sucked down as by a whirlpool into a bottomless depth. As I repeated the pronoun 'me' I felt as if one mask after another fell off until the actor behind these masks was stripped to his naked core.*

To be able to reflect upon the full nature of one's self, however, seems to require the cognitive skills and experience of a person with a mature nervous system. To become aware of oneself, one must go outside of his- or herself and ponder the self and, for example, analyze one's motives for behavior. This only becomes possible, according to Piaget,[2] at the stage of formal operations.

THE DESIRE FOR SELF-AWARENESS

The wish to become self-aware often has to do with the search for meaning in life and the desire to experience a choice in the process of who one is becoming. In other words, the question, "Who am I?" is necessary before one can truly be who one chooses to be.

Parents tell children how to act most often with good intention. Most children are socialized into becoming what their parents or guardians believe are good human beings who will live happy and productive lives. The influence of the family on one's self-esteem and self-concept is a very important topic that will be covered in more depth in Chapter 2.

The goal of health professional education is to assist students in becoming a certain way: *professional*. What does it mean to "be professional"? Much has been written elsewhere about that question. Suffice it to say here that any description of a professional would contain the integration of a body of knowledge and skills and the proficient and effective delivery of the same. In the profession of health care, proficient and effective delivery requires a "therapeutic use of one's self" while interacting with clients. Superior skill in the technology of the profession must be balanced with the art of relating to those who request our services in such a way that healing is facilitated rather than interfered with.

If health care consisted of "working on bodies" alone, perhaps a consideration of the self would not be necessary. But the fact remains that health care involves people interacting with people in such a way that what is not right is correctly analyzed and appropriately influenced so that it is changed to approximate more closely what is right. This analysis and influence takes place between human beings who have not just brought their bodies to us, but have brought their feelings, their fears, their hopes, their frustrations, their pain. Illness is meaningful only as it is lived, moment to moment. When we care professionally, we care for people living with their illnesses, not for broken bodies. Let's take a closer look at the nature of the "self," what it is, what it is not, how it grows and is influenced, and how it performs as we mature into healthy, more "self-actualized" human beings.

THE SELF

Human beings are tremendously complex organisms, capable of portraying various identities or roles depending on what the situation calls for or stimulates. Much study has been devoted

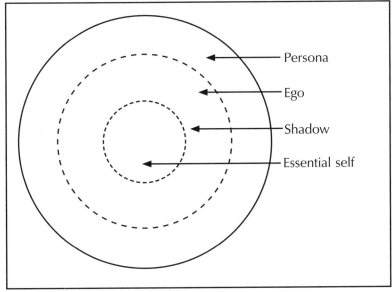

Figure 1-1. The Nature of Self.

to the manner in which we can divide ourselves into various parts or take on different roles and yet still remain essentially the same person, or "whole." Transactional analysis literature teaches about the "parent, adult, and child" in each of us.[3] We each portray various roles throughout the day, such as employee, boss, sister, brother, friend. Carl Jung, in his attempt to explore the nature of the unconscious, described archetypal elements present in all personalities. Among them were the persona, the shadow, and the self. Freud is famous for his explications of the ego, the id, and the superego. All of these now rather common terms were created to help explain the complex behavior of human beings.

The psychology literature informs us about the nature of the self and its role in human growth by way of Figure 1-1. This figure represents the various layers of a person, or the various aspects of a personality. The outermost layer is best described as the **persona**, or the public face each of us puts on in the world in order to appear in control, intelligent, witty, sensitive, and lovable. We act in the ways we believe are going to bring us love and recognition. But deep inside we know that the persona is really a mask. Underneath that mask is another aspect of ourselves that is filled with doubts and insecurities. Almost all of us are dissatisfied with living our lives totally from behind the mask. Each of us desires to drop our false fronts and to become who we truly are, to express ourselves more honestly, to be more truly ourselves and to be loved for it.

The second layer can be seen to be composed of the **ego**, or the center of the conscious mind as described by Freud, and the shadow, the unconscious, "natural" side of our personalities. The ego is the part of us that gets the job of living done. It is the force that gets us through school, that makes choices for us that are designed, as best we can know, to bring us happiness. It problem solves for us and helps us have the courage to act and the patience to wait. But the ego is made up of all kinds of misinformation about ourselves and about the world. Egos tend to be very protective; they tend to move us toward safety, toward the status quo. The ego believes in its own omnipotence. But it has to sustain that belief by using a lot of energy, and by ignoring many messages that would refute that omnipotence. The feeling of a godlike ego is an illusion. In fact, the ego is filled with erroneous ideas and fears about the world and about ourselves. Our egos tell us we're very intelligent one minute, and the next they tell us we're totally naïve and stupid. One minute they tell us the world is a wonderful, loving place and the next that it's a dangerous place.

Each of us tends to listen to the still, small voice of the ego when we have to make important choices, but we become very confused about what is important and true. That's because we tend to allow the voice of the ego to reflect what we've heard from important people in our lives about ourselves. If we heard, "You are so stupid, you'll never amount to anything" when we were young, we believed that for a time, until we had the power to prove that it wasn't true. As we achieved success, we told our egos, "See, I really am bright. I *can* succeed!" But instead of dropping the old data and incorporating the new, the ego holds onto the whole package and spits both messages at us at times when we feel most unable to modify that quiet voice.

The **shadow** is the unconscious part of this second layer. It is our inferior side, the part of us that wants to do all the things our ego tells us we can't do. When we say things like, "I wasn't myself," or "I don't know what came over me," we're acknowledging the presence of our unconscious shadow that tricks us into behaving in ways we say we abhor.

Underneath these outer 2 layers, at the center of the person, lies the rest of us, the "more" that the outer 2 layers can't fully incorporate: **the "self."** The self is the essence of the person, and incorporates both conscious and unconscious elements of the person into itself. I have my persona, I have my ego, I have my personality, I have my body, I have my possessions in life… I am my self. The self is the irreducible energy of my uniqueness. It is the thing that makes me absolutely unique in all the world, in spite of the fact that, for example, I have an identical twin sister, and probably thousands of people share my name. It is that marvelous essence of me that I approach as the masks are, one by one, stripped away in the search for what is undividable, what is at my core. It is the unfolding answer to the eternal question, "Who am I, really?"

The self is that energy that can linger for days before the moment of the "crossing over" into death of the physical body. Those who care for the terminally ill have often experienced the phenomenon that, for a time before the body stops functioning totally, it is more accurate to say that all that remains in the bed is a shell that looks like the person's body. The essence of the person seems to "come and go," little by little spending more time gone than present.

The self has to do with the energy inside each human that reincarnationists say is a piece of the deity that is never created or destroyed.[4] It is my "higher self." Christians would call it the "Christ self" within each of us. It exists for all time; it always has and it always will. And the task of human beings on earth is to house this energy as we grow and change, lifetime after lifetime, with the end goal of becoming more like God, like truth.

Jung says this about the nature of the self:

> *The self… can include both the conscious and the unconscious. It appears to act as something like a magnet to the disparate elements of the personality and the processes of the unconscious, and is the centre of this totality as the ego is the centre of consciousness, for it is the function which unites all the opposing elements in man and woman, consciousness and unconsciousness, good and bad, male and female, etc., and in so doing transmutes them. To reach it necessitates acceptance of what is inferior in one's nature, as well as what is irrational and chaotic. This state cannot be reached by a mature person without considerable struggle; it implies suffering, for the Western mind, unlike the Eastern, does not easily tolerate paradoxes. [The self] consists… in the awareness on the one hand of our unique natures, and on the other of our intimate relationship with all life, not only human, but animal and plant, and even that of inorganic matter and the cosmos itself. It brings a feeling of "oneness," and/or reconciliation with life, which now can be accepted as it is, not as it should be.[5]*

Thus, the self, once uncovered, seems to hold the real truth about us as human beings. It is our connection with the Truth, and it is out of this center of our existence that we come to feel at-oneness with our fellow human beings. It is the self that is able to cross over in empathy and experience and feel what a moment in life must be like for another person. It is the self that we return to as we quiet our working minds in meditation.

It is the self that allays our fears, that gives us true courage rather than braggadocio or false bravado; it is the self that feels the essential goodness of our humanness, in the face of our incompleteness; it is the self that grows in wisdom and becomes more as we mature, approaching the all-knowing goodness of Truth; it is the self that enables us to laugh at our egos and forgive the well-meaning unkindnesses visited upon us by parents and relatives as they tried desperately to get us to "act right" as children and thereby systematically helped to destroy our inborn connectedness with our true selves.

SELF-AWARENESS

Carl Rogers has said, "It appears that the goal the individual most wishes to achieve, the end which he knowingly and unknowingly pursues, is to become himself."[6] How do we become ourselves? How do we discover our true natures? How do we access the self? How do we get close to it, get right up next to it? It begins when we recognize the burning desire to be known for who we are, not for who we believe others want us to be. It begins when we are willing to shed the roles we've assumed in order to win attention and affection and acceptance, and instead commit to being truthful and honest. Often the first steps we take in this direction come with our challenges to our parents and the "rules of the house."

Self-awareness requires reflection in order to ascertain who we truly are. The ego will work overtime to tell you about yourself, but it takes time and an effort of a different sort to reflect deeper, to the messages of the true self.

Often we need help in this process, for our perceptions are unavoidably colored by the messages we heard when we were very young. To sift through unchallenged truths that were reinforced for years (for instance, all women are emotional, all men are insensitive) requires, for example, the perspectives of literature, art, and music and the professional preparation of counselors and psychologists to help us examine our habitual assumptions. The goal of growth of this sort is to expand the narrow, parochial views we held as children and become more aware of a wider world view that incorporates diversity, that trades black and white, dualistic thinking for the wonderful colors of ambiguity, free from the need to be "right," free from the fear of being "wrong." It is, in a sense, the search for truth that we're after as we mature in our world view. We want to enfold all possibilities rather than leave out information that might be critical for comprehending the complexities of ourselves, of our lives, of the world we live in. In the search for the self the goal becomes to give up beliefs that entrap us in negativity, doubt, and self-centered behavior and replace them with beliefs that enlarge our consciousness and help us feel compassion for our oneness with all of life, and sincere interest in the needs of those we serve.

EXAMPLE OF LACK OF SELF-AWARENESS

When we find ourselves distracted from the moment, or if we have never participated in self-awareness activities, patients can suffer from our insensitivity. A recently graduated physical therapist was having a particularly difficult day and was not taking a regular check on his emotions. He went into his patient's room and found the patient engrossed in a conversation with his nurse. The patient was trying to understand the various medications he was taking and their possible side effects. As the physical therapist waited for this discussion to be completed, he became more and more impatient, recognizing he was becoming more behind in his patient treatments for the day. Had he stopped for a second and taken a deep breath, he might have realized first of all that he was annoyed, but second, that this was an important conversation, and he had several choices available to solve his problem. But because he lacked self-awareness and tact, he saw the problem not as his, but as the nurse's. He interrupted the conversation rudely and stated, "Look, I've been waiting patiently here for 5 minutes. I am on a tight schedule, and I have to see this patient next. Please wrap this chat up and let me get to work, will you?"

This lack of self-awareness brought a negative energy into the entire situation, and this could have been completely avoided had the physical therapist, once he recognized his emotion of annoyance and impatience, reviewed his options, and invited the nurse and patient to help him decide when would be a good time to return, as this was obviously an important conversation that needed to continue, and the needs of the patient were more important than his schedule.

Very often the major goal of young people as they become socialized into acting professionally is to recognize that patient care is about patients, not about "me." Patients and their needs come first, and this may be a new perspective for young professionals to adopt. It's all part of growth and development into maturation.

SEARCH FOR THE SELF

This text is designed to help you examine your values, your beliefs, and your communication patterns in an effort to assist you in the search for your self and to broaden your world view. For it is from the self that we give health care of the highest quality. It is the self that has the capacity to see clearly, to display compassion in the face of threat or fatigue, that "crosses over" in empathy. It is the self that sets appropriate boundaries and refuses to attempt to have personal needs met by patients. It is the self that has unlimited patience and great understanding. It is the self that comprehends the need to be ethical and act with integrity. It is the self that has the desire and the capability to feel unconditional positive regard and a oneness with all living beings that cancels out judgement and prejudice.

It is the frightened ego, however, that pities and pretends that it is displaying compassion; it is the frightened ego that becomes impatient and defends itself rather than offering a healing response to the angry patient; it is the ego that needs to be puffed up and made to feel important at the expense of others' feelings. It is the frightened ego that requires our patients to do as we say, to get better, to thank us for helping them.

All of us want essentially the same thing: to be respected, to be treated with unconditional positive regard. But all of us want that positive acceptance of our whole being, not just of our persona, not just of our ego. We want others to love and accept us as we are wholly, in all of our incompleteness.

The more the ego tries to defend itself, the more difficult it is to catch a glimpse of ourselves, our essential natures. If you have been told that you tend to respond defensively to people, you developed this coping skill out of necessity. But it is not very useful in patient care. This will be a good opportunity for you to examine the messages you're receiving that make you feel as if you must defend yourself. Defensiveness always obliterates the truth. It is noisy and useless; it has no sense of humor at all. It is the mark of a person responding to life from an insecure ego, not the sign of a whole and integrated self, that might respond to criticism, for example, with, "I didn't know I was coming across that way. I'll take a closer look at my behavior now."

As health practitioners gain expertise, they find it becomes important to regularly take stock of one's feelings during the day. The emotions are key to what we experience and sometimes we find ourselves disassociating from people in response to feeling overwhelmed with work, or feeling insecure or angry with the system. Regularly experiencing our feelings as they arise in our day becomes an important component of practitioner well-being, and keeps us connected with ourselves, and able to focus on our patients, and the task at hand. Patients appreciate demonstrations of personal caring and responding with emotion to their stories and situations of the day. The expert clinician knows how to do this, and at the same time set appropriate boundaries that allow for therapeutic presence without burdening the patient with our feelings. The more connected we are with our own selves, the more connected we become with our patients and colleagues, and the higher the quality of our caring and efforts.[7]

SIGNS OF GROWTH IN SELF-AWARENESS

As people struggle to become more themselves, usually out of the painful realization that the masks they've been using are no longer bringing them happiness and love, Rogers[6] describes them as changing in noticeable ways.

They seem to:

1. Drop the defensive mask with which they have faced life, and begin to discover and to experience the stranger who lives behind these masks—the hidden part of self.

2. Emerge with a tendency to be more open to all elements of experience; growing to trust in one's organism as an instrument of sensitive living.

3. Accept the responsibility of being a unique person.

4. Develop the sense of living in life as a participant in a fluid, ongoing process, continually discovering new aspects of one's self in the flow of experience.

When we live daily with an awareness of our true selves, negative feelings are confronted and the beliefs behind them are analyzed and replaced with beliefs that are more positive and cosmic. Thus, we take responsibility for creating our own reality, moment to moment. No longer do we allow ourselves to get away with such beliefs as, "You make me so angry." We acknowledge that we make ourselves angry in response to someone, because of a belief we have about that person or that behavior. And then we search for a larger, more hopeful and understanding belief that will replace feelings of negativity.

CONCLUSION

The goal of this entire text is to assist you in learning more about your self, so that the way in which you relate to patients who come to you for help might be sensitive, compassionate, and free from prejudice and negativity. Central to this goal is the assumption that our true or essential selves reflect the essential goodness in all of us, and can be covered up by the persona, the many masks we wear and by the ego that sees the world through lenses that were originally set when we were very young and helpless. The behaviors that facilitate healing as we apply our technology are those behaviors and those underlying beliefs that bring about wholeness and oneness. Behaviors that interfere with healing result in fragmentation, discord, negativity. I believe that it is possible to grow such that the nature of our essential selves is accessible to us, and that, out of a connectedness with our essential selves, we are empowered to provide health care of the highest order. In that connectedness with our essential selves, we have the power to realize the fears and shortcomings of our egos, the falseness and manipulation of our personas. And out of that connectedness with our essential selves we can be the persons we were created to be—capable of unconditional positive regard for all humans. This is the greatest calling of the health care professional. It is a tremendously challenging task to grow to this goal. But the rewards are indescribable.

REFERENCES

1. Zaner R. *The Context of Self.* Athens, Ohio: Ohio University Press; 1981.
2. Piaget J. *The Construction of Reality in the Child.* New York, NY: Basic Books; 1954.
3. Berne E. *Transactional Analysis in Psychotherapy.* New York, NY: Grove Press; 1961.
4. Challoner HK. *The Wheel of Rebirth.* Wheaton, Ill: The Theosophical Publishing House; 1969.
5. Fordham F. *An Introduction to Jung's Psychology.* Baltimore, MD: Penguin Books; 1953.
6. Rogers C. *On Becoming a Person.* Boston, Mass: Houghton Mifflin; 1961.
7. Gordon GH. Giving bad news. In: Feldman MD, Christensen JF (eds). *Behavioral Medicine in Primary Care—A Practical Guide.* 2nd ed. New York, NY: McGraw Hill Medical; 2003:21.

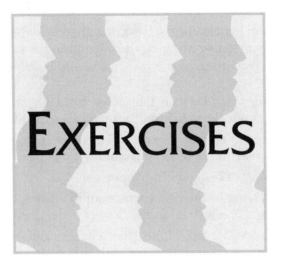

EXERCISES

EXERCISE 1: WHAT'S SO ABOUT ME?

On a separate sheet of paper that you can keep confidential, answer each of the following as honestly as you can for this moment. Allow at least half a sheet of paper for each question. Each question requires reflection, but jot down the first thing that comes to mind, then take time with each question to clearly communicate your awareness (or lack of it)! You may wish to complete the entire set over a period of a week or so, taking one or two questions at a time.

What's So About Me

Date:

1. I would describe myself as…

2. Others would describe me as…

3. I am proudest of…

4. I was most embarrassed when I…

5. I am most annoyed about myself when I…

6. I get angriest when…

7. Under severe stress, I usually…

8. Aspects of my communication that I want to keep and refine are…

9. Aspects of my communication that I want to change include…

10. What I want others to understand about me is that…

11. I'm most anxious that…

12. Characteristics of other people that impress me most include…

13. I protect myself when…

14. I would be willing to die in 6 months if…

15. I don't know how to say…

16. People are essentially (good, bad, neutral)…

17. Goals I want to achieve…

    a. With this course…

    b. In my lifetime…

Discussion

Once you've answered these questions, write a description about yourself from what you've discovered. Are you totally happy with yourself at this point? What would you change? What did you learn about yourself that will assist you in being a health professional? What may detract from your effectiveness? How aware are you of the messages from your ego, of your shadow? How aware are you of your self? Identify responses that have a negative aspect to them. What is the belief that you hold, that makes that answer true for you? What is an alternative belief that you also hold that would replace the negative one so that your response might be more positive and hopeful?

Example: I protect myself when I am criticized for being too unscientific, too naïve or idealistic. Negative belief: I lack the intellect to scientifically prove what I believe is true and important. Replacement belief: The scientific method holds one way of verifying what is true. The balance of logic and facts with intuitive knowing together frames a larger truth. I have proven skills as a scientist, and I have faith in my intuition. Both serve me well in my work.

EXERCISE 2: CLINIC WAITING ROOM EXERCISE

This exercise is designed to help you recognize nonverbal indicators of emotion, and thus keys to inner values, that are often subtle and overlooked, but when recognized can be of valuable importance in communication. The instructor writes one word describing an emotion on a 3-x-5 file card. Words such as: impatient, lonely, sad, eager, peaceful, relaxed, satisfied (see the Feeling Wheel for suggestions in the Preface to the First Edition) are used, and there is one card for each member of the class, and it is kept secret, known only to the holder of the card.

Three chairs are placed side by side in the front of the classroom to represent the waiting room in a clinic.

The exercise starts by having one person come forward, spontaneously, and his or her task is to act out the word on his or her card. Then another person comes forward and joins the first person, acting out his or her word. You can use verbal expression but you cannot use the word on your card. The goal of the rest of the class is to guess what emotion or behavior each person is representing. A third person then comes forward, spontaneously, and the first person gets up and leaves; so there are always 2 people interacting in the "clinic."

Once everyone has had a chance to play act their word, the entire class forms a circle for discussion, and guesses each person's word on their card. Discussion should be focused on the nuances that each person used to convey an exact meaning, for example to "depressed" in contrast to "sad." Finally, discussion should center on how this would be helpful to students in interaction with their patients, and even more importantly perhaps, in self-awareness. How does each student convey feelings of joy? Anger? Impatience? Fear? What about being a health professional is joyful, frustrating, fearful, and how would that look in your behavior? How will you know this?

EXERCISE 3: AUTHENTICITY/AUTONOMY SELF ASSESSMENT TOOL

Reflections from this exercise:

At this moment:

1. How in control of your life do you feel?

| 0 | 1 | 2 | 3 | 4 | 5 | 6 | 7 |

Totally help-
less, a victim

Total control
over my life

2. How in control do you expect to feel?

1 to 1 1/2 years from now

| 0 | 1 | 2 | 3 | 4 | 5 | 6 | 7 |

2 to 2 1/2 years from now

| 0 | 1 | 2 | 3 | 4 | 5 | 6 | 7 |

5 years from now

| 0 | 1 | 2 | 3 | 4 | 5 | 6 | 7 |

3. How well do you know yourself—who you really are and who you really are meant to be, unique in all the world?

| 0 | 1 | 2 | 3 | 4 | 5 | 6 | 7 |

Not a clue;
I constantly
surprise
myself

Very familiar
with who I
am and am
becoming

4. How well do you accept yourself as you are?

| 0 | 1 | 2 | 3 | 4 | 5 | 6 | 7 |

Dislike myself
very much;
difficult to
accept any
part of me

Very com-
fortable with
who I am,
how I am in
the world

5. What are some goals you have in order to obtain the "good life," a life that's good for you?

1.
2.
3.
4.
5.

EXERCISE 4: COLLAGE

With the use of any material, construct a collage that represents you as you know yourself at this moment. Your collage may be comprised of pictures and colors as is the traditional collage, or you may wish to use other materials to construct a less traditional "montage." Do not choose representations of your persona only. Search your heart for symbols of your true self, the part of you that you hold dear but that you do not readily reveal. Also, choose representatives of your ego and your shadow as well. Bring your creation to class wrapped so others cannot identify it. Gather in small groups, place one creation in the center of the group and observe it carefully, without speaking, for 2 or 3 minutes. Gather a private impression of what the creator was trying to convey. Then, in turn, offer observations that you perceive about the person for 5 minutes or so. After this anonymous discussion, identify the creator. He or she then responds to what was observed by classmates, what was "on target" and where classmates missed the mark. Finally, group members should share what each learned about this classmate before bringing forth the next creation.

EXERCISE 5: JOURNAL

At the conclusion of these exercises, begin a journal about yourself during this time. Journal entries are most useful in learning about yourself if they relate what you learned from the experience. Most of us confuse the concept of a journal with a diary. A diary is designed to record significant events in one's life. A journal is a letter to yourself, designed to stimulate reflection about an experience, rather than just recording the experience. One way to keep from simply recording the event is to begin each entry with the following phrases.

❖ What I felt during the exercise.

❖ What I learned about myself.

❖ So what? Significance or meanings of my learning.

Your journal should be kept in a book with a cover, on pages that do not easily become dislodged. Entries are to be written, ideally, following each exercise, but at the minimum following each chapter. Many find it useful to journal as a way of privately discussing the chapter and its personal significance, as well. Your journal is what you make it. Most university students are unaccustomed to this sort of activity, however, and some abhor writing. For a short time, make a commitment to this activity. Don't forget to use the Feeling Wheel which is in the Preface to the First Edition (on page xi). Remember, this journal is by you, for your personal use. Set aside the time on your calendar and once you get into it, the journal will become rewarding. Your course instructor may wish to see your entries now and again to be sure you are keeping up. In that case, confidentiality may become more limited. You will not be graded on your journal. Since it is a collection of your feelings and reflections, a grade would be wholly inappropriate. However, the value of the activity is such that your instructor may collect it to check your discipline with the activity and may comment on how well you reflected on the experience rather than simply describing what happened.

FAMILY HISTORY

Carol M. Davis, PT, EdD, MS, FAPTA

OBJECTIVES

1. To describe, in general terms, the role families play in the formation of identity and self-esteem.
2. To examine the development of a mature personality as described by Erikson.
3. To introduce the concept of the "false self" in relation to the "true self" as it develops in dysfunctional families.
4. To stress the importance of self-awareness to develop authenticity or the awareness of the "true self" as opposed to the "false self," and to stress the importance of the concept of authenticity to effective, mature helping.

It has been said that a clinician's most important tool is the effective use of self. Our personalities and our styles of relating have everything to do with how effective we are in facilitating the healing process. No one wants to be treated unkindly, least of all when we're not feeling well. Yet unkindness abounds in health care settings. If we would ask health professionals to assess their ability to relate effectively with people, few would admit to lapses in temper, prejudicial behavior, irritability, or cutting sarcasm. Yet these and other negative behaviors occur with great frequency.

More difficult to observe are such negative behaviors as lack of honesty, breaking confidences, lack of fidelity to one's colleagues, and causing a patient to become overly dependent on oneself.

You might ask, "Why be a health professional if you can't act in ways that are positive and assist healing?" Often clinicians are unaware of their behavior or its effect on others. Patients challenge our sensitivity and maturity in unique ways. Patients react out of the stress of their illness or pain, but practitioners, also, must work under stress, the stresses unique to health care. It requires great maturity and patience to respond in healing ways in less than ideal situations.

INFLUENCE OF THE FAMILY ON SELF-ESTEEM

Before reading any farther, turn to Table 2-1 and skim through each column. Which column best describes your perception of the family dynamics you grew up with? Place a pencil check beside the phrase in column 1, 2, or 3 that best describes your family for each item listed.

Each of us views the world from a unique perspective. I like to use the analogy of a pair of lenses to illustrate one's worldview. You and I can be looking at the exact same thing, but what I see and hear and feel and experience generally will be different from what you experience because my "lenses" are set differently from yours. We receive our lenses as small children. One's worldview evolves out of what one hears and experiences as a child growing up in a unique family unit. Indeed, we actually develop in the ways that our parents would have us develop because we are, to them, an image on their lenses. Even twins, growing up under the same circumstances, will develop differences in their lenses, based on what each chooses to attend to, to ponder, to emphasize.

Children are not little adults, as Piaget first clearly described.[1] Children have underdeveloped nervous systems and lack the capacity to move, think, and act in the ways that adults can. Children live in a land of make-believe, enjoy fantasy, and are egocentric. They are unable to handle abstract logic, and are very present oriented and concrete. If you ask a child which 1 of 2 parallel, identical pencils is longer, she'll say, correctly, that both are the same length. Then if you slide one pencil so that it is ahead of the other, though still parallel, and then ask, "Which pencil is longer?' she'll say the pencil that is ahead of the other is longer. In other words, children can't conserve information. Likewise, children are unable to come outside of themselves and view themselves, as we discussed in Chapter 1. Ask a child who has a brother if he has a brother and he'll say, "Yes." Ask him if his brother has a brother, he'll say, "No."[2]

Finally, children idolize their parents. Feelings of helplessness and dependence are coped with by believing that Mommy and Daddy are perfect and no harm can come to me as long as they are with me in life.

Erik Erikson[3] has developed a useful description of the development of personality (Table 2-2) that centers on the successful resolution of tension in a series of dialectical steps encountered by the growing person from birth onward. A certain degree of accomplishment is required with each stage as it is encountered, or the child will have to master the goal later. This is similar to the child who skips crawling, wherein critical movements necessary to accomplished gait remain absent. There is a certain level of suffering or pathology that results, even if one seems to be functioning adequately. Table 2-2 summarizes Erikson's theory of development. We will return to this theory in Section II when we discuss the development of effective helping behaviors.

Human beings are among the few living creatures born without the capacity to crawl, wiggle, or walk to a source of food. It might be said that we are 9 months in the womb and 9 (or more) months out, totally helpless to move about to a source of food or nourishment.

We lie there, like blobs, and must wail and cajole to get the attention of the big people around us in order to get our basic survival needs met. The fact that we are born totally dependent on others for our survival is a critical aspect of the development of our worldview, for who we are and how the world is for us depends totally on how we are responded to in our profound neediness and on what we hear others say to us and about us. As a child, I have no identity save what others say about me. It is obvious that the maturity of the parent, and the extent to which the child is wanted and anticipated have a great deal to do with how the parent responds to the child, and thus fosters or inhibits the development of a sense of self-identity and self-esteem.

Few of us grew up in ideal homes. Perhaps you think you are the exception. The fact is that we experience denial, and many of us have difficulty remembering the negative things about our childhood. Remember that little children all think that their parents are perfect. Adolescents give up those notions but replace them with strongly held mores to honor parents and respect them. If parents were emotionally or physically abusive to a child, the child will automatically believe it

Table 2-1		

CHARACTERISTICS OF FAMILIES

Open/Healthy	*Troubled*	*Closed/Unhealthy*
Open to change	Nothing can be done	Rigid, fixed, harsh rules
Flexible responses to each situation	What's the use?	Right vs wrong, no exceptions
High self worth	Shaky self-worth	Evasive responses
People are valued as individuals	Cover feelings of low self-control	Low self-worth, lots of shaming behavior
		Low ownership—blaming
Functional defenses	Use defenses to hide pain	No choice—react compulsively and rigidly out of fear
Uses defenses as coping skill with insight	Defenses more often deny real feelings	Short fuses
	Choice is lost	Lots of avoidance or rage
	Always smile or cry or complain, etc.	
Clear rules discussed	Unclear—Rules inconsistent	Edicts or no rules at all
Hours, respect for property, telephone use, chores, etc regularly negotiated	Depends on who is asked what day, which child, etc	Chaos—rules cannot be followed
People take risks to express feelings, ideas, beliefs	Not safe to express feelings or give opinions: "Don't rock the boat"	Denial of problems
		Ignore bizarre behaviors
	Can't disagree	No talk rule—even about serious problems, especially drinking, drugs
Can deal with stress, pick up on other's pain	Avoid pain	Denial of stress
	Do not see it in others	Can't cope with any more—glazed eyes don't see pain
Nurturing and caring for each other. Seek out those in pain to support, encourage	Sweep problems under the rug	Ignore basic need to be seen, acknowledged
	Pretend all is ok	Children become early helpers
Accepts life stages, welcomes them	Parents may compete with kids—growth is accepted painfully—don't talk about sex	Passage of time is ignored—change is feared—adults treated as children—children may try to act like adults
Celebrates growth—Sexuality, new friends, accomplishments	Try to keep children dependent	Children ridiculed, teased but try to become helpful
Either clear hierarchy or egalitarian—strong parental coalition—less need to control—can negotiate	Hidden coalitions across generations—parental coalition weak—rigid or shifting pattern of domination	Either upside down family—children may run it, or chaotic—no giving out of rules, or one parent in charge of all and can't cope
Affect is open	Negativism, low feeling, bickering, argumentative controlled mood, some feelings okay, some not, inconsistent acceptance of feelings	Cynicism, open hostility, violence, sadism—actually try to manipulate and hurt each other
Direct expression of feelings—all feelings are okay—anger is in context of awareness of other person		Only happiness is allowed
Considerate of others		

Table 2-2

PSYCHOSOCIAL THEORY OF DEVELOPMENT:
A SUMMARY OF ERIKSON'S EPIGENETIC STAGES OF DEVELOPMENT

Trust vs Mistrust (0 to 12 months)

From birth to approximately 1 year, this stage is the basis for all future development of personality. A feeling of physical comfort accompanied by minimal fear and uncertainty results in a sense of trust for the infant. The quality of the relationship with mother or maternal figure is more important than quantity of food or love demonstrations. Experiences with one's body are the first and primary means of social interactions for the baby; thus they provide the foundations for psychological trust. The issues involved in trust and mistrust are not settled for all time during this phase of life; they may arise again and again during development and later life. Later confrontation with trust may shake one's basic trust or provide another opportunity for further development if these needs were not met adequately the first time.

Autonomy vs Shame and Doubt (2 to 4 years)

As the child of 2 to 4 experiences the world around him, he begins to discover that his behavior can bring about certain results. Out of these encounters with reality grows a sense of autonomy. At the same time, the child has some conflicts about asserting independence or remaining dependent and in which situations. Exploring is a primary goal of this growing and increasingly coordinated physical being. It becomes more and more difficult to remain in a confined place. The child is occupied with activities involving retaining and releasing—manipulating objects, expressing himself, making new friends and letting them go, and bodily functions. The degree to which the child will allow others to regulate his behavior is regularly tested, leading to a greater sense of self-understanding and responsibility. Or in the case of over control, leading to shame and doubt.

Initiative vs Guilt (4 to 5 years)

During the fourth and fifth years, language development and locomotion have reached a sufficiently high level to permit expansion of imagination. Play activities are more interesting and companionship with peers is sought. There is curiosity and comparison with others around size and skill issues: who is the better tree climber, who is biggest or best at—almost anything. The child in this stage is into everything and seeks attention verbally and physically. Sexual curiosity and genital stimulation are apparent. Adult treatment of the curiosity will reinforce the initiative or result in shame and guilt. Because of a very active imagination, the child may feel guilty for the mere thoughts and for activities which no one has observed. The evolving conscience is becoming established and will ultimately control initiative. If the child's activities are perceived as a nuisance, whether motor or verbal, it may develop feelings of guilt over self-initiated activities which may last a lifetime. Healthy identification with parents, teachers, and peers help resolve some of the guilt problems.

Industry vs Inferiority (6 to 11 years)

Between the ages of 6 and 11, the child moves seriously into the world of competition, and the separation of work and play develops. The individuals having impact on the developing sense of self now include many other adults and a wider sphere of peers. As the lessons of work are learned, the child often needs to slip into the familial play world to bolster what may feel like flagging initiative. The developing industry evolves from efforts and achievement rewarded by significant others and leads to a sense of social worth. When the child learns social worth is linked to background of parents, color of skin, or the label on his clothes, identity with those conditions rather than self may result. These first four stages form the base upon which the adolescent builds a sense of identity.

continued

Table 2-2 (cont)

Identity vs Identity Diffusion (12 to 18 years)

During this stage of changes, the consistent task is striving to be oneself and to share oneself with something else. The beginning of separation from parents finally becomes a serious agenda. The adolescent experiences the need to be master of his own affairs and to be free of dependency. The emerging young adult is eager to know his abilities and to have the adult world recognize them as well. The adolescent also fears that the demands of adulthood will exceed the capacities to meet them. Time perspective vs time diffusion becomes the dilemma. When the adult world offers the adolescent responsibilities and privileges at an appropriate pace, commensurate with capacity and desires, there is resolution of some of the issues with a sense of time perspective, as opposed to urgency and hopelessness. The derivatives of the second stage of "autonomy vs shame and doubt" are reworked in the adolescent in the form of establishing a sense of self-certainty. When adult(s) can offer reinforcement appropriately to build the adolescent's self-esteem, feelings of inferiority diminish. The remains of "initiative vs guilt" reappear with the need to discover individualized and unique talents and interest. There seems to be a need to experiment with different roles and express initiative in different ways. If stymied in this dimension, it may seem easier to resolve the conflict by seeking behavior or roles in conflict with parents or the community—thus achieving a negative identity which is preferable to an "identity diffusion" which is experienced as being nobody at all. Most authorities agree that the period of adolescence brings with it an increase in psychic energy. The young person who uses these energies effectively can experiment in many ways and have experiences of achievement. If much of the energy is used to resolve feelings resulting from earlier unresolved crises, which often reappear at this time, then the rather fragile sense of self may be seriously threatened, with introspection interfering with concentration. The successful resolution of adolescent tasks and the development of a strong sense of identity may require many years beyond age 18. During this time, the young adult experiments with new behavior and may ignore some societal mores in the process. It is important for this process to work itself through, especially with talented and creative persons. Negative labeling may reinforce a temporary identity which, given time, will work itself into something else.

Intimacy vs Isolation

The first phase of adulthood comes into being after the adolescent has worked out a sense of identity. Sexual and psychological intimacies between two people while retaining one's own identity is the primary task of this stage. This goal is sought through forms of friendship, leadership, athletics, even combat. Unwillingness or inability to achieve intimacy will result in distancing oneself from others who pose a threat to identity. Achievement is characterized by the ability and willingness to share with another in mutual trust, to regulate cycles of work, and to participate in society in self-satisfying ways. This stage continues through early middle age.

Generativity vs Stagnation

The basic agenda of the middle years is aimed at guiding the next generation, whether in parenting or through employment and enjoyment situations. The critical question of this time occurs when the individual looks back to examine what has happened up to that time in life and whether it was good. If the individual turns inward and becomes self-absorbed, stagnation results.

Integrity vs Despair

The primary task of the later years is the acceptance of one's self and one's life. When the individual has experienced the feelings that accompany a share of the good things of life without being overwhelmed by its tragedies, disappointments, and frustrations, ego integrity is the result. There is acceptance of one's existence with full responsibility and commitment to a certain way of life and its values. Having experienced what is felt to be a full life, the individual can accept giving it up with "integrity." If on the other hand the person feels there has been little good from life and there are few prospects of any coming, there is a sense of despair often accompanied by fear of death.

Reprinted with permission from Ramsden E. Affective dimensions in patient case. In O. Payton, ed. *Psychosocial Aspects of Clinical Practice*. New York, NY: Churchill Livingstone; 1986.

was her fault, for she must have been bad. Part of maturation is to give up our idealized view of our parents. No parents are perfect. Ironically, however, the more abandoned the child was, the more she clings to the fantasy of how perfect her parents were. To idealize your parents is to idealize the way they raised you.[2] It is very important to look back at what was happening in your family when you were growing up as one mechanism to increase your awareness of your self and your worldview. What do you remember about the circumstances of your birth? Were you a wanted child?

Each child is born into a unique and complex family situation and encounters various challenges, as described by Erikson, as he or she develops day by day. If I, as a newborn, experience feelings of physical comfort, emotional calm, and joy at my presence, and if my needs are attended to with love and compassion, I will develop a sense of trust and the view that the world is essentially a warm and loving place. However, if, for example, something happens to my mother and I become a burden to others left to care for me, and people who are mourning the loss of my mother harbor resentment toward me for causing her loss, I will experience a different set of feelings and may believe that the world is uncertain and chaotic in nature. If I am born to a 15-year-old who still needs love and attention from her parents, and who has little love to give and should be giving it to herself, the situation becomes cruelly different. Very likely, she can't stand to hear me cry and may beat and smother me when I do. If that is the case, I will experience the world as a hostile place, and I will mistrust from the very first days of my life. This scenario is the genesis of violent adolescents out of control, so prevalent in our contemporary society.

And so we develop inwardly; we set our emotional lenses in response to the way our maturing nervous system takes in the information around us. At about age 2 we are confronted with the need to be toilet trained. This is reflected in Erikson's second stage, Autonomy vs Shame and Doubt (see Table 2-2). Some children are placed on the "potty" at 6 months, before head control occurs, let alone complete myelinization of the nerves. As the description on the table suggests, a critical learning at this stage is the child's appropriate and balanced willingness to allow others to regulate and control his or her behavior. Autonomy results in the feeling of success free from shame and guilt. Shame and guilt result when the child is unable to succeed and consequently allows the adult to over control his or her behavior. Only shame, or the feeling that "I am bad," can result when a child is placed on a potty and told to urinate when she doesn't even know what that means or how it feels to control that function because she cannot yet feel sensation in those nerves. However, when the child is fully ready for this learning, a marvelous feeling of success and pride results with being able to "make bubbles" in the water on command.

It is unrealistic to believe that each stage of development might be totally successfully conquered. Children will have successful resolution at times and will suffer unsuccessful resolution at times. The point that I want to stress is that the balance toward more successful resolution than unsuccessful has a great deal to do with parents and other adults who don't set children up to fail. Parents who do not parent well were, themselves, not parented well. Dysfunctional parents learned to be dysfunctional from the families they grew up in.

Current self-awareness is assisted by an attempt to remember (and to ask the help of others who watched one grow through) critical stages in development over the years. How we respond to the world today is greatly influenced by our sense of ourselves and the adequacy of our self-esteem. The development of a healthy self-esteem requires more successful than unsuccessful resolution of the tensions described by Erikson either as we mature, or later. As adults we can examine our growing up experiences, gain insight into our dysfunctional views and consciously change our distorted worldview, or correct our lenses, to give us a more true and accurate focus of the world and of ourselves. However, we usually enter into this examination only because we're experiencing emotional pain or we're bored with our lives.

HEALTHY OR OPEN FAMILIES

Healthy families interact in ways that have been described as "open" in contrast to the rigid or "closed" functioning of troubled or dysfunctional families (see Table 2-1). A family functions to provide a safe and supportive environment for all of its members to learn basic values, to grow and become more fully human. In healthy families, members feel empowered to adapt to change and feel supported in coping with the stresses of the world both outside the home and within. The stress inside the home is usually perceived to be less than the stress faced outside in the world, except in transient phases of family crisis. Individuals are recognized as being unique and having worth. There is value to the family unit, and there is open communication where members feel free to speak their opinion, but do so with concern and caring for others. In sum, family members feel safe, supported, encouraged, and appreciated. Roles and responsibilities of members are flexible but clear. People function well day to day and in crisis. Finally, quality time is shared by parents and children and is enjoyed.[4]

Sadly few of us grew up in ideal situations, and very few of us received all that we needed to mature as healthy, fully functioning, mature, true selves.

DYSFUNCTIONAL OR CLOSED FAMILIES

Charles Whitfield believes that many people grow up in families that stifle the development of the true self and instead cultivate in the child a false or "codependent" self.[5] Children need to feel as if they are safe and protected at all times. They need to feel free to ask questions, to run and play, and to know that the boundaries that parents set for them are fair and consistent. Children need to feel as if they can be children, learning and growing without fear of being ridiculed or punished cruelly for making mistakes. Children need to be invited to feel their feelings and to put words on them so that they can learn gently how not to be impulsive and controlled by their feelings.

Dysfunctional families, however, respond to the neediness and dependence of a child in ways that interfere with the development of authenticity. In the dysfunctional family, children are to be seen and not heard. They do not feel free to make mistakes but feel that if they are not "right" they will be called stupid. "Children are virtuous when they are meek, agreeable, considerate, and unselfish."[5] Adults assume the role of authoritarian masters, intent on breaking the child's will at any cost, or they tend to absent themselves totally from parenting, escaping in alcohol, work, mental illness, or travel. Children, who think of their parents as perfect, soon begin realizing that they are not free to act naturally, or to be a child, and so adopt another way of being, usually that of comforting and nurturing the parent. The child thus becomes parent to the parent. As a result, a false self emerges in the child. According to psychologist Alice Miller,[6] the persistent denial of the true self and true feelings takes its toll in the development of the coping mechanisms of depression or feelings of grandeur, neither of which is facilitative to a realistic view of the world or to healing.

HEALTH PROFESSIONALS' SELF-ESTEEM

It has been said that many people enter the health professions for a variety of poor, though unconscious, reasons. Among those reasons might be a need to be depended upon, a need to control people, and a need to get one's natural attention and affection needs met. Some may be looking for emotional healing themselves by way of making life easier for others. Few people are conscious of these motives, however. Nonetheless, they act in ways that are responsive to their unconscious needs and thus do things that are harmful, in the long run, to patients and are contrary to the healing process. These are the characteristics of "early helpers."

Dysfunctional families breed early helpers. One example of a dysfunctional family is one where one or both parents are addicted to alcohol. It is estimated that "28 to 34 million children and adults in the United States today grew up or are presently being raised in alcoholic homes."[6] The literature that has developed from the Adult Children of Alcoholics (ACOA) movement in the United States has shed needed light on the distorted worldview of the adult who grew up in a home where one or more of the parents were not able or willing to parent. This circumstance encourages the development of the "false self," stifles the successful resolution of the tensions described by Erikson, and contributes to chronic low self-esteem and feelings of being, if not "very bad," never good enough. All children experience shame, but children in dysfunctional families take on shame as part of their identity. Children in dysfunctional families are never free to be children; they have to be grown-up and helpful, and it seems as if, since this is a difficult task indeed, they're always doing something wrong. Shame is different from guilt. Whitfield[5] describes shame as "the uncomfortable or painful feeling that we experience when we realize that part of us is defective, bad, incomplete, rotten, phony, inadequate or a failure." Thus guilt says, "I made a mistake;" shame says, "I am a mistake."

Self-esteem can be viewed as the extent to which we are able and willing to "own" our essential goodness (our true self) in the face of our own incompleteness or lack of perfection. More than simply self-acceptance, self-esteem includes pride in the promise of ongoing growth and change with maturity, the hope of a richer, more peaceful and congruent life as a result of honest, day-to-day struggle. Children reared in dysfunctional families feel the shame of never being quite good enough, rather than feeling confidence and pride in doing the best they can. Because they were ridiculed and punished just for being, they grow up repressing hurtful feelings, thus believing they had a marvelous family life as a child. Underneath the repressed feelings lie severe self-esteem problems that must be admitted and talked about in order for one to identify the "lenses." Feelings of shame must be identified and confronted and replaced with a more humane, realistic acceptance of one's own imperfections and essential goodness.

Parental dysfunction may or may not be due to alcohol or drug dependence. The critical factor seems to be how well the parent was present for the growing child in such a way as to encourage the natural curiosity of the child, the natural desire to learn and grow and explore the world, how well the parent nurtured and protected the child, and how safe and free from potential harm the child felt.[5] When the parent absents him- or herself from those responsibilities, for whatever reason (drug dependence, workaholism, depression or mental illness, absence of a good model for parenting), the child starts parenting the parent, and an "early helper" emerges. A common description given by children from dysfunctional families is that they feel that they were a burden, they feel that they were being bad when they simply showed natural curiosity or asked questions. In fact, it was their very existence that seemed to bring unending pain and suffering to their family.

Children are not meant to be parents. When they take on this role, they take on a false self, and authentic feelings of curiosity, fear, and need become repressed, covered by feigned feelings of bravery and affection in an attempt to please the needy parent. Common characteristics that materialize from the distorted worldview and false view of the self that then emerge include:

- ❖ Fear of losing control.
- ❖ Fear of feelings that seem overwhelming.
- ❖ Fear of conflict.
- ❖ Fear of abandonment.
- ❖ Fear of becoming alcoholic or drug dependent.
- ❖ Fear of becoming dependent on another person for survival.
- ❖ Overdeveloped sense of responsibility.
- ❖ Feelings of guilt and grief.
- ❖ Inability to relax and have fun spontaneously.
- ❖ Harsh self-criticism.
- ❖ A tendency to lie, even when it's not "necessary."

- ❖ A tendency to let one's mind wander, to lose track of a conversation, to figuratively "leave the room." Denial and/or the tendency to create reality the way you want it to be, rather than the way it is.
- ❖ Difficulties getting close to people, with intimacy.
- ❖ Feelings of vulnerability, of being a victim in a harsh world.
- ❖ Compulsive behavior, tendency to become addicted to things that alter mood.
- ❖ Comfort with taking charge in a crisis; panic if you can't "do" something in a crisis.
- ❖ Confusion between love and pity.
- ❖ Black and white perspective—all good or all bad.
- ❖ Internalizing—taking responsibility for others' problems.
- ❖ Tendency to react rather than act.
- ❖ Experiencing stress-related illnesses.
- ❖ Overachievement.

In spite of all of the above, children have a marvelous ability to survive and cope.[7] Children from dysfunctional families are the "heroes" in health care, the ones who, at great personal sacrifice, go above and beyond the call to fix things for everyone else and are praised and admired for it. They thrive on rescuing others and on creating order out of chaos. And, very often, these are the people others admonish to "lighten up," for they take every aspect of their lives very seriously.

As Miller points out, having a worldview that necessitates the above coping behaviors, the behaviors of a false self (not the true self), inevitably leads to depression and often to the desired comfort of addiction as well.[6] Addictive behavior is repeated; habitual behavior is designed to bring comfort and to take attention away from experiencing what appears to be the negative, intense feelings of the true self that attempt to break through in a given situation. For all the comfort that the addiction brings, the dependence it brings on chemicals (often depressants), on experienced "highs," or on a kind of numbness simply reinforces a denial and continues to reinforce the false self, making the authentic or true self even more difficult to locate. Whenever the true self is blocked, our life energy, our authenticity, and our capacity to truly respond to the question, "Who am I?" are blocked. We cannot grow and become who we were created to be. We are stuck like a mouse on an exercise wheel.

CODEPENDENCE

For many young people, addictive impulses are focused not only on drugs and alcohol, but on another person—a potential source of affection to help ease the pain of never feeling as if one received enough authentic recognition, affection, and unconditional love as a child. Discomfort emerges when one nervously admits that he or she cannot live without the other person, the dependency has become so great. Since the true self of the person has been lost long ago, it is the false self that has fallen in love and proceeds to do its best to please the other, indeed, to live for the other, much as it did for the parents. This phenomenon of living for (being addicted to) the happiness and well-being of another person is termed codependence. In fact, codependency is experienced with more than just a person. It has been described as "...an exaggerated dependent pattern of learned behaviors, beliefs and feelings that make life painful. It is a dependence on people and things outside the self, along with neglect of the self to the point of having little self-identity."[5] The person demonstrating codependent behavior looks outside himself or herself to discover what he or she wants, needs, or believes in for identity, security, power, and belonging. They look outside themselves to feel whole and to get what is missing inside. The codependent person often says yes when he or she means no.

Greeting cards do us a great disservice when they express this pathological view with sentimentality such as, "Even before I knew what my needs were, you were there to help me. You alone taught me the meaning of true love." These are leftover fragments, or memories of immature needs, from our totally dependent infant. Adults must mature and take responsibility for knowing what their needs are, and set an appropriate course to get them met, beyond destructive dependence on others. The goal of maturation is to develop autonomy, self-control, and interdependence on others.[8] One's identity, power, self-worth, and individuality must be experienced as coming from within.

THE NEED TO KNOW OURSELVES

The mature healing professional must know him- or herself well, as stated in Chapter 1. He or she must be aware of behaviors that will result in harmful dependence on patients for getting personal needs for intimacy met. The end goal of all healing is the restoration of independent function for the highest and deepest quality of life possible for the patient. Patients who depend on us for this function never feel able to make it on their own. We foster this destructive dependence when we, ourselves, depend on our patients to meet our needs for attention, affection, and/or power and authority.

Self-awareness helps us to identify if our lenses need resetting, cleaning, or replacing. It is very difficult to help others effectively if we need help ourselves. Help is available, through the insights gained in this course, through reading the excellent literature now available for those who grew up in dysfunctional families, from counseling, from participation in stress groups and 12-step groups such as Al-Anon, Overeaters Anonymous, Narcotics Anonymous (NA), Alcoholics Anonymous (AA), and Adult Children of Alcoholics (ACOA) that meet in all the major cities in the United States. The goal of seeking help is always to become acquainted with the true self that was repressed many years ago. In this process, one gains insight into the distortion of his or her lenses, and then often, for the first time as an adult, clearly discerns that there are choices in behavior and that many of the choices one has habitually made in the past have contributed to a chronic feeling of chaos and victimization. Another goal would be to identify negative shame-based beliefs and replace them with more accepting, cosmic beliefs as described in Chapter 1.

The groups listed above were formed by people who realized that compulsive behavior and addictions serve to blunt one's awareness of the true self. In order to rid oneself of addictions, support is necessary. These groups are devoted to helping people heal from their addictive behavior and live authentic and genuine lives in the search for the true self, lost long ago in an effort to cope with the unfair stress of childhood.

SELF-AWARENESS THROUGH ACTION

The exercises for this chapter are designed to help you review your family history, your growth and development, the messages you received and the values you adopted from growing up in your particular setting and circumstances. Try to withhold judgement on what you remember and experience. Remember, feelings are—they exist. Feelings are neither bad nor good, appropriate nor inappropriate; they just are. However, what we do with our feelings, how we respond to them is open to our evaluation and choice. Being aware of our feelings is the first step. No family is perfect, and parents often parent the way they were parented. Use these exercises to gain insight into your experience and to set goals for your personal growth that will help you become a mature healing professional.

CONCLUSION

The next chapter will discuss values in more depth. We develop our values initially by learning what to value from significant people in our lives, but a value cannot be said to be our own until we accept it for ourselves and act on it. In your journal, reflect on your values that you "caught" from significant people in your life. How many of them can you say you have truly reflected upon or tested and have adopted as your own? Do you hold any values that would be perceived as negative? By whom? How does that make you feel?

REFERENCES

1. Piaget J. *The Construction of Reality in the Child.* New York, NY: Basic Books; 1954.
2. Bradshaw J. *Bradshaw On: the Family.* Deerfield Beach, Fla: Health Communications, Inc.; 1988.
3. Erikson EH. *Identity, Youth and Crisis.* New York, NY: WW Norton; 1968.
4. US Department of Health and Human Services. *Identifying Successful Families: An Overview of Constructs and Selected Resources.* Washington, DC: Department of Health and Human Services; 1990.
5. Whitfield CL. *Healing the Child Within.* Baltimore, Md: The Resource Group; 1986.
6. Miller A. *The Drama of the Gifted Child.* New York, NY: Basic Books; 1981.
7. Malone M. Dependent on disorder. *MS Magazine.* 1987;15:50.
8. Greenberg LS, Johnson SM. *Emotionally Focused Therapy for Couples.* New York, NY: The Guilford Press; 1988.

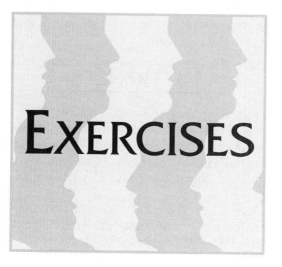

EXERCISES

EXERCISE 1: MAGIC CARPET RIDE

This exercise is best carried out with the instructor reading the instructions to a group. It is intended to help participants remember what it was like as they were growing up in their families. The magic carpet is a symbol for a ride back into time and memory. Thus, this is a type of guided imagery exercise followed by personal reflection on the content, which concludes with a group discussion where participants are able to share with one another, at their own level of comfort, what insights they gained.

Instructor

"So, sit back in your chairs, feet flat on the floor, and breathe deeply three times, each time feeling more and more relaxed. Concentrate on your breathing, have your mind go blank as you focus on the air going in through your nostrils, and back out through your mouth. With each breath you feel more and more relaxed. (Pause)

"I want you to go back in time when you were a little child in elementary school. (Pause)

"You are inside your house, with your family all gathered together; your parents are there, or those who reared you, and any brothers and sisters are also there. (Pause)

"People are having a conversation. (Pause)

"What are they talking about? (Pause)

"Now ask them to stop talking for a second because you want to ask each of them an important question. Starting with the adults, ask each one, in turn, to tell you something about you. Listen carefully to the descriptions each gives you and pay attention to the feelings each person seems to display as each answers your questions. (Pause for 2 or 3 minutes)

"As you get ready to leave the group, say goodbye to each person and come gently forward in time to the present, opening your eyes slowly as you return. (Pause)

"Before talking, write down the names of each person with whom you spoke, then jot down what each told you about yourself, and the feeling or attitude conveyed in that message, and how that made you feel. (Pause for 2 or 3 minutes)

"Now choose one person to share your experience with. Remember, your fantasy was a very private adventure. Some of what you remembered you may decide to keep private. You choose, carefully, the extent to which you want to reveal things about yourself and your family. (Pause 5 minutes for discussion in twos or threes)

"Now return to your written comments. Search each message for the values that underlie each. For example, if you heard from your mother, "You're so messy! I wish you'd clean up your room," you might discern that she values neatness or obedience to her values. "You're so helpful" naturally leads one to the value of helping or perhaps altruism, unless said with sarcasm. Then search for the message behind the message. Perhaps what was meant was, "I wish you'd stop interfering in my life by always trying to do things for me."

Large Group Discussion

1. List and discuss various messages and feelings. How many heard essentially negative messages about themselves? How many essentially positive? How many half and half?

2. How many people live up to the description heard from one or both parents? Negative or positive? Give examples.

3. List and discuss values inferred from messages.

Conclusion

Record what you learned and felt about the exercise in your journal. Explore the impact that the messages you heard have on your current self-esteem. How do you feel about yourself today, in general? How does that relate to the messages heard? Was this exercise a positive or a negative one for you? What made it so?

EXERCISE 2: FAMILY GENOGRAM

A genogram is a map of a family for several generations. It is a very useful picture that reveals multigenerational patterns (Figure 2-1).

1. Draw your genogram for at least 3 generations. Label anything that seems important to you. See if you can locate pictures of family members to go with the circles and squares on your page.

2. Try to identify any addictions, family tension or conflict, or incidents of children parenting their parents. What patterns emerge? What do you now know about yourself that you failed to see before? What stories are important enough to be handed down? Who/what is the family proud of? What secrets does the family hide from others?

3. Discuss your genogram with 2 other people in your class that you choose. Each of you should take 5 minutes to describe the people represented and 25 minutes to discuss the family dynamics as you understand them.

4. Perhaps questions came up for you about various family members' lives and habits. Write to relatives asking them to fill in the missing pieces to help you better understand your heritage.

Figure 2-1. Family genogram.

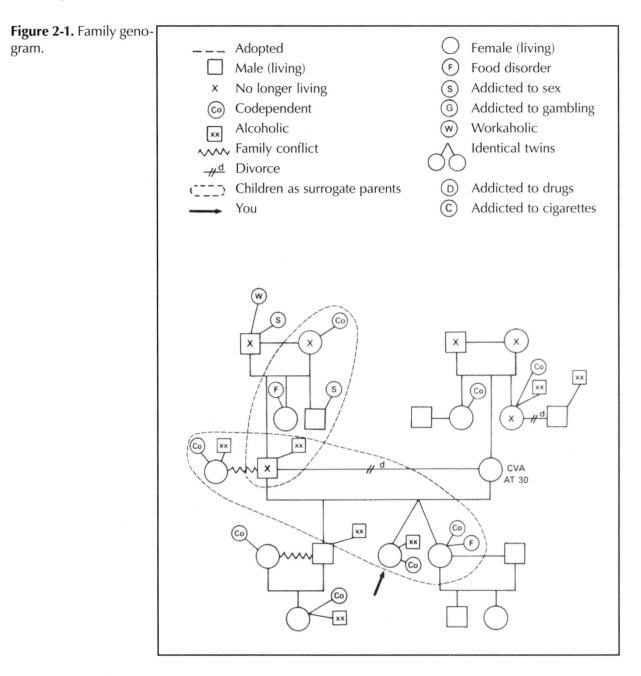

5. Remember, with this exercise in particular, the importance of confidentiality. Nothing revealed should ever leave the classroom. Be worthy of the trust placed in you as others take the risk of discussing private and sensitive material with you.

6. Keep a journal about your feelings and your awareness from this exercise. Can you identify behaviors that you've developed from your family that may interfere with mature healing? Comment on any and problem solve ways in which you might be able to work through those behaviors.

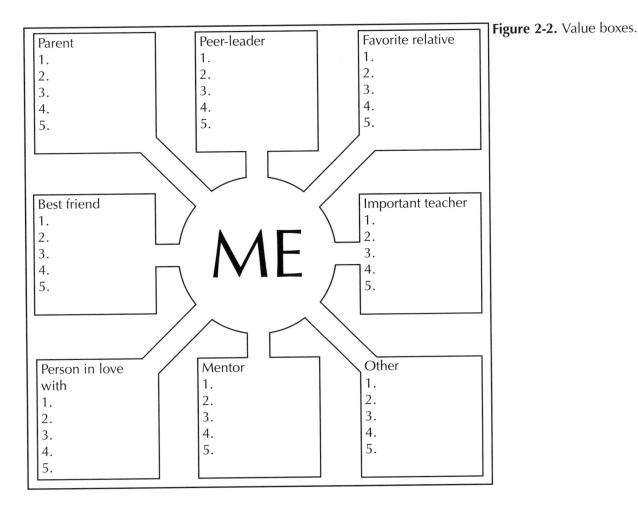

Figure 2-2. Value boxes.

EXERCISE 3: VALUE BOXES

1. Figure 2-2 is a diagram of 8 boxes surrounding a circle that represents you. Each box represents a significant person in your life. Envision a person that corresponds to the descriptor at the top of each box and place that person's initials in the upper right corner. If there is no one who meets that description right now in your life, cross out the descriptor and simply put another important person's initials there. One person should not appear in 2 boxes.

2. Now list 4 or 5 things you perceive each person would want you to value. What do they count on you for? What demands do they place on you? What do they want you to do, think, be? What do they want you to value?

3. Now look for similarities from various people. Is there a value that is repeated often? List it below the diagram to the right as a recurring value.

4. Underline each value that you want for yourself, and place those values in the center circle.

5. Now list the conflict areas to the lower left of the diagram. What do others want for you that you do not desire?

6. What values seem most important to you?

VALUES AS DETERMINANTS OF BEHAVIOR

Carol M. Davis, PT, EdD, MS, FAPTA

OBJECTIVES

1. To define and examine personal and professional values and to explore the role they play in determining behavior.
2. To emphasize the importance of critical thinking or reflection to the formation of one's values.
3. To examine the values that underlie behaviors that interfere with healing and those that enhance healing.
4. To distinguish between being morally aware and morally conscious.
5. To distinguish between nonmoral values and moral values.

The process of professional socialization is a process of growth, of becoming a professional person. Ideally that growth is holistic and permeates our selves at deep levels. We realize we have grown and learned when we can observe changes in our behavior. Most obviously, we know more as we become professional. We incorporate an entire new body of knowledge and skill and use much of it daily in our professional care, but we also develop different attitudes and values as we grow professionally. In other words, professional growth involves changes in our knowledge, our skills and our attitudes, values, and beliefs.

All people, after a certain age, can be said to have values. Some of those values were examined in Chapter 2. Consequently, you're now more aware of some of the values you learned and adopted or "introjected" from your family. It is very appropriate for family members to help us grow as children by teaching us what to believe and value when we are too young to choose critically for ourselves. Babies are not born with values. We appreciate this when we eat at a restaurant with a 4-year-old who has not yet been socialized adequately and runs around the room playfully throwing food at people.

Sometimes we introject the values of our parents so completely that we don't even know what we value or why. The story is told of a young couple starting life together cooking a special ham dinner for guests. As one partner prepared the roast, he cut the 2 ends of the ham off before putting it in the oven. His wife chided him for wasting so much meat, and he defended himself by saying that his mother taught him always to cut the ends off. "Why?" she asked. He responded that he didn't know, but he thought it was very important; probably something to do with the proper cooking and circulation of juices.

The next time they visited his parents' home, the new wife asked her husband's mother about cutting the ends off the ham. "Oh, yes," she replied, "My mother always taught me to do that. It's critical to the cooking of the meat."

Still not satisfied, Grandmother was called on the phone. "Grandma, tell our new daughter-in-law why it's so important to cut the ends of the meat off the ham before cooking it!" Grandma replied, "Oh, that old trick. It's just a habit I got into. When I first married, we didn't have a big enough pot to fit the meat in, so I just trimmed the ends. After awhile, it just became a habit, I guess."

So it is with some of the values we "catch" from our parents, without thinking about them. Cutting off the ends of ham is not a good example of value-based behavior, but the analogy is important. A clear definition of value-based behavior follows shortly.

Carl Rogers'[1] research indicated that immature people, in an attempt to gain or hold love, approval, and esteem, place the locus of evaluation of values on others. They learn to have a basic distrust for direct experiencing as a valid guide to appropriate behavior. They learn from others what values are important and adopt them as their own, even though they may be widely discrepant from personal experience. Because these introjected values are not based on genuinely experienced personal feelings, they tend to be fixed and rigid, rather than fluid and changing.

Rogers[1] disclosed a list of what he termed the commonly adopted or "introjected" values and their associated beliefs found very often in the subjects from the United States that he studied in the 1950s and 1960s:

1. Sexual desires are mostly bad. *Source*: Parents, teachers, the church.
2. Disobedience is bad. To obey is good; to obey without question is better. *Source*: Parents, teachers, the church, the military.
3. Making money is the highest good. *Sources*: Too numerous to mention.
4. Aimless, exploratory reading for fun is undesirable and lazy. *Source*: Teachers, the educational system.
5. Abstract art is good. *Source*: "The sophisticated people."
6. Communism is all bad. *Source*: The government.
7. To love your neighbor is the highest good. *Source*: Parents, the church.
8. Cooperation and teamwork are preferable to acting alone. *Source*: Companions.
9. Cheating is clever and desirable. *Source*: The peer group.
10. Coca-Cola, chewing gum, electric refrigerators, and automobiles are utterly desirable. *Source*: Advertisements. (This is still reinforced by people in many parts of the world.)

Clearly this list reveals that commonly held values reflect the cultural mores of the time a half century ago. As we enter the 21st Century, it is much more difficult to find broadly held cultural values than it was 50-plus years ago when the United States was emerging from the great Depression and World War II. Individualism has become even more valued, sometimes to the detriment of the society as a whole. What values can you identify that are broadly held halfway through this first decade in the new century? Surely the commonly held sanctions against killing and abuse hold true. The entrepreneurial spirit and creativity are quite honored. Unfortunately, the value of making a lot of money as an end, no matter what means is employed (as long as you don't get caught breaking the law) seems to prevail. "Having a lot" in these times is mistaken for self-worth and intrinsic value. The health care system has seen a decline from a service profession to a business, as an economic driven health care system took shape in the mid-1990s. Universal access to health care no longer seems valuable to those in charge of making the rules. Perhaps we're getting ahead of ourselves. Let's take a closer look at what constitutes values.

DEFINING VALUES

What is a value? Values have been defined in many ways, but in general, the term value refers to an operational belief which one accepts as one's own and which determines behavior. Morrill[2] is far more specific, however, and defines values as:

❖ Standards and patterns of choice that guide persons and groups toward satisfaction, fulfillment, and meaning.

❖ Constructs that orient choice and shape action.

❖ Concepts that call forth thought and conduct that have worth, that lead (under the right conditions) to the fulfillment of human potential or to the discovery of a variety of types and levels of meaning.

❖ Concepts that are not themselves beliefs or judgements but come to expression in and through thought.

❖ Concepts that are not themselves feelings or emotions, but they inevitably involve desires and fears; cannot be defined as deeds, but are always mediated through specific acts.

Thus values orient our choices and inspire our actions. Since this is a text devoted to developing appropriate professional ways of being, it becomes critical to examine and clarify the values you now hold in relation to the values that form ethical and sensitive professional caregiving.

VALUES VS NEEDS

Values can be distinguished from needs, which also influence our behavior. If I am thirsty, without thinking much about it, I get something to drink. Needs push us into behaving in certain predictable ways. Abraham Maslow[3] outlined in detail a theory of human behavior based upon a hierarchy of needs. However, for behavior to be value-based, I must reflect upon the choices I have and act according to my reflection. Thus, need behavior is more automatic and driven, whereas value-based behavior takes place upon reflection.[4] Implied in this distinction is the idea that value-based behavior is more mature, less impulsive, especially when compared to behaviors that are based on the more basic or lower level needs.

Clearly, cutting off the ends of the ham does not represent value based or reflective behavior, but represents an introjected behavior based on the tendency to distrust one's own experience as a guide. Perhaps the value underlying this behavior was to follow the example of elders in spite of logic. Indeed, 2 generations of the family distrusted their own experience—and so it goes in our families.

MORAL VS NONMORAL VALUES

The professional socialization process requires the clarification and prioritization of currently held values, and the adoption of new values that are consistent with the values of the profession. Deciding how to prepare ham or what clothes to wear to a party is a decision-making process of a different sort than deciding whether a patient is a good candidate to receive an above-knee prosthesis. The differences are important. The first category is an example of personal choice or preference; the second is a professional decision. Both personal and professional choices can be based on reflection of values, but professional choices are not the same as value preferences. The first is a choice that bears little consequence for the chooser if the less-than-best decision is made. However, the decision about the prosthesis has profound consequence for another person if the less-than-best decision is made.[5]

Values that lead to personal preference are termed **nonmoral values**; values that have to do with the way we relate to and interact with fellow human beings are termed **moral values**.[6] Moral values such as compassion, trust, justice, honesty, love, confidentiality, and faithfulness to one's professional colleagues form the heart of a profession's value structure. Moral values take on more importance than value preferences and must be regarded with greater seriousness because the needs of human beings are more important than what food or music or hairstyle we prefer.

PROFESSIONAL VALUES

Professionalism is grounded in core values. In days past, professions assumed that new members would automatically "pick up" professional values and behaviors, but this is no longer the case.[7] The American Physical Therapy Association (APTA) has identified 7 core values that, to them, comprise professional behavior: accountability, altruism, compassion/caring, excellence, integrity, professional duty, and social responsibility.[8] These values are accompanied by behavioral indicators that describe what one would see if the physical therapist were demonstrating the core values in their daily practice. Even a cursory look at these values reveals that they might be universally held values, rather than unique to physical therapy alone, and so I include them here.

1. **Accountability**: Active acceptance of the responsibility for the diverse roles, obligations, and actions of the physical therapist including self-regulation and other behaviors that positively influence patient/client outcomes, the profession, and the health needs of society.

2. **Altruism**: The primary regard for or devotion to the interest of patients/clients, thus assuming the fiduciary responsibility of placing the needs of the patient/client ahead of the physical therapist's self-interest.

3. **Compassion/Caring**: Compassion is the desire to identify with or sense something of another's experience; a precursor for caring. Caring is the concern, empathy, and consideration for the needs and values of others.

4. **Excellence**: Practice that consistently uses current knowledge and theory while understanding personal limits, integrates judgement and the patient/client perspective, embraces advancement, challenges mediocrity, and works toward development of new knowledge.

5. **Integrity**: The possession of, and steadfast adherence to, high moral principles or professional standards.

6. **Professional duty**: The commitment to meeting one's obligations to provide effective physical therapy services to individual patients/clients, to serve the profession, and to positively influence the health of society.

7. **Social responsibility**: The promotion of a mutual trust between the profession and the larger public that necessitates responding to societal needs for health and wellness.

VALUES CONFLICTS

There are times when the behavior of health professionals comes into direct conflict with patients' behavior. The moral or interpersonal values that the profession espouses, for example, in its Code of Ethics or its Core Values statements, and the behavior observed in many hospitals often seem far removed from each other. Often the behavior exhibited in conflict situations is not value-based, or based on reflection, but is impulsive and defensive.

Values conflicts are always rich in their lessons for learning, though many of us shy away from them because we are afraid of doing the wrong thing. In tense times, most of us want someone to "tell us what to do."

A moral dilemma exists when we don't know what choice to make from two or more conflicting choices, thus we have difficulty choosing which value should have priority. Chapter 4 focuses on the examination of ethical dilemmas and their resolution, but a brief example here will illustrate this point. Respect for life is the central value for advocates of a woman's right to choose abortion as well as for those opposed to abortion. The difference in opinion and belief of these 2 groups is not the value of life, but the importance of the mother's life or the fetus' life. The antiabortionists claim the primacy of the fetus' life above all considerations; the reproductive-freedom advocates claim the primacy of the mother's choice for the quality of her life and resist outside interference with her right to choose.[5] Likewise, those who favor capital punishment value the lives of those who might become victimized over the life of the person convicted of murder.

The set of moral norms adopted by a professional group to direct value-laden choices in a way consistent with professional responsibility is termed a code of ethics. One might follow the code without internalizing it, introjecting it just as one did in younger years with parents' values. For a code of ethics to function as a set of professional moral values, one must reflect on it and decide that it, indeed, forms a values complex around which one is willing to organize professional choices. Thus, as stated previously, reflection is necessary to the internalization of values to make them truly one's own, whether personal or professional. Those who make the smoothest transitions into professional practice are likely to be those whose personal values and priorities greatly overlap with the values inherent in their chosen professional practice. Given that one's basic human survival needs are met, the more one reflects on one's choices and upon which choices result in the good and meaningful life, the more one is apt to experience consistent reward from choices made.[6]

VALUES THAT DETRACT FROM A THERAPEUTIC PRESENCE

Often patients end up needing the help of rehabilitation professionals because of impulsive, poor choices reflecting an immature and inconsistent set of values that have been introjected, but not clarified or claimed as one's own. An example might be the young man who comes to physical therapy needing relief from low back pain incurred from lifting a heavy railroad tie while showing off in front of some young women and men he decided he needed to impress. Many patient problems in movement and function are not the result of "fate" but result from a lifetime of choices that reveal little attention or value to behaviors that preserve physical and emotional health. Thus, it sometimes becomes difficult to avoid becoming judgemental, and as professionals, we sometimes feel resistance to treating people who have not practiced wellness behaviors and have become, for example, obese, or are chronic smokers.[5]

Professional ethics demand that, when a feeling of criticism and negative judgement of a patient occurs, we must be aware of it and consciously work to not let it interfere with our commitment to compassionate, quality care. Common behaviors that reveal difficulty in this task include the following.

1. Acting cool or aloof, obviously paying more attention to other patients.

   Underlying value: Prejudice or indifference.

2. Overly criticizing the patient so that he or she feels as if nothing is right.

   Underlying value: Prejudice, perfectionism, rigidity.

3. Treating the patient as an object rather than a person with feelings of pain, worry, and insecurity.

   Underlying value: Depersonalization.

4. Treating the patient as if he or she were a child, incapable of understanding or making wise choices.

   Underlying value: Patronizing, adopting an air of condescension.

5. Being unable or unwilling to help the patient in treatment; leaving the patient alone most of the time.

    Underlying value: Indifference or prejudice.

6. Making fun of the patient in his or her presence and/or behind his or her back.

    Underlying value: Depersonalization.

7. Telling others things the patient shared in confidence.

    Underlying value: Breaking confidentiality.

8. Refusing to let the patient work on his or her own; constantly supervising and instructing.

    Underlying value: Fostering dependence. Getting own need to be needed met from patients.

9. Guessing what is best to do. Refusing to find correct and best treatment alternatives. Acting on habit.

    Underlying value: Refusing to recognize and act based on one's own limits of knowledge.

10. Always fitting the patient in as if everything else is more important.

    Underlying value: Selfish interest over needs of patients.

11. Refusing to listen to patient's story of pain and difficulties dealing with pain and dysfunction.

    Underlying value: Importance of defending oneself against personal feelings of fear and insecurity around pain and possible addiction.[5]

Most of us would read this list of behaviors and say to ourselves, "I'd never act like that!" But in fact, as much as we would not ever want to act in ways that interfere with healing, when we are unclear of our values, or, more important, when we are not in touch with our feelings, when we don't know ourselves, we often end up doing and saying things, especially under stress, that we regret later. These regretful behaviors stem, in part, from impulsive and immature needs to be spontaneous and egocentric, and arise from feelings of criticism, and the judgement that our patients don't deserve our help. Perhaps they grow out of unrecognized fears such as not knowing the right thing to do or perhaps they stem from not having clarified the values underlying a therapeutic presence.

THE VALUES THAT REINFORCE HEALING

Essential to a "therapeutic use of self" is the capacity to feel compassion for those who need our help. Compassion is quite different from pity, wherein I feel sorry for this poor person (and secretly feel smug and am thankful that this is not my problem). Compassion in a mature health professional is a value that is fueled with imagination and the ability to envision what is possible from the other person's perspective. When we truly value our patients as human beings, we express behavior based on moral values that enhance healing, such as sincere and active listening, a desire to treat patients as adults, in charge of their own lives and capable of making wise and appropriate decisions for themselves. We treat what they say with confidence and respect; we attend to them with interest and obtain their informed consent for therapeutic procedures. We convey to them that their choice to come to us was well-founded, and that we will help within clearly set boundaries and expectations. In other words, we work to be able to sincerely feel genuine positive regard for all of our patients and relate to each with sensitivity to their uniqueness.

When we become professionals, we gain many things, but we also give up some things. One of the things we give up is the right to walk away from people we would rather not treat. What patient would be your most dreaded? Would it be the rapist? The child abuser? The alcoholic? The person who is HIV positive or has AIDS? When we judge our patients, we can't help but treat them as less than human. What is required is a sense of oneness with all human beings, regardless of the mistakes they may have made. Deciding that the mistakes you have made are far less "evil" only distances you from your patient.

As professionals, we also give up the right to say whatever we feel at any moment. We give up the right to speak and act impulsively, and we take on the responsibility to act in accordance with Core Values and the Code of Ethics, or, in similar terms, to act according to the moral values that facilitate healing. No longer may we claim the luxury of spontaneous outbursts or selfish indifference. No longer may we put our own needs before the needs of our patients. No longer may we be run by unclear values or fears that have not yet been examined and resolved.

Professional rehabilitative care requires problem solving that is proactive, based on scientific data and demonstrates a consistent, conscious value of choosing behavior that is conducive to healing. As a professional clinician, you must become an informed reasoner. You must learn to value the systematic gathering of facts and compassionate relating to people who come to you for help. You must value taking the time to reflect on your behavior and choose to act in ways that reinforce healing. Central to this process is the courage to examine carefully your values and the values of healing and to make a commitment to change behaviors that interfere with effective and compassionate care. Feedback from others is important, but at this point in the text, you are asked to focus on self-examination.

DEVELOPMENT OF AN ETHICAL CONSCIOUSNESS

We are not born with the knowledge of the right thing to do; we develop the ability to solve moral problems in conjunction with cognition. There are 3 common approaches to teaching children the right thing to do.[2] The most common is the objectivist approach, or legalism, which asserts that to do the right thing is to obey the rules. The "rightness" of the value is within the value itself; therefore, it is always right, for example, to love people, to act justly, honestly, and with compassion. Organized religion teaches this approach to values education. To do the right thing, one should obey the higher authority, do as the Bible says, follow the Torah, the Koran, or the Ten Commandments, etc. However, objectivism offers little help in reconciling the contradictions that can be found in the Bible or resolving the dilemma, for example, between honoring your parents and following your own conscience in developing your career when your choice and the choice your parents would have you make are at odds. Likewise, objectivism fosters the development of a moral belief system based on outside authority. For these reasons it does not adequately serve the purpose of dilemma resolution in health care.

Ethical subjectivism, or values clarification (examined briefly in the exercises) offers an alternative that approaches ethical relativism.[9] Ethical relativism is the view that each person's values should be considered equally valid. Subjectivism suggests that one examine the conflicting values to make sure that each is, indeed, a value. If a belief or idea does not meet true "value" status, it is relegated to a position of less importance than a true value. To satisfy the definition of "value," so Raths and colleagues suggest, a value must satisfy the seven criteria listed in Table 3-1.[9] The content of a value, so important in objectivism, becomes secondary to the process of determining if something is, indeed, a value.[9]

How well does subjectivism assist us in making value-based decisions? It probably doesn't make that much difference if one begins treating patients at 8 am or 8:30. People will (and often do) argue the importance of their priorities, but nonmoral values or value preferences are just that, relative preferences. Moral values present a different story. In fact, moral relativism renders an ethical code meaningless.[6]

Thus in a moral or ethical dilemma in which one must choose between doing the loving thing and following the rules, it does little good to use a subjectivist approach, clarifying if both compassion and justice fit the criteria of a value. What is needed is a way of weighing the relative goodness of each value in the situation. Thus both subjectivism and objectivism fall short of informing us clearly how to decide between two conflicting values, which is the better to choose.

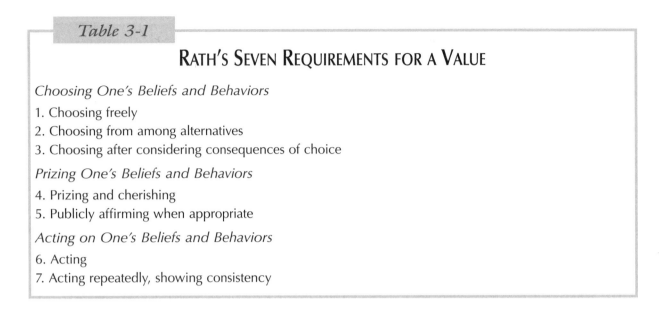

Table 3-1

RATH'S SEVEN REQUIREMENTS FOR A VALUE

Choosing One's Beliefs and Behaviors

1. Choosing freely
2. Choosing from among alternatives
3. Choosing after considering consequences of choice

Prizing One's Beliefs and Behaviors

4. Prizing and cherishing
5. Publicly affirming when appropriate

Acting on One's Beliefs and Behaviors

6. Acting
7. Acting repeatedly, showing consistency

Carol Gilligan[10] and Lawrence Kohlberg[11] both have developed theories that assist us in our task. Their theories each fall under the category of contextualism, in which they assert that, as people develop their ability to think, they also develop their ability to reason about the right or best thing to do in a given situation. This approach to dilemma resolution has been termed contextualism, because the context of the situation provides the key information in deciding the right thing to do in that situation. Certain values are, as the objectivists suggest, always going to assume great importance, but the key to resolving the dilemma is to collect all the pertinent data about this particular situation and then weigh alternatives for the best thing to do, according to the best and most mature debate. How do we discover the most adequate reasoning, the most mature debate? Developmental psychology and philosophy inform us here.

DEVELOPMENTAL ASPECT OF MORAL DECISION-MAKING

Developmentalists, in general, assert that as people grow and change, they pass through predictable stages in which new behaviors are formed and stabilized. The maturation process consists of a progression through a series of passages or stages that reflects the increasingly sophisticated changes occurring in a person's nervous system. Thus children are not "little adults" and should not be treated as such, nor be asked to act like adults before they know what that means.

Perhaps the most famous developmentalist, Jean Piaget,[12] suggested that as cognitive abilities develop, the ability to know the right thing to do also develops. Piaget suggested 4 stages of development of a moral conscience: amoral (ages 0 to 2), egocentric (ages 2 to 7), heteronomous (ages 7 to 12), and autonomous (ages 12 and over) (Table 3-2). Kohlberg based his work on that of Piaget and further refined the stages based on research conducted around the world.[11] Kohlberg suggests 6 stages men and boys go through in developing a mature moral consciousness (see Table 3-2). Earliest and most immature is the punishment and obedience stage in which that which is wrong is that for which I get punished. Tables 3-2 and 3-3 illustrate the progression of stages through stage 6, an autonomous stage of knowing the right thing based on a decision of conscience in accord with self-chosen, well-thought-out ethical principles appealing to logical comprehensiveness, universality, and consistency and that flow from the basic principle of justice.[11] When faced with dilemmas, Kohlberg observed that people did not just work out the right answer for themselves by guessing

| Table 3-2 | | | | |

DEVELOPMENT MODEL COMPARISON

Piaget's Moral Development Model	*Kohlberg's Moral Development Model*			
	Level	**Orientation Stage**	**Characterized By**	**Personally Stated As**
Amoral stage— Ages 0 to 2				
Egocentric stages— ages 2 to 7—lacks morality, bends rules and reacts instinctively to environment	*Preconventional*	1. Punishment and obedience orientation 2. Instrumental relativist orientation	Satisfying one's own needs	I must obey the authority figure or else…
Heteronomous stage—ages 7 to 12—based on total acceptance of a morality imposed by others	*Conventional*	3. Good boy-nice girl orientation	Conformity to social conventions and expectations	I probably should because everyone expects me to.
		4. Law and order orientation	Respect for authority and society's laws	I ought to because of duty to obey the rules.
Autonomous stage—age 12 and over—based on an internalized morality of cooperation	*Postconventional or autonomous*	5. Social contract orientation	Conformity to the ever-changing values and demands of society	I may because of my role in society, but I often question the relative values of society.
		6. Universal ethical principle orientation	My conscience holds me responsible for doing what is right.	I will because I know it is the right thing to do.

Reprinted with permission from Piaget J, Kohlberg L. Comparison of the stages in two models of moral development. In: Francoer, RT. *Becoming a Sexual Person.* New York: John Wiley and Sons; 1982:673.

or by trial and error. Rather, depending on their age and maturity, they appealed to a category of reasons outlined in the stages in Table 3-3. As you can see, both Kohlberg and Piaget believed that children progress from a total abdication to an outside authority to an autonomous stage wherein they make their own choices.[11,12]

Carol Gilligan,[10] also a contextualist and student of Kohlberg, reacted to the fact that Kohlberg only studied men and boys and then generalized his theory to girls and women. Kohlberg stated that girls and women get "stuck" in stage three: Good boy-nice girl orientation that reveals conformity to social expectation, because girls are socialized to stay at home and tend the house, yielding to the decisions of the man in the house. Right is that which pleases others.

Gilligan's work challenges the rigidity of this assumption.[10] In her studies of how girls, college women, and housewives perceive the same set of moral problems outlined by Kohlberg, she reveals

---

Table 3-3

KOHLBERG'S STAGES OF MORAL DEVELOPMENT

1. Preconventional Level

Child is responsive to cultural rules and labels of good and bad or right and wrong as they relate to physical consequence of action (reward of punishment).

Stage 1: Punishment and obedience orientation

Avoidance of punishment and unquestioning deference to power valued in their own right, not in terms of respect for underlying moral order supported by punishment and authority (Stage 4).

Stage 2: Instrumental relativist orientation

Right actions are those that satisfy one's own needs. Reciprocity is not a matter of loyalty or justice, but of "You scratch my back and I'll scratch yours."

2. Conventional Level

Maintaining the expectations of the individual's family, group, or nation is valuable in its own right, regardless of consequences.

Stage 3: Interpersonal concordance or "good boy-nice girl" orientation

Good behavior is that which pleases others and is approved by them. Behavior is often judged by intention. One earns approval by being "nice."

Stage 4: "Law and order" orientation

Right behavior consists of showing respect for authority, following the rules, doing one's duty, and maintaining the given social order for its own sake.

3. Postconventional, Autonomous, Principled Level

Clear effort to define moral values and principles that have validity and application apart from authority of groups or other persons holding these principles.

Stage 5: Social contract, legalistic orientation

Right actions are defined as those that have been critically examined and agreed upon by the whole society. Emphasis placed on procedural rules for reaching consensus in the face of relativism. Aside from what is constitutionally and democratically agreed upon, what is right is a matter of personal values and opinion. It is possible to change the law when it is to the benefit of society. Outside the law, free agreement and contract are the binding elements of obligation (the "official" morality of the US Government and Constitution).

Stage 6: Universal-ethical principle orientation

Right is defined by the decision of conscience in accord with self-chosen ethical principles appealing to logical comprehensiveness, universality, and consistency. The basic universal principles are those of justice, of the reciprocity and equality of human rights, and of respect for the dignity of human beings as individual persons, no matter which nationality, race, color, or creed.

---

that women "appear to frame moral problems in terms of conflicting personal responsibilities rather than conflicting rights and the concept of justice."[10] Thus, as a function of social conditioning, adolescent boys may well focus first on achievement and self-identity, and much later focus on developing a value of intimacy and friendship, while girls do just the opposite. Both genders have the same ability to mature to higher stages of moral conscience; that is, girls and women do not simply stop maturing morally at stage 3. However, girls and women seem to mature, not linearly as Kohlberg's scale illustrates, but horizontally, in netlike fashion, favoring the higher importance of relationship over abstract goals such as social justice and achievement.

MORAL AWARENESS VS MORAL CONSCIOUSNESS

To be morally aware is to know what the dictionary says about, for example "compassion," and to be somewhat aware if your behavior fits that description at any given time. To be morally conscious, however, is to examine how compassion weaves its way through your behavior, how it influences you in your various decisions, how you feel about compassion with regard to justice, for example, in a moral dilemma. Thus moral consciousness represents a deeper way of knowing and thus a firmer commitment to consistency in moral behavior, or the way we interact with other human beings. The goal of this text is, at the least, to confirm your moral awareness, and ideally, to help stimulate a moral consciousness that is consistent with quality, compassionate health care. Knowing the right thing to do does not guarantee doing the right thing. But it is a major first step. Pellegrino[13] suggests that quick self-examination on the effectiveness of one's therapeutic presence might be accomplished by answering these three questions truthfully:

1. Do I listen and not only respond to, but satisfy the fundamental questions each person who is ill and anxious brings to me?
2. Can I accept the patient for what he or she is, not for what I think he or she should be?
3. Can I handle my authority in a humane way that respects the life and values of the patient?

To be able to answer yes to any of these questions requires that we continue to grow as persons as we become professionals. The value of a lifelong commitment to growth and increasing moral consciousness insures a meaningful and peaceful professional as well as personal life.[13]

AWARENESS THROUGH ACTIVITY

The exercises are designed to help you further analyze important personal values you currently hold, to help you learn which of your values you value most, or what is your highest order value. A visit to a clinic or patient care area where you will be asked to make careful observations of behavior and to comment on the values that seem to underlie it will help sensitize you to the stresses of patient care and will illustrate various kinds of interactions that take place with patients. Finally, a "forced choice" exercise will pull out some introjected values that you may not even be aware you hold.

REFERENCES

1. Rogers C, Stevens B. *Person to Person—The Problem of Being Human*. Lafayette, Calif: Real People Press; 1967.
2. Morrill R. *Teaching Values in College*. San Francisco, Calif: Jossey-Bass; 1980.
3. Maslow A. *Motivation and Personality*. New York, NY: Harper and Row; 1954.
4. Beck C. A philosophical view of values and value education. In: Hennessy T, ed. *Values and Moral Development*. New York, NY: Paulist Press; 1976.
5. Davis CM. Influence of values on patient care: foundation for decision making. In: O'Sullivan S, Schmitz T. *Foundations of Rehabilitation*. 4th ed. Philadelphia, Pa: FA Davis; 2004.
6. Wehlage G, Lockwood AL. Moral relativism and values education. In: Purpel D, Ryan K, eds. *Moral Education—It Comes With the Territory*. Berkeley, Calif: McCutchen; 1976.
7. Hensel WA, Dickey NW. Teaching professionalism: passing the torch. *Acad Med*. 1995;73(3):179-185.
8. American Physical Therapy Association. *Professionalism in Physical Therapy: Core Values*. Available at: www.apta.org. Retrieved July 14, 2005.
9. Simon SB, Howe L, Kirschenbaum H. *Values Clarification—A Handbook for Teachers*. New York, NY: Hart Publishers; 1972.

10. Gilligan C. *In a Different Voice.* Cambridge, Mass: Harvard University Press; 1983.
11. Kohlberg L. The cognitive development approach to moral education. *Phi Delta Kappa*; 1975: 670-677.
12. Piaget J. *The Construction of Reality in a Child.* New York, NY: Basic Books; 1954.
13. Pellegrino ED. Educating the humanist physician—an ancient ideal reconsidered. In: *Fostering Ethical Values During the Education of Health Professionals.* Proceedings of a conference of the Society for Health and Human Values. Philadelphia, Pa; 1975.

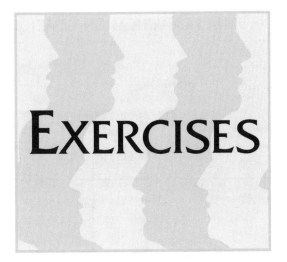

EXERCISE 1: VALUES CLARIFICATION CHART

Values shape and orient our choices, and so one way to examine our values is to examine our choices and to see if those choices have been made after reflection. On the next page is a chart that helps you explore things that can be said to be of value to most people. In addition to inquiring about the manner of choosing the item and its underlying value, the chart, taken from Simon, et al.[9] also asks us how positive we feel about the item and its value. The Values Clarification theorists claim that, in order to be a true value (as compared to a hope or aspiration or goal), it must meet these seven criteria of choosing, prizing, and acting:

Choosing (Table 3-4)
1. Chosen freely
2. Chosen from among alternatives
3. Chosen after thoughtful consideration

Prizing
1. Cherish it
2. Publicly affirm it

Acting
1. Do something about it
2. Consistently act on it in life as pattern

Table 3-4

VALUES CLARIFICATION CHART

Item	What Makes It Valuable? Underlying Value	Choosing			Prizing		Acting	
		1	2	3	1	2	1	2
1. Something I'm saving money for. *Vacation cruise*	*Meet new people Relaxation Stress relief*	✓	✓	✓	✓	✓	✓	✓
2. Most important thing I did last year.								
3. Something I quit doing recently.								
4. My dream vacation—no restrictions.								
5. One thing I'm proud of.								
6. A risk I'm glad I took.								
7. Something I learned to do in the past few years.								

A. Complete the chart on your own.

B. Discuss with 1 or 2 other classmates for 10 minutes.

C. Journal about what you learned.

EXERCISE 2: VALUES PRIORITY

Life Planning Handout—Value in Life?

Name_____ Date _____

Age _____ Year in College_____ Years living away from parents' home _____

1. Read through the entire list. This is not a semantics test, so feel free to cross out the definition and add your own if you wish.
2. Circle each item's level of importance to you.
3. After completing item 2 above, pick out and list in the spaces provided the 5 items that you feel are the most important to you and the 5 items that are the least important.

ACHIEVEMENT (Accomplishment; results brought by resolve, persistence, or endeavor)
        Not very important   Important   Very important

AESTHETICS (Appreciation and enjoyment of beauty for beauty's sake, in both arts and nature)
        Not very important   Important   Very important

ALTRUISM (Regard for or devotion to the interest of others; service to others)
        Not very important   Important   Very important

AUTONOMY (Ability to be a self-determining individual; personal freedom; making own choices)
        Not very important   Important   Very important

CREATIVITY (Developing new ideas and designs; being innovative)
        Not very important   Important   Very important

EMOTIONAL WELL BEING (Peace of mind, inner security; ability to recognize and handle inner conflicts)
        Not very important   Important   Very important

HEALTH (The condition of being sound in body)
        Not very important   Important   Very important

HONESTY (Being frank and genuinely yourself with everyone)
        Not very important   Important   Very important

JUSTICE (Treating others fairly or impartially; conforming to fact, truth, or reason)
        Not very important   Important   Very important

KNOWLEDGE (Seeking truth, information, or principles for the satisfaction of curiosity)
        Not very important   Important   Very important

LOVE (Want, caring; unselfish devotion that freely accepts another in loyalty and seeks the other's good)

| Not very important | Important | Very important |

LOYALTY (Maintaining allegiance to a person, group, or institution)

| Not very important | Important | Very important |

MORALITY (Believing and keeping ethical standards; personal honor, integrity)

| Not very important | Important | Very important |

PHYSICAL APPEARANCE (Concern for one's attractiveness; being neat, clean, well-groomed)

| Not very important | Important | Very important |

PLEASURE (Satisfaction, gratification, fun, joy)

| Not very important | Important | Very important |

POWER (Possession of control, authority of influence over others)

| Not very important | Important | Very important |

RECOGNITION (Being important, well-liked, accepted)

| Not very important | Important | Very important |

RELIGIOUS FAITH (Having a religious belief; being in relationship with God)

| Not very important | Important | Very important |

SKILL (Being able to use one's knowledge effectively; being good at doing something important to me or others)

| Not very important | Important | Very important |

WEALTH (Having many possessions and plenty of money to do anything desired)

| Not very important | Important | Very important |

WISDOM (Having mature understanding, insight, good sense, and judgement)

| Not very important | Important | Very important |

Five Least Important: **Five Most Important:**
1.   1.
2.   2.
3.   3.
4.   4.
5.   5.

(Directions: Number 1 = Favorite value of the 5 listed. Transfer numbers to summary table on next page.)

The Five-Sort Value Inventory

1. ( ) Achievement
   ( ) Altruism
   ( ) Justice
   ( ) Religious Faith
   ( ) Wealth

2. ( ) Altruism
   ( ) Autonomy
   ( ) Loyalty
   ( ) Power
   ( ) Recognition

3. ( ) Creativity
   ( ) Love
   ( ) Pleasure
   ( ) Recognition
   ( ) Wealth

4. ( ) Aesthetics
   ( ) Justice
   ( ) Pleasure
   ( ) Power
   ( ) Wisdom

5. ( ) Altruism
   ( ) Honesty
   ( ) Love
   ( ) Physical Appearance
   ( ) Wisdom

6. ( ) Achievement
   ( ) Aesthetics
   ( ) Health
   ( ) Honesty
   ( ) Recognition

7. ( ) Achievement
   ( ) Autonomy
   ( ) Physical Appearance
   ( ) Pleasure
   ( ) Skill

8. ( ) Autonomy
   ( ) Emotional Well Being
   ( ) Health
   ( ) Wealth
   ( ) Wisdom

9. ( ) Honesty
   ( ) Knowledge
   ( ) Power
   ( ) Skill
   ( ) Wealth

10. ( ) Achievement
    ( ) Emotional Well Being
    ( ) Love
    ( ) Morality
    ( ) Power

11. ( ) Aesthetics
    ( ) Autonomy
    ( ) Knowledge
    ( ) Love
    ( ) Religious Faith

12. ( ) Aesthetics
    ( ) Loyalty
    ( ) Morality
    ( ) Physical Appearance
    ( ) Wealth

13. ( ) Creativity
    ( ) Health
    ( ) Physical Appearance
    ( ) Power
    ( ) Religious Faith

14. ( ) Health
    ( ) Justice
    ( ) Love
    ( ) Loyalty
    ( ) Skill

15. ( ) Aesthetics
    ( ) Altruism
    ( ) Creativity
    ( ) Emotional Well Being
    ( ) Skill

16. ( ) Emotional Well Being
    ( ) Justice
    ( ) Knowledge
    ( ) Physical Appearance
    ( ) Recognition

17. ( ) Altruism
    ( ) Health
    ( ) Knowledge
    ( ) Morality
    ( ) Pleasure

18. ( ) Morality
    ( ) Recognition
    ( ) Religious Faith
    ( ) Skill
    ( ) Wisdom

19. ( ) Emotional Well Being
    ( ) Honesty
    ( ) Loyalty
    ( ) Pleasure
    ( ) Religious Faith

20. ( ) Achievement
    ( ) Creativity
    ( ) Knowledge
    ( ) Loyalty
    ( ) Wisdom

21. ( ) Autonomy
    ( ) Creativity
    ( ) Honesty
    ( ) Justice
    ( ) Morality

Value Inventory Rating Summary

To summarize the results of the previous exercise, enter the numbers you recorded (for the first set of 5) in the first box of each of these values below. Each value occurs 5 times, so when you are through recording all 21 sets of 5, you will have 5 entries for each value. Add those 5 numbers across. The Totals column will then give you some ideas of the respective weights you give to the values involved. Remember, the lower the number in the Totals column, the higher that value ranks in your priorities.

						TOTALS
1. Achievement						
2. Aesthetics						
3. Altruism						
4. Autonomy						
5. Creativity						
6. Emotional Well Being						
7. Health						
8. Honesty						
9. Justice						
10. Knowledge						
11. Love						
12. Loyalty						
13. Morality						
14. Physical Appearance						
15. Pleasure						
16. Power						
17. Recognition						
18. Religious Faith						
19. Skill						
20. Wealth						
21. Wisdom						

Top 3 values:
1.
2.
3.
Are you surprised? If yes, why? If no, why not?

EXERCISE 3: ENVIRONMENTAL CRISIS

This is another exercise designed to help you learn more about the values you learned at home, some of which you may not have given much thought to but accept as true and often believe everyone accepts them as true.

The Situation

You are a young health professional in a moderately sized metropolitan hospital that has an entire unit devoted to the care of patients with kidney disease. The Kidney Unit can accommodate 5 people at a time on dialysis and is the only unit within a 500-mile radius that has dialysis capability. At times there are scheduling difficulties, at which time a committee is called together to help resolve decisions of priority. The committee is made up of health personnel from the hospital and community, and of lay people from the community. You are on that committee.

The community in which you live and work has had a crisis. A toxin has leaked into the water supply for the city and has made over half of the citizens terribly ill. Those most vulnerable to the toxin are people with kidney disease. Ten people lie near death (within 1 hour) unless their blood is dialyzed. There are only 5 machines.

The committee has been called together to decide who should receive priority. It is impossible to save the lives of all of the victims, but you must make the decision of which 5 will be saved.

Your group has only minimal chart information about the 10 people and 30 minutes to make the decision. Your group realizes that there is no alternative to making this choice if 5 people are to be saved. With no decision, all 10 people will die.

Here is what you know about the 10 people:

1. Bookkeeper, male, 31 years old
2. Bookkeeper's wife, 30, 6 months pregnant
3. Second year medical student, male, African American
4. Famous historian and author, 41 years old, female
5. Hollywood actress, 50 years old
6. Biochemist, 35-year-old female
7. Rabbi, 54-year-old male
8. Olympic athlete, shot put, 19-year-old male
9. College student majoring in health profession other than medicine, female
10. Owner of a topless bar, 56-year-old male, prison record

Instructions

1. Read the situation carefully.
2. Working alone, decide the 5 people who are to go on dialysis. You have 10 minutes to make your personal decision.
3. At the instructor's signal, join with 3 others in the room and, working as a group of 4, decide on the 5 people to receive dialysis. You have only 20 minutes to make your decision. Argue strongly for your ideas and opinions. The future of these people's lives depends on your group decision. Make sure your group is satisfied with the final list. Agree with other group members only if they truly convince you that their idea is better than yours.
4. Decisions by majority vote are not permitted. Every member of your group must agree with, and be committed to, the decision.

Table 3-5

VALUES AS DETERMINANTS OF BEHAVIOR

Group	1	2	3	4	5	6	Total
Bookkeeper							
Bookkeeper's wife							
Medical student							
Historian							
Hollywood actress							
Biochemist							
Rabbi							
Athlete							
Health professional student							
Topless bar owner							

5. Group discussion: At the end of 30 minutes, 1 member of each group comes forward and places a mark in the data summary box on the board in the front of the room (Table 3-5). Discuss as a group.

   a. Why you decided on each person. What were the assumptions you made that convinced you and others of the worth of each person's life?

   b. What process did you go through to decide? Once you accepted the responsibility for the decision, was it difficult to decide on the final 5? Who in the group was most convincing? How vocal were you in arguing for what you felt was right?

   c. What values emerged as you decided on the worth of a person's life and the opportunity for that person to continue living? Where did those values come from? When your decision was challenged, were you surprised that someone placed a different value higher than yours? Or did you assume most everyone would agree with you?

   d. After reflecting a few minutes, comment on this exercise and what it teaches us about the nature of stereotype, labeling, and prejudice. How might this affect our decisions as clinicians?

Did anyone suggest that every life has equal value and, therefore, recommend a lottery? How do you feel about that idea?

Journal about what you felt as you completed the exercise and what you learned about yourself with regard to what you believe is true and worthwhile, and what you learned about your style of arguing for what you believe in. What are you feeling?

EXERCISE 4: CLINICAL FIELD TRIP

This is an exercise designed to deepen your understanding of the nature of health care behavior and, specifically, of patient-clinician interaction. Read over the questions below carefully and then visit a facility where patients are being treated by health professionals from the profession you've chosen. Visit as an observer only, as a "fly on the wall" and carefully make observations from which you'll respond to the question asked. Once the questions are answered, journal about what you learned and felt with this experience.

1. What pleased you about what you saw?
2. What bothered you?
3. How did this experience impact on your choice to be a health professional?

Clinical Interaction Observation

1. Observe the environment. Describe how things are ordered, how things appear, and comment on possible underlying values.
2. Is efficiency a value? How do the patient care professionals perform or function in relation to wise use of time?

The patient/practitioner relationship is one of the major influencing factors affecting the success of treatment. This relationship is based upon the establishment of sound, professional judgement. No two practitioners approach the patient in exactly the same manner. With experience, you will develop your own personal style of rapport. By observing interactions between experienced health professionals and their patients, you will be better prepared to form your own approach to patient interaction.

Use the following questions as a guide to direct your attention to specific aspects of patient treatment. You will be concerned primarily with the verbal and nonverbal communication which exists between practitioner and patient.

Attending Skills

1. What did the practitioner do to attend to the patient's personal needs and/or comfort before, during, and after treatment?
2. How did the practitioner maintain the patient's dignity during treatment?
3. Did the practitioner seem to really listen to the patient's description of his or her illness/disability as it is "lived" by that person?

Communication Skills

NONVERBAL BEHAVIOR

1. Did the practitioner exhibit any personal mannerisms/behavior that might have added to or detracted from gaining the patient's confidence?
2. Could you add and explain why any additional behaviors might have been effective?
3. Was the practitioner a good listener? What behaviors make you say that?
4. Did the practitioner maintain eye contact while talking with patients? If not, did it seem to detract?
5. Were practitioner and patient at the same eye level for most of the time? Comment.

VERBAL BEHAVIOR

1. Describe and comment on the practitioner's voice quality as he or she communicated with patients (soft-spoken, brusque, rapid, etc).
2. How did the practitioner seem to motivate the patient? Was the method effective?

Summary

❖ What impressed you most about your visit?
❖ What impressed you least?
❖ What did you learn that you didn't know before?

(Adapted from course material developed by Marilyn DeMont Phillips, PT, MS)

IDENTIFYING AND RESOLVING MORAL DILEMMAS

Carol M. Davis, PT, EdD, MS, FAPTA

OBJECTIVES

1. To describe professional ethics and to distinguish among ethical situations, ethical problems, moral temptation, and true ethical dilemmas.

2. To describe the various factors that should be considered in making a sound ethical decision.

3. To compare discursive or principled ethical reasoning processes with nondiscursive aspects of ethical reasoning.

4. To outline the difficulties inherent in using the principles and rules of traditional biomedical ethical reasoning alone in resolving dilemmas.

5. To offer the Realm-Individual-Process Situation (RIPS) model for ethical problem solving that incorporates traditional discursive ethical reasoning with nondiscursive elements such as story, virtue, discernment, and meta-beliefs, and applies these to individual, institutional, and societal dilemmas.

Ethics is the study of morality. Moral decisions are decisions about what is right and wrong, or better and best, to do in a situation. *Descriptive ethics* discusses the moral systems of a group or culture, *normative ethics* deals with establishing a moral system that people can use to make moral decisions, and *metaethics* is the study of the meanings of ethical terms.[1] *Bioethics*, or biomedical ethics, is the application of ethics to health care.

Why should health professionals have to consider the ethical? Practitioners are faced with several decisions each day. Most health professionals place great importance on making sound clinical or therapeutic decisions in their practice. At times, the legal ramifications of a clinical decision become apparent. But less seldom do practitioners consider the ethical or moral implications of their decisions unless they come face to face with a difficult moral dilemma, one that is not easy to resolve with confidence.

ETHICAL DECISIONS ARE A PART OF CLINICAL DECISIONS

Whereas clinical decisions are based on weighing and considering facts (eg, given these lab values and these symptoms, the diagnosis seems to be X) moral decisions are based on weighing and considering values, so there is no such thing as a *true* or *false* moral decision. But just as it is highly important for health professionals to make the right clinical decision, it is assumed that practitioners would rather act ethically than not, choosing the highest or best moral alternative in a value laden dilemma.

Clinical decisions, no matter how purely factual they seem, still deal with people making decisions about what is best and true for other people. Few clinical decisions, especially those that deal with alternative treatment choices, are void of a moral component, for most clinical decisions necessitate weighing the value of various outcomes. Different people may place different importance on the values aspects of any decisions.[2] Value-laden ethical decisions, like factual clinical decisions, are better made if they are made thoughtfully and rationally, not based solely on intuition or the emotion of the moment.

ETHICAL SITUATIONS, PROBLEMS, AND DILEMMAS

There are 3 major kinds of ethical decision-making opportunities in clinical practice: **ethical situations**, **problems**, and **dilemmas**. **Ethical situations** contain important values or duties, but require no problem solving, no difficult decision making, yet ethical action is part of the situation. Many ethical decisions are simple to solve. In the same or a similar situation, the majority of people would do the same thing such as refusing to assist, indeed, trying to prevent, a depressed person from taking his own life.

Then there are **ethical problems**. **Ethical or moral temptations** fall into this category, where we know what we should do but do not want to do it, often because we stand to profit, or self-interest takes precedence over doing good for others (or beneficence).

More difficult ethical decisions, **dilemmas**, deal with which is better and which is worse—do I continue to treat (and bill) this terminally ill patient even when my treatment is of little benefit, but my visit seems to make a big difference in the quality of his day-to-day existence? This example might be seen to be a struggle between the ethical principles of beneficence (contribute to the good of each patient) and distributive justice (just distribution of limited resources to those who would benefit most).

The choice of the right thing to do is very unclear since acting on one moral conviction means breaking another.[1] For example, as a physical therapist, if I act on behalf of my patient recovering from a stroke but in a plateau stage, and document that he is still progressing with physical therapy, I am not telling the truth, for he has gone into a stage where progress is not obvious each day. However, if I tell the truth, the best interests of my patient are compromised, for the third-party reimbursement will be withdrawn, and he will not be able to pay for therapy. If this happens, in my professional opinion, he will regress. This illustrates a dilemma where beneficence, acting in the best interest of my patient, means breaking a moral conviction to tell the truth. Which is the higher moral alternative? How do I decide?

Some would say that the most difficult of all moral decisions in health care have to do with allocation of scarce resources. Who deserves to receive help and on what do we base our decision?[2] The above situation may illustrate the third party payers' reply to the question of distributive justice, that is, only those who are showing regular change—either improvement or decline—should be reimbursed for physical therapy services. If they want to continue with treatment, they will have to pay for it out of pocket.

WHAT DO WE DO WHEN FACED WITH NOT KNOWING WHAT TO DO?

When faced with an ethical decision, what choices do we have? We could ignore it, we could follow our ideas or perceptions of "current custom," (what "everyone else would do in this situation"), we could ask our superior what to do, we could search for a policy that speaks to our problem, or a rule to follow, we could do what feels emotionally best or right, we could follow our perception of the dictates of our religion, we could follow our perception of the dictates of our family rules, or we could apply traditional methods of ethical dilemma resolution in the search for the best moral alternative.[2]

This last suggestion is advocated in bioethics, of course, but unfortunately, many health professionals choose one of the former alternatives and "hope for the best." Ethical dilemma resolution has not received the attention in professional curricula that clinical decision making has received. Many health professional educators feel very uncomfortable teaching students how to decide the best moral alternative, for there is no one principle that binds us, there is no absolute dictum against which we can measure the adequacy of our moral choice as being best.

BIOMEDICAL ETHICS VS EVERYDAY ETHICS

What issues come to your mind when we speak of biomedical ethics or health care ethical decisions? The press favors reporting life and death moral dilemmas that deal with issues that reflect the increasing impact of high technology on health care: organ transplants, fetal tissue research, euthanasia, and abortion, for example. Granted, these ethical dilemmas are important, and we all benefit from studying the ethical treatment given these issues from ethicists who help direct us in our own decision making. Our task is to read the various arguments and to decide which argument and conclusion seems to match our own evaluation of the best alternative, both in terms of logical soundness and consistency and in terms of what we feel in our hearts is the highest moral alternative.

Many bioethicists would tell us that our hearts should have nothing to do with this problem solving, for our hearts contaminate our reasoning with subjectivity that cannot be substantiated with logic.[3] This would seem more acceptable if we were robots dealing with robots. Because we are people, health professionals dealing with the everyday issues of deciding the best thing to do with people who are our patients and their families, it is impossible for many of us to find comfort solely in the rationalistic discursive resolving of dilemmas according to principles alone. The compelling facts of each situation, our own personal priorities, our personal knowledge of the individuals and situation involved, and our own personal integrity developed over time by making decisions and weighing the consequences, will all come into play to help us decide which is the best decision in this particular situation, with the limited information we have in this moment.

Rarely do we deal with life and death ethical problems of euthanasia day to day. The ethical dilemmas we face day to day have to do with trying to do the best thing for our patients within the organization or institution of health care delivery, created mainly to meet the needs of great numbers of people, not individuals. These dilemmas often have to do with maintaining or improving the quality of a single patient's life. In discussing quality of life in the nursing home, the well-known ethicist, Arthur Caplan,[4] says it this way:

> *In one sense the disproportion of time and energy spent discussing transplants, artificial hearts, and other issues of high technology, acute care medicine, is appropriate. Matters of when and whether life should be maintained are of fundamental ethical importance, but the seemingly small stakes involved in the nursing home context—setting mealtimes and bedtimes, use of the phone, the right to keep personal property in one's night-stand—should not lull anyone into thinking that daily life in a nursing home lacks either ethical content or importance.*

A survey of the most common ethical issues faced by physical therapists in New England reported in 1980 listed issues such as which patients should be treated, the obligations entailed by that decision, who should pay for treatment, and what duties are incumbent on physical therapists as they relate to physicians and other professionals.[5] In 1996, Triezenberg published data that indicated that there was a shift in most common ethical issues toward concerns about overutilization, supervision of support personnel, informed consent, protection of patients' right to confidentiality, justification of appropriate fees, truth in advertising, preventing sexual misconduct and abuse, maintaining clinical competence, ethical guidelines for the use of human subjects in research, and inappropriate endorsement of equipment and products by physical therapists.[6] Interestingly, a panel of experts listed what they felt would be future ethical issues within the next 10 years (1995 to 2005). That list included: response of physical therapists to environmental issues of pollutants and health hazards associated with specific treatment modalities (eg, fluoremethane spray effect on the ozone layer), employment discrimination, duty of physical therapists to report misconduct in colleagues, defining the limits of personal relationships in physical therapy, encroachment on practice, utilization of treatments not validated by research, use of advertising, and sexual and physical abuse of patients by physical therapists and those whom they supervise.[6]

FOUR COMPONENTS OF ETHICAL ACTION

The ability to make a mature moral or ethical decision requires 4 behaviors that are often viewed as progressing developmentally: **moral sensitivity**, **moral judgment**, **moral motivation**, and **moral character**[7] (Table 4-1).

Table 4-1 illustrates simply knowing the best or right thing to do does not insure that a person will do it. Most difficult of all of the components is moral character or moral courage. Moral sensitivity, judgment, and motivation can be encouraged and taught, but standing up for what you believe in the face of adversity requires self-discipline, impulse control, and resistance to fear of rejection and losing one's position, status, acceptance, or job.

INGREDIENTS OF A MORAL DECISION

A moral statement says that, in situation X, person Y should do Z. Thus, a moral statement includes: what should be done (Z), who is to do it (Y), and the conditions under which the statement is applicable (X).[2] Most decisions made each day in health care are working decisions based on the facts of the situation. The decision is subject to modification or even reversal when more facts become known. Decisions have to be provisional when each day brings new facts to bear. This is the reality of day-to-day health care. "Our task then," according to Francoeur, "is to collect as much information as possible and then refer to the principles involved and choose the highest or best moral alternative in light of the situation at hand."[8]

Let's take a look at discursive or principled ethical reasoning and see how it can guide us in deciding the highest or best alternative, and then look at nondiscursive methods that will help us discover our own "metabeliefs," which underlie and influence our final decisions about what truly is right and best in each situation.

TRADITIONAL BIOMEDICAL ETHICS

Traditional discursive or principled ethical reasoning requires adherence to 4 levels of thinking: 1) the *particular ethical decision* will be made by 2) favoring an *ethical rule* which 3) sits within an *ethical principle* which 4) evolves out of an *ethical system*.[8]

Table 4-1

FOUR COMPONENTS OF MORAL ACTION

Moral Sensitivity

Ability to interpret a situation correctly and appropriately.

Awareness of how our actions will affect others.

Awareness of all possible lines of action and their effects on others and self.

Ability to imagine various scenarios with limited facts.

Ability to role play and take the other's part.

Moral Judgement

Judging which action is right or best, wrong or worst.

Judging which line of action is more morally justified given the facts.

Grasping the importance of the context of the situation which will point to the higher, more caring, more morally justified value.

Moral Motivation

Prioritizing moral values over personal values.

Wanting to care, do the beneficent thing over self-interest.

Moral Character

Having the strength of your convictions, courage, and persistence in overcoming distractions, pressures, and obstacles, no matter how large.

Having implementation skills, focus, and ego strength: "Here I stand. I can do no other." (Martin Luther)

Resisting fatigue, the morality of the day, the morality of expedience.

Having self-discipline, impulse control, and skill to act according to one's highest goals.

Resisting the need to be approved of, liked.

Ethical systems grow out of how we tend to view the world, or, in the terminology of Chapter 1, how we "set our lenses." We try on and adopt points of view about right and wrong as we grow up and follow the dictates of higher authorities such as our parents and church authorities.

Two ethical systems predominate: 1) ends- or results-oriented systems that say that the best way to decide the right thing to do is to act to bring about the best result, the maximum good, (teleological systems), and 2) duty- or principle-oriented systems or deontological systems that say that the proper decision should not simply be decided by the results. The highest moral alternative should be situated in principles or rules known to be right whether they serve good ends or not.[2] In sum, in deciding the best thing to do, does the end (commonly the greatest good) most of the time justify the means, or do the means need to be carefully weighed without primary concern for the outcome?

An example of a behavior that stems from a teleological or consequential way of looking at an ethical problem (ends are the most important) would be to act so that the greatest good can be brought about for the greatest number. That which is best is that which benefits everyone. Individuals come second to the good of the group. Hospital and nursing home administrators often make decisions based on this principle, for example when all patients are required to go to bed at a certain time for the convenience of the staff. Another question that could be asked to weigh the good of an action from this perspective would be, "Would I be satisfied with the consequence of this action if it were done to me?"

On the other hand, duty-oriented ethicists would look to ethical principles, which are those general and foundational truths, laws, or doctrines used by deontological ethicists to generate ethical rules about how to act in certain situations, <u>regardless of the consequences</u>. Many principles exist, and in each situation we appeal to the most relevant and appropriate principle to generate the highest moral action.[8] Previously we described ethical dilemmas that seemed to be related to the principles of beneficence, truth telling, and distributive justice. We had to decide whether telling the truth or loyalty to the patient was the highest moral alternative in the context of the situation.

MORAL PRINCIPLES AND RULES OF PROFESSIONAL CODES OF ETHICS

Four moral principles, and 3 rules that stem from those principles, make up the foundational ethical framework for the professions (law, theology, and medicine), each one of which provides service to the community.[8] A scan of most Code of Ethics documents will reveal ethical standards based on the following principles and rules:

Autonomy—Do that which enables the patient's/client's right to choose for one's life and to voice that choice for as long as possible. Informed consent, or the freedom to act on one's own behalf and to implement one's free decision, is a right situated in the principle of autonomy.

Beneficence—Do that which is best for your patient or client. In fact, professionals are obliged to act in the best interests of the patient, when the benefit to the patient outweighs harm it may cause the professional. At first glance, it may seem as if beneficence and nonmaleficence are the same, but they are not.

Nonmaleficence—Above all, do no harm. Do not do anything that: may cause injury; disable or kill a person; or undermine the person's reputation, property, privacy, or liability. In all cases, prevent any harm from happening. This principle is often the one that is cited as the higher alternative to not allowing a patient to die because removing life support is seen as causing harm rather than allowing a natural event to occur (allowing death to take place rather than stopping it). The key question to be answered is, by your action are you preventing harm (an untimely death), or preventing death from taking place when it is inevitable and no semblance of meaningful life is probable.

Justice—Act with fairness to all:

❖ *Distributive justice*: Equal distribution of goods (attention, service) to all members of a group. (All qualified drivers with disabilities receive the same sticker to be used on their cars for parking privileges).

❖ *Compensatory justice*: Act to make up for past injustice (affirmative action)

❖ *Procedural justice*: First come, first served, or alphabetical order most common procedures used to be fair to several.

The 3 ethical rules that follow from these 4 principles include:

1. **Veracity**—from autonomy and beneficence. Tell the truth; do not lie. Most often this rule is challenged with the question of just how much of the truth should the patient hear, and when.

2. **Confidentiality, Privacy**—from beneficence. Moral obligation to keep confidential all information concerning patients/clients even if not specifically requested by the patient or client, except when doing so would bring harm to innocent people or to the patient or client personally. In addition, patients or clients have the right to keep private information not relevant to care.[8]

3. **Fidelity**—from beneficence. Actions should at all times be faithful not only to one's patient or client, but to one's fellow colleagues. Criticizing the opinion of a colleague to a patient or family members undermines the whole of health care. When you disagree with a colleague, you can simply say that you have formed a different opinion.

In sum, these principles and rules serve as a beacon to all health professionals when confronted with a moral dilemma. Due to the nature of the professions (bound in service), these values turn out to be the higher ones in principled decision-making. At times we are confronted with a patient who requests one thing (autonomy), and we feel it is not in his or her best interest to comply (beneficence). Then we must guard against paternalism, or choosing for the patient what is best because we think we know better. Instead we must strive to inform the patient so that he or she can make the best decision for him- or herself. And then we must do what we can to ensure our patients' right to choose for themselves, even if we disagree.

Most often, unfortunately, the common dilemma is between autonomy or beneficence and self-interest, in other words, moral temptation, which becomes disguised or rationalized.[9] For example, the physical therapist may say that 10 or more treatments are necessary to meet the functional goals set for the patient in order to ensure the income from those visits, whereas if the patient had been placed on an adequate home program, those visits may not have been necessary. The extra income is a self-interest decision that would be rationalized as necessary treatment for quality care. This decision was far more common a decade ago than it is today, and in part, poor judgements such as this (multiplied by millions) is what helped push the pendulum of reimbursement to the other, highly unfair, extreme. Currently, it is the exception, rather than the rule, to be reimbursed fully by third-party payers for care that is given.

ADVANTAGES AND DIFFICULTIES WITH THE UTILIZATION OF PRINCIPLES

When one is face to face with having to decide which is the highest moral action to take in a given situation, it helps to be freed up from the intensity and confusion of spontaneous feelings. This is true whether we're deciding a "true" biomedical dilemma such as distributive justice—who should be treated and who should not, or a day to day dilemma such as the head nurse who has to decide whether the dying patient on the unit can have a visit from his grandchildren from out of town who arrived after visiting hours were over.

Utilizing a reflective problem-solving process that takes into account all of the given facts and uncovers all of the principles and rules that might apply is a way to rise above the subjective moment in an attempt to articulate an objective and defensible rationale for your decision. Trying to discern the best rule or principle, or the highest moral action is often the most difficult decision, especially when you have limited information and must act right away.

We've stated that a teleologist will adopt the point of view that the facts should be weighed and the action that is best would be the action that benefits the greatest number. (The head nurse decides that the visit of young grandchildren might be disruptive to other patients—the greatest number—and decides not to allow it.)

The duty-oriented person will refer to a list of principles and pull out all of those that seem to bear on the case, and weighing the facts, decide which principle is the highest in this situation. (The head nurse decides that beneficence, contributing to the good of the patient, is more important than worrying about future decisions if all patients ask for this privilege and the chaos that might result [justice].)

THE DIFFICULTIES OF PRINCIPLED DECISION-MAKING

Edmund Pellegrino, a well-known medical ethicist, asks, "Is there a set of obligations which bind all who practice medicine?"[10] Is there one rule, or set of rules, that health professionals will find almost always is the highest moral alternative in health care? This task of deciding would be made simpler if there were. Put simply, adherence to principles doesn't always work because people disagree about which principles are most acceptable. Gilligan posits that "the way people define moral problems, the situations they construe as moral conflicts in their lives and the values they use in resolving them are all a function of their social conditioning."[11] Thus, even recognizing a problem as having an ethical aspect to it has a lot to do with how we were brought up, and how we view the world, how our "lenses are set."

NONDISCURSIVE APPROACH TO ETHICAL DILEMMA RESOLUTION

"While acknowledging the power of such rational systems, nondiscursive ethicists, however, challenge the narrowness of a strictly applied, formal system of ethical reasoning."[12] Nondiscursive ethicists do not claim that discursive ethics are too theoretical or difficult to carry out. Rather their complaint is that theories, principles, and rules alone promote a formalized, purely objective, cognitive way of thinking that is excessively rational and unbalanced. Too often principles are in conflict. Nondiscursive ethicists attempt to balance the process of dilemma resolution by incorporating such aspects of thought as imagination, virtue, character, role, power, discernment, and liberation in their search for an adequate method to decide the highest moral alternative.[13]

The Importance of a Person's Story

The final ethical choice (even the decision of which theory seems more compelling), ends vs means, derives from within a personal moral narrative, developed over time, that we all inherit. Robert Nash believes that to restrict ethical decisions to rules and principles alone "sends out the false message that a person's story is irrelevant to (or worse, destructive of) the 'proper' formation of a moral self."[13] A person's story is a "moral necessity because it provides one with the ethical skills to form one's life truthfully, committedly, and courageously… Objective discursive systems allow for rational, step-by-step deliberation and decision-making. However, the individual's moral intentions and motives originate in, and are formed by, significant people and events in the individual's life."[13]

The key perspective in discussing the nondiscursive aspect of dilemma resolution is to make clear that a choice of the highest moral alternative can be seen to be seated in a rather consistent system of values that can be uncovered by proving one's moral convictions in a deliberate fashion, or by writing a personal ethical autobiography. Once this story is better understood, important questions of character and virtue (What kind of a person am I? and What kind of a person should I be as a health professional?) can be brought up to the light of day. Health professionals must be helped to recognize the way they have set their lenses so that they can adjust to a more professional perspective. For example, if what emerges on self-examination is a preoccupation with self-interest or a fear-laden perspective that takes precedence over autonomy, nonmaleficence, or beneficence, which are critical to professional health care value decisions, then the health professional must realize that decisions he or she makes very often will not be with highest concern for the welfare of the patient.

Deontology and teleology both presume personal integrity. Principled ethicists believe that one develops moral character and integrity by making rule-based decisions justified by ethical principles. Nondiscursive ethicists insist that moral character and integrity consist of more than this. Being moral requires constant training as a child and young person, and that training is more than applied ethics. "Integrity is the life-long outcome of actions that shape particular kinds of character… and the character that develops is like the narrative of a good novel; it gives a coherence to ethical decisions, and forces individuals to claim their actions as their own."[13]

As we learned in the previous chapter, cognitive developmental psychologists such as Kohlberg favor a type of training to be moral.[12] They maintain that children are only able to learn how to make higher or more adequate ethical decisions as they develop their cognitive reasoning skills. Moral developmentalists advocate teaching children how to reason morally by teaching them how to solve moral problems. The best moral decisions, according to Kohlberg, are those that are logically consistent and admit to fewer exceptions, respect the dignity of all persons, and aim toward just treatment of all people regardless of the law, or of the person's race, creed, color, gender, or sexual orientation. Finally, cognitive developmentalists such as Kohlberg and James Rest offer a method of testing that developmental level of moral consciousness of a person by asking them to comment on the moral aspects of a dilemma that they identify as being most relevant.

In this way, subjects reveal whether they have progressed in their reasoning to an understanding of moral principles or if they remain "stuck" in simply obeying the law or doing that which is socially appropriate.[12]

VIRTUE ETHICS—THE DEVELOPMENT OF INTEGRITY OR CONSISTENT MORAL BEHAVIOR

What kind of a person should I be? Integrity is built from a continuum of choices, some important enough to be remembered, some almost habitual and unreflective. Each time a student cheats in class or a citizen cheats on reporting income for tax purposes, that choice to behave unethically, no matter what the rationale, wears away at the development of integrity. Choice is not only about what to do in a given situation; choice in making moral decisions is about who I want to become. The key question in self-examination is this, "How does a truthful examination of my moral actions fit my moral image of myself?" Do I claim to be a person of virtue and integrity but choose to participate in gossip, judge others with prejudice, lose my temper, break my promises if I believe they're stupid promises, hurt people under the guise of trying to "help" by being honest, or lie when it is expedient to my goals? Answering truthfully requires our lenses to be set to listen carefully to the essential self; the ego must be still. For the ego, the pragmatic goal seeker will act to get ahead and rationalize that action so that it sounds acceptable, even clever.

How does this detrimental pattern of choice make sense? It makes sense if, in my autobiography I remember the moral axioms of a parent who repeated such phrases to me as "Get them before they get you;" "If you don't look out for yourself, no one else will;" "People get what they deserve;" "The only thing that matters is who wins;" "The winner is the one with the largest or most possessions or salary;" and "Life is hell and then you die, and they throw dirt in your face." This pattern of negative choices also makes more sense today in light of commonly reported ethical lapses by our national and state elected and appointed leaders who most often publicly claim to be highly moral. The moral dictum of "do and say whatever you think will get you re-elected" is the behavior we read about continually. Our country seems to have slipped into a period of the morality of personal gain and expediency, with the emphasis on not being caught. Only now are we waking up to the fact that one result is that we are destroying the planet we live on in the name of personal gain and technological "progress."

Fear-based axioms such as "get them before they get you" are often behind this behavior, and, over time and with repeated exposure, this negativity will seat itself in one's conscience. Feelings of guilt and shame will then surface when you feel someone is out ahead of you, or is better than you are in class, or when you feel as if you've acted naively or allowed yourself to be taken advantage of.

In a conflict over altruism or beneficence vs self interest or personal gain, it will be difficult to act for the good of your patient when to do so makes you feel as if you've been taken advantage of. Very often, day-to-day ethical decisions are made by deferring to policies and procedures as a way to assuage guilt. For example, a day-to-day decision of what to do about a walker, paid for by the patient but left behind after her discharge to a nursing home, may not be seen as an ethical decision if one refuses to deal with this mistake because she's "too busy with more important things."

"It's just too bad that the walker was left behind. Thanks for the donation to the department. I don't have time to chase down discharged patients. They're not our concern once they've left this facility." This treatment of a decision ignores the ethical aspect entirely. Selfish concern over the value of one's time vs concern over returning property to its rightful owner and then "passing the buck" by claiming that it's not your fault or problem are attempts to brush away the inadequacy of this mistaken choice.

Thus one's character, built up over the years by listening to important moral statements and making little decisions day after day, will dictate even whether a clinical decision has a moral component to it or not. If a *value-laden decision* is not even recognized, *the process of solving the dilemma for the highest good will never even begin.*

In other words, being moral means: 1) being able to identify the moral aspect of a problem; as well as 2) being a certain kind of person who wants to be able to reason adequately; and finally 3) doing the right thing. Virtue ethicists claim that virtues such as compassion, generosity, fidelity, graciousness, justice, and prudence should be cultivated in people so that doing the right thing becomes consistent with one's character.[14] A person will choose one's ethical behaviors more wisely if he or she chooses in accordance with commonly held virtues. Virtue ethicists argue about which are the most important virtues, of course. Karen Lebaqcz argues that the virtues of fidelity and prudence should be central to the professions. Fidelity to clients includes trustworthiness, promise keeping, honesty, and confidentiality; prudence has to do with "an accurate and deliberate perception that enables professionals to perceive realistically what is required in any situation."[15]

DISCERNMENT AS A VIRTUE

The common criticism of virtue theory is that cultivating virtue in one's being does not dictate that one will act virtuously in all instances. One might argue that a virtuous person, by definition, would tend to act in a virtuous way, but character traits alone are not enough to ensure the highest moral action.[16]

However, if one has reflected on one's values, has paid attention to moral choices, and has developed integrity and compassion over time, it becomes easier to act with moral consistency, and inconsistencies serve to stir one's conscience in a way not as available to the morally unaware. As Table 4-1 suggests, moral character is more assured following moral sensitivity, judgment, and motivation.

The concept of the *discernment* is integral to the development of character in that discernment is that ability to assert that there is more than objective rationality to moral decision-making. Thus, by introducing the whole topic of nondiscursive aspects of moral dilemma resolution in this chapter, I am acting on the quality within me of discernment. I believe that the best truth to be found is found *within* the human decision-maker, within the essential self, and every moral decision is a decision that should combine the best of logic and rational methods with attention to the various impulses and movements that occur within a deliberative consciousness.[13]

What is required in day-to-day ethics is a balance of heart and head, founded in a virtuous moral character that places the good of our patients foremost. Ethical decision-making should never be reduced to subjectivity and feelings or intuition alone. The nondiscursive aspects of moral decision-making are not meant to replace the discursive, but to add to it to approach a balance with head and heart. Attention to the nondiscursive elements in a moral decision helps one to gain a personal understanding of the moral life. It is in paying attention to this aspect of moral reasoning that one can decide, for example, "when one is willing to make or break a promise, when to tell only the truth, to decide what one is willing to die for."[13] Further, to learn to live the consistent and good moral life is one reason why, I believe, we are all here on this earth.

THE ETHIC OF CARE

The ethic of care suggests we do what is most important to preserve the integrity of the therapist patient relationship.[17] To care for the patient is to have regard for his or her views, interests, and cultural mores, to hold warm acceptance and trust for the other, rather than doing good simply because beneficence dictates it. Sensitivity to the deepest values and concerns of the patient in the context of his or her life situation is what drives the decision-making. Obviously to follow an ethic of care requires moral sensitivity and judgement, discernment, and excellent interpersonal skills. Clinicians must listen carefully to the initial history and the patient's description of the problem, and the meaning that this has in the person's life. The current economic pressures of the health care system commonly place restrictions on the ability of the therapist to engage with patients in such a way as the ethic of care requires. The institutional constraints on caring have to be confronted as an ethical situation for therapists to be able to practice without feelings of conflict or doubt, but once this is done, the quality of one's practice can be anticipated to improve.

ETHICS AND THE LAW

As a general rule, ethics provide higher standards of the best or "right" thing to do than do state laws. Laws are created to protect the citizens of the state from unsafe practice; ethics bind a professional to the highest form of care.

With regard to the laws of health care practice, each state in the United States has statutes called "practice acts" that guide the limits of professional obligation and responsibility for professionals in that state alone. The statute itself is accompanied by a document, usually referred to as Rules, that further clarifies the statute. The Rules can be clarified and changed more easily than the statue itself, which was created by the lawmakers of that state for its citizens.

Changes in health care management are occurring so rapidly that health care professionals are constantly having to refer to their practice acts to ascertain what is within and what lies outside the scope of their practice, as well as the scope of practice for paraprofessionals such as physical and occupational therapist assistants.

When no specific law exists to cover an action that ends up in the courts, in the past, the court (the judge) ruled according to interpretation of the facts of the case and his or her interpretation of the practice act. However, in recent years, courts have been holding health professionals to a higher standard than the state practice act dictates.[18] For example, in spite of the fact that not all physical therapists are members of the APTA, which binds its members to a Code of Ethics for proper practice, the court is starting to accumulate case law decisions that all physical therapists are professionals who should be held to this Code of Ethics standard.

MANAGED CARE

In many cases, corporate health care, managed competition, capitation, and prepaid health organizations (PPOs) have been limiting patient access to physical and occupational therapists, and limiting the therapists' choice of and duration of reimbursed treatments. Under managed care, physical therapists have both professional obligations to patients and may have contractual obligations to managed care organizations (MCOs). It is important that health care professionals be able to carefully analyze their patients' needs and use sound moral reasoning and ethical dilemma resolution skills to decide on the appropriate actions for the good of the patient, and for justice or appropriate fairness when there is a shortage of professional care available.

Remember that until recently managed care corporations had no moral obligations to their clients—the patients. Managed care is a business only. In the eyes of the law, MCOs do not practice health care. The primary duty of the health care professional is always to the patient, and secondarily to the business contract. This can result in ethical distress when you know the best thing to do but are prohibited from doing it by the organization within which you practice. For example, if, under capitation agreement, the MCO provides coverage for only 6 visits and the goals set for the patient at the initial evaluation cannot be met in such a short time, the health professional can be held liable for abandonment if his or her response is to discharge the patient short of the agreed upon goals with the comment, "Your MCO told me I had to stop care." Business cannot dictate to a health professional when to discontinue treatment.[18] Professionals are obligated to provide needed care. Likewise, professionals have the right to maintain an adequate financial base of practice, and thus should seek private or other reimbursement from the patient.

Case law now indicates that the court's expectations are for the professional to carry out the duty to continue to serve the patient pro bono, or without compensation. Thus each practice needs to develop a policy or guide outlining how it will determine the incidence and limits of pro bono care, and beyond that, the care of the patient who cannot pay but requires treatment should be transferred to colleagues who have pro bono capacity at that time.[18]

Currently, several state legislators in the United States Congress are drafting legislation that will offer protections for consumers enrolled in managed care plans, as well as health care professionals providing their care. For example, some states now have state statutes that permit consumers to sue their managed care organizations when less than adequate care has occurred.

When health care as a service is managed as if it were a business, where profit is the primary reason for its existence, a conflict is bound to emerge. We have seen the concept of facilitating the healing of the whole patient or client all but disappear from health care. Business executives with their eyes on the bottom line dictating to health care professionals who they can treat, for how long, and what is reasonable to charge, strip health professionals of their ethical foundations. The very definition of a profession's autonomy requires that professionals are the only ones who can make those judgments, and they are morally obliged to make them, not with profit in mind, but with service for those in need.[9]

It is important that you, as a young health care professional, stay current with local, state, and federal guidelines on health care practice and reimbursement, and learn how to resolve the ethical dilemmas that result in these unstable times. Some predict that the negative impact of business on health care will become even more restrictive to providing quality care before improvements begin., but some benefits have occurred as a result of this shift toward managed care. Although the savings in health care costs are far less than were predicted, the current trend has resulted in isolated areas of cost containment, as well as a greater shift of the burden of care to patients and their families. This results in more responsibility on the part of patients for their health, for prevention, and for maintenance of their own care.

Above and beyond all trends and reimbursement mechanisms, when the interests of the patient and the professional collide, always remember that beneficence and autonomy ethically must outweigh self-interest.[9] If professionals were engaged only in business, there would be no dilemma. Health care professionals are bound by codes of ethics of service, not profit, that mandate advocacy for our patients who come to us because we have both the education and the commitment to help them.

RIPS PROFESSIONAL ANALYSIS MODEL FOR RESOLVING ETHICAL PROBLEMS

Professional behavior requires fulfilling a role in society in relationship to individual patients or clients, in relation to the institutions and organizations in which we practice, and in relation to society as a whole. In the past, resolving ethical dilemmas concentrated on one aspect of this complicated relationship alone—the relationship with individual patients or colleagues. While all ethics is interpersonal, the most compelling dilemmas we deal with in this new century often concern our relationship with our organizations and institutions and with society.[19] In truth, to be ethically competent, we must be able to resolve all kinds of ethical situations taking into consideration the context of the situation (the realm), the individual process involved (moral sensitivity, judgment, motivation, and courage) and the kind of ethical situation that is before us—an issue, problem, temptation, or dilemma.[20]

Dr. Laura Lee (Dolly) Swisher from the University of South Florida has developed a model of analysis that combines the work of Jack Glaser[21] in the realm arena, James Rest[7] in the individual process arena, and Ruth Purtilo[21] in the ethical situation arena and has termed it the RIPS Model of Analysis, or the Realm-Individual Process-Situation Model.[20]

The ethical rules of veracity or informed consent or confidentiality are well worked out at the individual level, but when it comes to the systems, policies, and procedures of organizations and institutions, or the cultural dictates of society, it becomes far less clear as to how to act. Swisher explains that each of the realms, at best, tries to promote the good and encourages moral behavior, but each realm will differ on definitions, on priorities, on authority, and on what data are meaningful in coming to the decision of what is best and right in a given situation. In other words, ethics gets more complicated as you move beyond the concerns of individuals, and you cannot resolve organizational and societal ethical distress and dilemmas with individual modes of action. The inability of a person in a wheelchair to access an entrance to a public building is, in part, an issue of justice (individual), but it requires policy changes beyond simply changing the rules (organizational and societal). Likewise, the unwillingness of Medicare to reimburse for treatment based on faulty research or inaccurate reimbursement formulas goes far beyond veracity. Policies and procedures, authority, laws, and bureaucratic customs all converge on decisions of federal reimbursement, and "organizational and social problems demand strategies and solutions appropriate to that realm."[20]

SOLVING THE ETHICAL PROBLEM: A SUGGESTED PROCESS

Ethical issues, problems, and dilemmas occur frequently, and require different problem analyses and solutions. The most difficult problem to resolve is a dilemma, when two or more ethical principles conflict with each other in a given situation and it is unclear what the best or highest moral action would be. Several processes for dilemma resolution have been suggested in the literature.[1-3,6,9,10,16,17-22] I suggest the following problem-solving method be applied to solving *all* ethical situations including ethical dilemmas. It incorporates rule-based method (deontology) with consideration of the consequences (teleology) and attends to nondiscursive elements (virtue theory and the ethic of care), as well. This method is an adaptation of the work of Seedhouse and Lovett,[23] and the work of Swisher with the RIPS model.[20]

1. Gather all the **facts** that can be known about this situation.

2. Decide which **realm** is primary: individual, organizational, or societal (Table 4-2).

3. Then decide the **process** that seems to be called for: sensitivity, judgment, motivation, or character (see Tables 4-1 and 4-2).

4. Decide what level of ethical **situation** is involved: issue, problem, temptation, distress, or dilemma (see Table 4-2).

5. If the situation is within the realm of **organization, institutional or societal efforts** for resolution should focus on identifying needed policy and systems changes. Suggest the values that are involved and the policies and procedures that contribute to the ethical problem. Tackle the problem at the individual process level required—sensitivity, judgement, motivation, or courage (see following example). Very often intervention consists of writing letters to Congress, publicly demonstrating, and other methods aimed at raising sensitivity to unjust and immoral laws and policies.

6. If the situation is a **true ethical dilemma** at the individual level then proceed to decide which ethical *principles* are involved (eg, beneficence, nonmaleficence, justice, autonomy, confidentiality, veracity, and/or fidelity).

Table 4-2		
RIPS FRAMEWORK TAKEN FROM THE WORK OF SWISHER		
Realms	*Individual Process*	*Situation*
Individual	Moral sensitivity	Issue
Organizational	Moral judgment	Problem
Societal	Moral motivation	Dilemma
	Moral courage	Distress
		Temptation

Adapted from Swisher LL. Realm-Individual Process-Situation (RIPS) Ethical Analysis Model. In: Arslanian LE, Davis CM, Swisher LL. *Ethics From the Trenches: Everyday Ethics and the Real World.* Presentation at the APTA Combined Sections meeting, Nashville, TN, February 2004.

7. Clarify your professional *duties* in this situation (eg, do no harm, tell the truth, keep promises, be faithful to colleagues, etc). Duties such as these are often outlined in one's Code of Ethics.

8. Describe the general *nature of the outcome desired*, or the consequences. Which seems most important in this case, an outcome that is most beneficial for the patient, for the family, for your colleagues?

9. Describe pertinent *practical features* of this situation—one or more of the following: disputed facts, the law, the wishes of the others, resources available, effectiveness and efficiency of action, the risk, your Code of Ethics and Standards of Practice, the degree of certainty of the facts on which you base your decision, the predominant values of the others involved (which may or may not coincide with the values predominant in health care in the United States).

When all of the pertinent aspects that go into this particular decision are laid out before you, then you must use your discernment to decide which action is the highest moral alternative. You should be able to justify your decision by explaining both your ethical reasoning process and your conscious weighing of one value over another in this situation, based on what you know about your moral character, the virtues, traditions, and beliefs that frame your choices in life and your professional ethical mandates.

APPLICATION OF THE SUGGESTED PROBLEM-SOLVING PROCESS

Let's take an example first of an ethical situation that involves the expectation of a kickback or gift in exchange for referring patients. An occupational therapist certified in hand therapy visits a local orthopedic hand surgery practice with information about her skills and her practice in hopes of educating the physicians and office staff about the benefits of referring their patients to her for rehabilitation. She is told by the receptionist that unless she was prepared to offer regular golf outings at the local country club, she could not compete with the local physical therapist who got there before she did, even though he was not board certified.

This surely is an ethical problem. Let's apply the problem-solving process to it. The **facts** are that a highly qualified hand therapist would like to receive referrals from an orthopedic surgery practice, but she is told she must give a kickback or pay for the referrals in competition with another therapist who at face value seems less qualified to help the patients than she is. Another fact is that kickbacks are against the law, but unlike pharmaceutical manufacturers and medicine, exactly what constitutes a kickback, and what constitutes an "expense associated with promoting one's business" has not been clearly delineated by either physical or occupational therapy organizations.

Going to Table 4-2, we decide that the principle **realm** involved here is organizational. The ethical situation is between the occupational therapist and the orthopedic practice or the organization. The **individual process** required is one of moral courage, or implementation. The OT is motivated to want to work for change but will need the courage to report this infraction and still remain in her mind a viable therapist in the community. The **situation** would be one of distress. She may be tempted to just look away and not make waves, and thus protect her business, but she knows that what is going on currently is unethical and illegal and not good for patients. She knows what she must do, but she has to work up the courage to do it. She has to report the physical therapist and the orthopedists to their state boards of practice. So this is not an ethical dilemma at all, but a very uncomfortable ethical distress.

Now let me illustrate how I would use this process to solve a dilemma. One rather common ethical problem that occurs in spinal cord rehabilitation facilities is the dilemma of what to do when a mentally competent patient refuses beneficial treatment. (We already know that this is at the realm of the individual.) First, the facts:

Alex is a 23-year-old patient with a cervical fracture and spinal cord lesion at the level of C6-7. He has had a surgical fusion and is medically stable and ready to begin rehabilitation, but he refuses to allow others to transfer him from bed to begin the process of tolerating sitting. Testing has revealed normal intelligence and a suspected level of grief and depression following this accident. No active motion has yet been seen below the level of the lesion. The nurses have had problems with his refusal to eat, the physical and occupational therapists have been unable to get him out of bed, and the social worker has been unable to engage him in discussion about his depression. He lies in bed with the covers over his head and says, "Leave me alone, I want to die." The physician on the case refuses to take Alex's desires seriously but also shows little compassion or sensitivity, and he commands the orderly to bodily remove Alex from the bed and wheel him to physical therapy. The other members of the team, while not wanting simply to yield indefinitely to Alex's depression, believe that the physician's order is inappropriate and are struggling with what to do. They feel a strong pull of loyalty to other members of the team, including the physician, but resist the "command" to force Alex to comply. They feel a loyalty to their patient, but believe his depression blocks him from making the best decisions for himself at this time.

APPLICATION OF THE PROBLEM-SOLVING METHOD

1. Gather all of the facts.
   a. Cervical lesion, complete, at C6-7.
   b. Young man, 23, no committed relationship to a partner. Family—father, mother, sister—supporting and visit regularly.
   c. Completed 2 years of college. Proven intelligence. Taking a year off to "find himself." Risk taker. Athlete.
   d. Accident occurred showing off by diving into shallow water of friend's pool at a party late at night.
   e. From family history, suspected addiction to alcohol, history of risk-taking behaviors.
   f. Family has excellent health insurance.
   g. Friendly, bright personality; strong previous desire to contribute to society. Active in "Big Brothers," Boy Scouts.
   h. Without conferring with the team, the physician has ordered that they act in a way that seems to many to be abusive and insensitive to the patient's hopefully temporary feelings of depression and hopelessness.

2. Decide which realm—**individual**—between the team, the patient, and the physician.

3. Decide which process is required. Well, it's not moral sensitivity. The team understands and recognizes the problem. But they do *not* know what the best thing to do is, so this requires a process of **moral judgment**.

4. Decide which situation is present. There is no moral temptation really. The team genuinely does not know what is best to do. This is a problem that seems to come to the level of a **dilemma**. To act in fidelity to the physician who believes he is doing the best for the patient will be going against what the team believes is beneficial for the patient.

5. Organizational or societal issues at work here are not primary, so we go to...

6. **Ethical principles** involved: Decision of allowing the patient to have his freedom to act in his own interest, *autonomy*, vs acting in a way to convince the patient to get motivated to begin rehabilitation—*beneficence*—contributing to the overall benefit of the patient. But the other factor is: what is the action that is most beneficial? The doctor's demand to bodily force the patient to comply with a rehab plan may be the end desired, but the means does not seem to be justified. Above all, do no harm (*nonbeneficence*) is an issue, and a logical question would be: what harm might result from physically forcing the patient to comply? Fidelity to one's professional colleague seems to be less important than do no harm.

7. Clarify your duties in the situation. If I am the physical therapist I have a different specific duty than if I am the social worker, occupational therapist, recreation therapist, or nurse. But each of us has the duty to act in such a way that the patient is supported in overcoming his natural depression and becoming invested in hope for a new life. Once Alex gets beyond his depression and understands at the deepest levels what his choices will be living with quadriplegia, then his decision to live or die will be his to make, free of interference. Right now he doesn't have all of the facts, and his depression keeps him from even considering what those facts might be and how important they are to his decision. In other words, his depression renders him mentally incapable of deciding adequately in his own best interest. My duty as a health professional is to contribute to the team's individual and collective effort to support Alex through his depression and to help him learn what he can expect from life living with quadriplegia. I am also obliged to be faithful to my colleagues so that we are united in our approach and work together for a good outcome, but I cannot be faithful to a plan that might cause the patient harm. The physician's order is not one that I can readily follow, so the desire to do no harm and the patient's beneficence seem more important than fidelity to my colleague, the physician.

8. Describe the general **nature of the outcome desired**. I want Alex to become involved in rehabilitation and to learn what it is like to be as independent as possible with his quadriplegia, without having to go through the humiliation of being bodily forced to participate in rehabilitation.

9. Describe pertinent practical features of the situation.

   a. *Disputed facts*—1) It is permissible to insist that patients not yield to depression by bodily forcing them to go to rehab. The end justifies the means. This fact can be disputed, as well as, 2) Alex is taking up someone else's bed who wants to be involved in rehab, and someone else "deserves" the rehab bed more.

   b. *Wishes of others*—1) Family wants everything done for Alex, as soon as possible. 2) Mother has little tolerance for son's depression. Concurs with physician's order. Father asks for patience and perseverance, plus treatment of depression.

   c. *Resources available*—Rehab beds are in demand, but money is not an issue for the family.

   d. *Risk*—Forcing Alex to be involved in rehab could cause injury to body or emotions. Also, it may backfire, causing more resistance.

e. *Degree of certainty of facts*—The most uncertain of the facts concerns the nature of the cervical lesion—what will Alex's physical and emotional deficit look like in 6 months, in a year? How debilitated will Alex be, and how independent can we hope he can become? How successful will he be in reforming his core self-worth and values so that he might live a fulfilled life as a patient with a disability? Likewise, we are uncertain just how long Alex's depression will last. But even with the uncertainty of the future, the fact now is that he is physically ready to participate in rehab. Also certain is the fact that rehab cannot take place successfully without Alex's cooperation.

Decision.

1. Meet with the team physician to discuss unwillingness to carry out the order to force Alex to go to rehab.

2. Confer with the psychologist, physician, nurse, and/or social worker and agree on a plan to systematically confront Alex's depression in a supportive way, with the goal of helping him through it in as timely a way as possible. Commit as a team to giving him the time he needs.

3. Once rehab has begun, practice beneficence and "guarded" paternalism while Alex is gaining a sense of himself with his new identity, and then be careful to relinquish any paternalism as Alex becomes able to cognitively and emotionally make decisions for himself, even if the health care team and/or family disagree with those decisions.

CONCLUSION

Two things seem obvious at this point. Moral decision making takes time, and I may not have considered aspects of this situation that seem quite apparent to you. What if the physician becomes enraged that the team has not followed his instructions and threatens to have each one fired? Sometimes moral stances come to this level of confrontation, but not often. When one's integrity is challenged, moral temptation seems to become more compelling. It helps to have systematically thought through your decision to avoid this lapse in moral judgement.

I hope you would see that the systematic process itself works to raise the decision-making process up out of the murky waters of intuition and subjectivity alone, and I could defend this decision as the best, or highest decision I could make at this time with the facts that I have been given. To go back on this decision because of a threat would weaken my integrity. I would hope that the situation would not come to that end, but if it did, I would be confident in my discernment and would, I hope, remain committed to my decision.

The exercises that follow will first give you a chance to discover more clearly the qualities of your discernment by asking you to write your moral autobiography, and then you will be given the opportunity to practice ethical dilemma resolution using the suggested process. Remember, you've been making personal moral decisions all of your life. Now what is asked of you is to search for the values, beliefs, stories, myths, and parables that have informed those choices in a consistent way, and how well will that way serve you now as a health professional? What changes must you make, if any, to remain true to a commitment to therapeutic presence and healing? Don't forget to journal about your discoveries.

REFERENCES

1. Purtilo RB, Cassel C. *Ethical Dimensions in the Health Professions*. Philadelphia, Pa: WB Saunders; 1981.
2. Brody H. *Ethical Decisions in Medicine*. Boston, Mass: Little Brown and Co; 1981.
3. Cahlahan S. The role of emotion in ethical decision-making. *Hastings Center Report*. 1988;June/July.

4. Kane RA, Caplan AL. *Everyday Ethics—Resolving Dilemmas in Nursing Home Life.* New York, NY: Springer Publishing; 1990.
5. Guccione AA. Ethical issues in physical therapy practice. *Phys Ther.* 1980:60(10):1264-1272.
6. Triezenberg HL. The identification of ethical issues in physical therapy practice. *Phys Ther.* 1996; 76(10): 1097-1106.
7. Rest JR. Background: theory and research. In: Rest JR, Narvaez D. eds. *Moral Development in the Professions.* Hillsdale, NJ: Lawrence Erlbaum Associates; 1994:1-26.
8. Francoeur RT. *Biomedical Ethics—A Guide to Decision-Making.* New York: John Wiley and Sons; 1983.
9. Pellegrino E. Alturism, self interest and medical ethics. In: Mappes TA, Zembang JS, eds. *Biomedical Ethics.* 3rd ed. New York, NY:McGraw Hill; 1991.
10. Pellegrino ED, Thomasma DC. *A Philosophical Basis of Medical Practice.* New York: Oxford University Press; 1981.
11. Gilligan C. In a Different Voice. Cambridge, Mass: Harvard University Press; 1983.
12. Kohlberg L. The cognitive development approach to moral education. *Phi Delta Kappa.* 1975;June:670-677.
13. Nash RJ. Applied ethics and moral imagination: Issues for educators. *Journal of Thought.* 1987;Fall:68-77.
14. Pence GE. *Ethical Options in Medicine.* Oradell, NJ: Medical Economics; 1980.
15. Lebaqcz K. *Professional Ethics: Power and Paradox.* Nashville, Tenn: Abingdon Press; 1985:87-99.
16. Purtilo RB. *Health Professional and Patient Interaction.* 4th ed. Philadelphia: WB Saunders; 1990.
17. Noddings, N. *Caring: A Feminine Approach to Ethics and Moral Education.* Berkeley CA: University of California Press; 1992.
18. Scott R. Challenges in professional ethics. *Symposium of Annual Scientific Meeting,* APTA. June 1997.
19. Purtilo RB. A time to harvest, a time to sow: ethics for a shifting landscape. Thirty-first Mary McMillan lecture. *Phys Ther.* 2000;80:1112-1119.
20. Swisher LL. Realm-Individual Process-Situation (RIPS) Ethical Analysis Model. In: Arslanian LE, Davis CM, Swisher LL. *Ethics From the Trenches: Everyday Ethics and the Real World.* Presentation at the APTA Combined Sections meeting, Nashville, TN, February 2004.
21. Glaser J. *Three Realms of Ethics: Individual, Institutional, Societal: Theoretical Model and Case Studies.* New York: Rowman and Littlefield; 1994.
23. Seedhouse D, Lovett L. *Practical Medical Ethics.* New York, NY: John Wiley and Sons; 1992.

SUGGESTED READING

Banja JD. Ethics, outcomes, and reimbursement. *Rehab Management.* 1994; Dec/Jan:61.
Clancy CM, Brody H. Managed care. Jekyll or Hyde? *JAMA.* 1995;273:338-339.
Curtain LL. Why good people do bad things. *Nursing Management.* 1996;27:63-65.
Grimaldi PL. Protection for patients or providers? *Nursing Management.* 1996;27:12.
Hiepler MO. *Lawsuits against HMOs and gatekeeper physicians.* Presented at the Sixth Annual Symposium on Managed Care, San Francisco, Calif, May 9, 1996.
Hiepler, MO. *Managed Care: A Revolution in Progress—Lawsuits Against HMOs/Gatekeeper Physicians.* Conference Recording Service. Berkeley, Calif. HFM96-3.
Palermo BJ. Capitation on trial. *California Medicine.* 1996;7:25-29.
Purtile RB, Jensen GM, Brasic-Royeen C. *Educating for Moral Action. A Sourcebook in Health and Rehabilitation Ethics.* Philadelphia: FA Davis; 2005.
Rodwin MA. *Medicine, Money and Morals.* New York, NY: Oxford University Press; 1993.
Salladay SA. Rehabilitation, ethics and managed care. *Rehab Management.* 1996;Oct/Nov.
Stahl DA. Risk shifting in subacute care. *Nursing Management.* 1996;27:20-22.
Zwerner AR. Capitation empowers doctors. *California Medicine.* 1996;7:29.

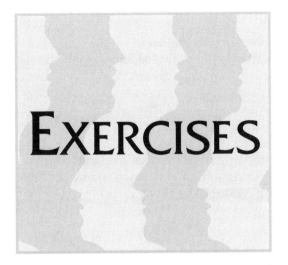

EXERCISES

EXERCISE 1: WRITE YOUR MORAL AUTOBIOGRAPHY

People reveal themselves in telling stories. We all have stories to tell about ourselves, our lives growing up, the choices we had to make, close calls we've had, funny incidents where we were caught off guard, a great (or terrible) date, a wonderful concert or movie, a great time with an old friend.

Carol Christ writes in *Diving Deep and Surfacing*:

> *When meeting new friends or lovers, people reenact the ritual of telling stories. Why? Because they sense the meaning of their lives is revealed in the stories they tell, in their perception of the forces they contended with, in the choices they made, in their feelings about what they did or did not do. In telling their stories, people speak of parents, lovers, ecstasy, and death – of moments when life's meaning seemed clear or unfathomable.*

One most important aspect of your story is your perception of how, growing up, the values of your family provided a sense of orientation for you—that perhaps became a taken-for-granted set of boundaries against which you played out your life, against which you had to contend, the currents in which you learned to swim, the forces that helped you to define yourself. In this way, those values provided a sense of meaning. They grounded you in powers of being that enabled you to challenge the obstacles of the world, to become who you are now.

Think back to when you were a child. You may want to interview parents and grandparents for more information.

1. What were the rules of the family? Where did those rules seem to come from? The Bible? The church? From ancient wisdom passed down?

2. What do you remember being punished for? What were your siblings punished for? Were you punished, or would you say you were "disciplined?" What is the difference to you?

3. What were you praised for? What were you encouraged to do? How did that make you feel?

4. Were there certain favorite virtues that were emphasized? For example, always refer to older people as Mr. or Mrs., always do your best, always tell the truth. Get good grades? Go out for sports?

5. What were the family rules for making decisions, or did that remain a mystery?

6. What do you remember being most emotional about? Did you have a favorite cause? Have you ever participated in a march for a cause or in any actions of civil disobedience? Would you, if you were challenged to? Why or why not?

Recount any major moral decisions you remember making. Write a story of the development of your moral consciousness. What values do you see as most important and how, from your story, do you know this? Does this have implications for your choice of profession?

EXERCISE 2: EXAMINE YOUR CODE OF ETHICS

Locate a copy of your profession's Code of Ethics. Analyze the Code statements to determine the values and ethical principles that are most esteemed by your profession. Next examine the Code, and its accompanying rules for what seems to be missing. What would you wish the Code and Rules would speak to that is not present? Are the directions for moral action specific enough for your guidance? Why not?

EXERCISE 3: EXAMINE YOUR STATE PRACTICE ACT

Locate a copy of the practice act for your profession and it's accompanying rules. Outline the scope of practice allowed by the act. What are you able to do, and what are you prohibited from doing? What guidelines are given with regard to delegation of care to aides and assistants? What might you be asked to do by an uninformed superior that would not be legal? What might you be asked to do that is legal but not ethical? How would you respond?

EXERCISE 4: VALUES DISCOVERY
(Adapted from the work of Dr. Elsa Ramsden, EdD, PT)

List the values you believe are the prominent values in society (for example, freedom of speech, more is better). Then list the values which were prominent in your family (for example, go to church on Saturday or Sunday, perfection is important). List the values you hold dear as an individual (for example, respect for others). (Refer to exercises at the end of Chapter 3 where you listed your values.)

Next list the values you found to be most important in your profession (eg, above all, do no harm, confidentiality). List the values you have observed in an area where patients are being treated by fellow professionals (eg, first come, first served). Finally, list what you perceive to be one individual's values as he or she practices your profession with patients (eg, confidentiality, beneficence).

Compare and contrast each set of values to your individual values. How well do they fit? What values listed can be located in your Code of Ethics? Which values are not contained in your Code?

EXERCISE 5: ETHICAL DILEMMA RESOLUTION

Below are several day-to-day ethical situations faced by health professionals. Choose one. Go through the process to solve it as illustrated in the chapter.

1. A physical therapist colleague in private practice admits that he charges less money for patients who pay with cash because he never records this income for tax purposes. You have been working for this therapist for 6 months, and in order to keep your job, he is asking you to adopt the same system and offers you a cash bonus of $5000 at Christmas because you deserve the money more than the IRS. Personal circumstances make this the only place where you can practice and still fulfill your family responsibilities. You are the only person in your family employed at this time, and you are supporting 2 children and an elderly mother.

   a. Look at Figure 4-2. Is this an individual, organizational, or societal problem?

   b. What kind of ethical situation is described here: an issue, problem, distress, temptation, or dilemma?

   c. Finally, what kind of process is required on the part of the physical therapist: moral sensitivity, judgment, motivation, or courage?

What should this physical therapist do? Why?

2. You have agreed to "fill in" for a home care therapist for 2 weeks. At 4 of the 5 patient's homes in one day, as you evaluated and treated according to your standards, the patients have made comments that the other therapist never did any of this kind of therapy. It becomes apparent to you that the therapist you are filling in for is giving no professional care. You are scheduled to move out of this town as soon as this 2-week time period ends to another state. If you report this person, you would need to return to the state to testify, but the state would pay your expenses to do so.

   a. Look at Figure 4-2. Is this an individual, organizational, or societal problem?

   b. What kind of ethical situation is described here: an issue, problem, distress, temptation, or dilemma?

   c. Finally, what kind of process is required on the part of the physical therapist: moral sensitivity, judgement, motivation, or courage?

What should this physical therapist do? Why?

3. At 4:45 a woman in severe pain walks into the physical therapy department with a referral from her physician to be evaluated and treated for severe low back pain. The physical therapist in charge (and the only one present) had stayed late to see patients well after the usual closing time of 5:00 for the past week. Further, the day care center had called just before the woman walked in, stating that the therapist's 6-month-old daughter was very sick, with severe vomiting and diarrhea, and they were very worried about her. The therapist's wife is out of town. The therapist tells the patient, "I'm sorry, we're closed for the day, and I must leave. You'll have to come back in the morning." The woman bursts into tears and says she doesn't even know if she can make it home, she is in such pain.

a. Look at Figure 4-2. Is this an individual, organizational, or societal problem?

b. What kind of ethical situation is described here: an issue, problem, distress, temptation, or dilemma?

c. Finally, what kind of process is required on the part of the physical therapist: moral sensitivity, judgment, motivation, or courage?

What should this physical therapist do? Why?

4. You are treating a woman who recently had a stroke. Her insurance allows for payment for only 10 treatments. What ethical implications are there when you cannot achieve agreed upon functional goals in 10 treatments? What is your professional responsibility? What is your legal responsibility? What would you do to resolve this problem short of refusing care? How might you go about working to change this organizational limitation from the insurance company? Would you do it? Why or why not?

EXERCISE 6: CONSIDER THE FOLLOWING TWO CLINICAL CASES AND RESPOND TO THE QUESTIONS BELOW

Mrs. A. is a 75-year-old patient sent to physical therapy outpatient service for chronic low back pain. Her symptoms were consistent with chronic degenerative changes in the lumbar spine, she has a history of osteoarthritis, and her most recent x-ray revealed bone thinning in the femoral neck and lumbar spine. Three weeks ago her husband of 55 years died after a long bout with COPD and lung cancer. She lives alone, and most of the day she is in pain, which is only slightly relieved with ibuprofen. She is hoping that you will confirm the seriousness of her problem and advocate for stronger pain medication from her physician. Once before she took a muscle relaxant that helped her pain tremendously, but she cannot get the physician to prescribe it until you evaluate her problem and give a report.

Mrs. B. is a 75-year-old patient sent to physical therapy outpatient service for chronic low back pain. Her symptoms were consistent with chronic degenerative changes in the lumbar spine, and she has a history of osteoarthritis. Her most recent x-ray revealed bone thinning in the femoral neck and lumbar spine. Three weeks ago her husband of 55 years died after a long bout with COPD and lung cancer. She lives alone, and most of the day she is in pain, which is relieved with percoset. She admits to you that she is probably addicted to her pain medication but that she desperately needs it now to help with her grief over her husband's death. She asks you to keep her confidence and not tell the physician that she is taking percoset, as he prescribed it for her husband.

1. List the clinically relevant similarities between these 2 patients

2. List the clinically relevant differences between these 2 patients.

3. What more do you need to know for:

Mrs. A?

Mrs. B?

4. What is the essential ethical difference between these two clinical problems?

    a. Look at Figure 4-2. Is this an individual, organizational or societal problem?

    b. What kind of ethical situation is described here: an issue, problem, distress, temptation, or dilemma?

    c. Finally, what kind of process is required on the part of the physical therapist, moral sensitivity, judgment, motivation or courage?

5. What would you do for Mrs. A? What would you do for Mrs. B?

This second section is composed of 11 chapters devoted to examining ways in which we interact with our patients and our colleagues. Chapter 5 introduces this topic with an examination of the nature of effective helping—what makes help helpful? If you've ever felt victimized by a well meaning person who insists on helping you when you don't want to be helped, you've experienced help that is not helpful. The characteristics of helpful help and the characteristics of effective helpers are both examined. The concepts of compassion and empathy are explored in relation to effective help. Empathy is distinguished from its similar interactional processes such as sympathy, pity, identification, association, and self-transposal. This chapter concludes with a closer look at the values that are conducive to helpful help, thus conducive to healing.

Chapter 6 introduces the development of a package of skills: problem identification, active listening, and "I" statements. Use of these techniques establishes a way of communicating effectively in the helper-helpee relationship. These skills also will assist you as you learn to be assertive in the face of tension. Chapter 7 presents assertiveness skill development and Chapters 8 and 9 prepare you for patient/client interaction by teaching you specific skills and knowledge to gain rapport.

Chapter 10 helps you to apply all that you've learned in conducting a "helping interview." Chapter 11 teaches you how to teach patients and their families. Chapter 12 offers knowledge and insight about our patients and clients with disabilities and how we can relate to them in the context of their situation with therapeutic presence. Chapter 13 provides a primer on human sexuality and essentials we all must know in order to communicate about this important area of function and expression in our patients.

Section II continues with Chapter 14, in which we examine the particular characteristics of effective interaction with those who are dying. Death is, for most of us, an uneasy reality that we would rather not have to consider as a natural part of our lives on earth. Depending on our profession and specialty, many of us will be called upon to care for those who have a limited time left on earth. It is helpful to have considered in advance the actions that are most caring and healing, and to be aware of potentially hurtful or harmful ways of communicating in these situations. However, even more important, considering our own limited time on the earth, we become intensely more aware of ourselves, of our priorities, of the attitudes and values that underlie a life of quality. Once you've experienced the readings and activities in Chapter 14, you should know much more than just how to communicate in a healing manner with the terminally ill. You will know more about yourself.

Chapter 15 concludes this section and the text itself. In this chapter we examine the concept of burnout, or the professional exhaustion sometimes experienced by health professionals, especially when they are confronted with problems that seem unsolvable or goals that seem unreachable. The final advice this text can offer you is that, when you are communicating well with your patients and colleagues, and taking a regular personal inventory of your feelings and the issues in your life as the journal process of this text has facilitated, burnout will be less likely to occur. The first step to preventing burnout is recognition of the problem. Nonetheless, emotional stress is, at times, inevitable. The key is to interrupt the process before it escalates. This chapter will help develop habits that will assist you in that process.

THE NATURE OF EFFECTIVE HELPING:
Empathy and Sympathy vs Pity

Carol M. Davis, PT, EdD, MS, FAPTA

OBJECTIVES

1. To describe the ideal overall aim of helping.
2. To explore the behaviors that interfere with effective helping.
3. To distinguish among sympathy, pity identification, self-transposal, and empathy.
4. To describe the characteristics of helping communication.
5. To reveal the characteristics of effective helpers.

When someone needs help, no matter what the nature of the help needed, we can assume that something's not right, something is interfering with day-to-day function and growth. Those of us in the healing professions have devoted our lives, for the most part, to helping those who need help in understanding and overcoming illness or disability. Some of us, however, are more concerned with working with people who are, essentially, well but need help in becoming more fit, or need help in preventing illness or injury. Whatever the problem, health professionals have devoted their professional lives to helping people overcome whatever is blocking them from living functionally useful and productive lives.

What should the overall aim of helping be? When we were small and needed help, we searched out whomever we felt could fix the problem and make us feel better. As children, we lacked the skills to solve our own problems, and so we depended on our mothers and fathers, or some capable adult to take charge. Unlike children, adults require a different sort of helping, for when someone constantly tries to "fix it," we often become resentful and angry and feel helpless and dependent. It is an important sign of maturity when we prefer to complete tasks, solve problems ourselves, and take pride in our individual accomplishments.

There are times, however, when we feel particularly alone and helpless and we may appreciate that "fixing" kind of attention and help offered by a friend. Remember the comment from a previous chapter that greeting cards emphasize this common human need in phrases like, "Before I even knew my own needs, you were there with a loving heart to respond." But this sentiment fails to acknowledge the more enduring need for adults to feel self-sufficient and capable of identifying and solving their own problems.

The overall aim of mature helping is to always make the helpee self-sufficient and to assist the helpee in achieving a more effective relationship between self and others and between self and the world.

We have discovered in previous chapters that our behavior is an expression of our values and our beliefs. Those who believe they are called to help others whether they want help or not can become annoying at the least and obstructive to others' development at the worst. Not all help is helpful. Many of us have laughed at the turmoil that can occur when a well-meaning person tries to open a door for us and actually blocks our way. At the other end of the continuum, however, is the well-meaning friend or parent who takes great care in telling us what to do in a given situation, then abandons us with indifference, refusing to support us until we comply with the advice given. "You asked me. I told you. You did what you wanted. Now I will have nothing to do with you." This is not very helpful.

As was pointed out in Chapter 2, helpers who have grown up in troubled homes and thus developed parenting skills too early bring immature ideas about the nature of effective help into adulthood. A few familiar characteristics of "unhelpful helpers" include an over-concern with matters that are none of their business, a need to be told how helpful, indeed, how *irreplaceable* they are to the functioning of a group, and a need to have others depend on them as if their very self-worth revolved totally around their ability to fix problems for others. Sadly, it often does.

The important truth in this matter is that no person can take responsibility for another person. We can only take responsibility for ourselves. Exceptions exist, of course, with children and with people who, for whatever reason, have lost the ability to be adequately in charge of their own lives (eg, those with certain mental illnesses, those with brain dysfunction). For most of us, the world exists for us the way we see it, the way we think about it. No one outside of us can make us happy or unhappy unless we allow it. Circumstances exist the way they are, but we have a choice as to how we think about them.

Effective helping usually has, as a primary component, a problem identification and problem-solving process. As health professionals, we learn important knowledge, skills, and values that we offer to assist those needing help to understand the nature of their problem(s) and to act in ways so that the problem is solved and a return to normal function and quality living is facilitated. *Our goal must always be to help the helpee become self-sufficient once again.* We must provide the conditions for our patients to identify their own goals around their health problem, provide the knowledge and skill to advise them on the wisdom of their desires, and then to help them get their needs met.

Patients may come to us with or without a diagnosis, but, contrary to common practice in most medical environments, the diagnosis serves as little more than a place to start in the helping process. The key questions remain: What are the problems from the patient's perspective? And what are the patient's goals in the healing process? Effective helping includes not merely a provision of information and therapeutic procedures, but involves helping the patient with the discovery of personal meaning as well.

THERAPEUTIC USE OF SELF

Central to this perspective on helping is therapeutic communication and the therapeutic use of one's self. How you view yourself will markedly affect your communication. Remember that the self-concept acts as a screen through which we view the world. Most of us have felt the discomfort of interacting with a person who continually apologizes for him- or herself, who distorts what we say out of feelings of insecurity, who responds with negativity and self-contempt. Each of us holds many varied opinions and ideas about ourselves, but our essential self-worth forms the core around which those ideas merge, and negative self-worth is one of the most important factors that needs to be changed in order to communicate from a healing perspective. Section I of this text focuses on the development of the ideas about the self, and how our feelings of self-worth evolve. This chapter focuses on the nature of effective communication in the helping process.

THERPEUTIC COMMUNICATION

Certain identifiable elements characterize therapeutic or healing communication. In the practitioner-patient interaction, the practitioner:

❖ Speaks—Communicates not just with an expression of ideas but with the ability to translate those ideas from an inner conviction to an outer clarity. Self-awareness enables the speaker to voice articulately well-thought-out ideas regarding the role of the patient in the healing process.

❖ Is fully present—Is totally focused on the patient and his or her ideas about the problem. Does not get lost in memories of "patients past" or possible future problems. Allows the interaction with the patient to command his or her full attention.

❖ Listens—Listens with the whole self, with the "third ear" in order to ascertain the patient's meanings and goals. Clarifies interpretations of what is heard. Resists categorizing or projecting personal beliefs and values. Resists giving quick advice, telling the patient what to do.

❖ Develops trust—Resists trying to influence the patient; instead, asks questions only to ascertain the truth about the problem as the patient perceives it. Communicates that the patient is worth listening to, that he or she has important information to add to this process. Resists assuming a priestly or parental role that conveys that the patient is dumb and that he or she is smart. At the same time, however, conveys the values of expertise and confidentiality and never neglects the opportunity for informed consent so that the patient feels that trust has been appropriately placed.

Thus the art of professional helping in the healing professions centers around the therapeutic use of oneself by way of a style of humanistic communication that places the patient in a position of informed equal, inevitably responsible for any positive outcomes in the helping process.

Health professionals:

❖ Listen, clarify, ask; never assume or make quick judgements.

❖ Identify problems with the patient, evaluate.

❖ Hypothesize causes.

❖ Treat through therapeutic measures and education.

❖ Reevaluate.

❖ Readjust to the new state and begin again until goals are reached.

A CLOSER LOOK AT INTERPERSONAL INTERACTION PROCESSES

At the heart of listening with the "third ear" is the process of self-transposal, which is often confused with empathy.[1] Empathy (Figure 5-1) is very often used interchangeably with several other interaction terms. Each term has a unique meaning, and it is helpful to understand and be able to distinguish among them. The terms most commonly used interchangeably with empathy include sympathy, pity, identification, and self-transposal. Of these, pity and identification often are not appropriate to the healing process. Let's take a closer look at each of these interactive processes.

When I *sympathize* (Figure 5-2) with you, I feel similar feelings about something outside of us along with you. I can feel joyful about your success, or I can feel sadness about the bad news that my patient received today. This is sympathy, or "fellow feeling." It is very commonly felt in health care, and it is totally appropriate in the healing relationship with patients.[1]

Pity (see Figure 5-2), on the other hand, rarely, if ever, is appropriate. When I pity my patient, I feel sympathy with condescension. "You poor thing," conveys an inappropriate inequality between myself and the other person; I lift myself up to be better than the other, and in that process, I

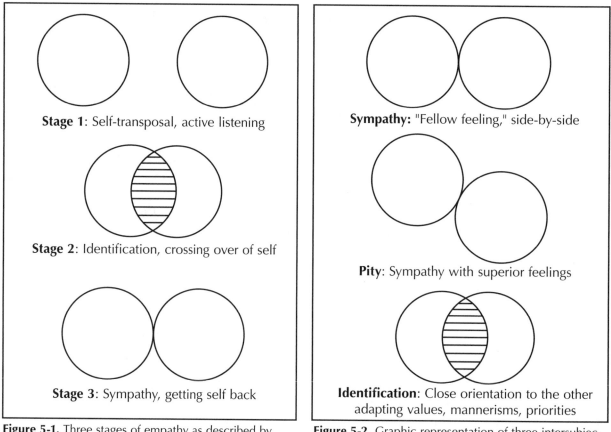

Figure 5-1. Three stages of empathy as described by Stein.

Figure 5-2. Graphic representation of three intersubjective processes.

demean the personhood of the other. Granted, pity may draw us to help others, but to help with condescension gives the message to the patient that you are judging him or her to be "pitiful."[1]

Identification (see Figure 5-2) can interfere with healing communication as well. When I identify with my patient, I begin to feel at one with him or her and in that process, I often lose sight of the differences between us. For example, just because we both have the same last name, or we both come from similar backgrounds, I may forget that he or she might have different values than I do. I may assume my patient feels as I do about wanting to know everything there is to know about a disease or disorder, or I may project that my patient is at her best in the morning and schedule her before noon. I forget to ask, to clarify. As a result, I confuse my meanings and values with those of my patient; I project my values onto the patient and act in ways that make the patient less important, less relevant to the healing process. In addition, as I identify, or become one with the patient, I risk losing my own perspective, which weakens my therapeutic objectivity, and I often become very subjective in the information I convey. Identification with patients often leads to an over-friendliness with patients and an inappropriate sharing of personal information that can interfere with the therapeutic nature of the relationship. I'll expand on this more before the end of this chapter.

Self-transposal is a cognitive "thinking of myself" into the position of the other. It is the process most often confused with empathy, putting myself in the other's place, or more commonly, walking a mile in another person's shoes. In his earlier writings, Carl Rogers refers to this as empathy, but in truth, self-transposal merely sets the stage for empathy to occur. In self-transposal, I listen carefully and try to imagine what it must be like for the patient to be experiencing what he or she is describing.[1]

Empathy as Unique Among All Interactive Processes

The process of *empathy* was first fully described by Edith Stein.[2] In her scholarly work, published in the 1930s, Stein characterizes empathy as absolutely unique from all other forms of interactions, distinguishable from other intersubjective processes first by the fact that we never empathize; empathy happens to us. It "catches" us. It is given to us much like true forgiveness; when it finally comes, it seems to be given to us. We can want to forgive, and try to forgive, but when the forgiveness finally comes, there is a sense in which we haven't done a thing except allowed it to come.

Second, empathy takes place in 3 overlapping stages (see Figure 5-1). The first stage is the cognitive attending to the other, or self-transposal, as described above. We listen carefully in an attempt to put ourselves in the place of the other. The second stage, following just a millisecond after, is, by far, the most significant. This is the "crossing over" stage, wherein we feel our selves crossing over for a moment into the frame of reference, or the lived world of the other person. We feel so at one with the other, we forget momentarily that we are 2 separate beings. This is the identification stage of empathy.

The third stage resolves the temporary confusion, as we come back into our "own skin," and feel a special alignment with the other after having experienced the crossing over.[2] This third stage resembles sympathy, or "fellow feeling." Thus empathy can be described as a momentary "merging" with another person in a unique moment of shared meaning. Elsewhere, I describe this process in more depth as it occurs within physical therapists for their patients.[1]

When empathy occurs, helping professionals need not lose their therapeutic objectivity, as so many fear, in getting "too close" to their patients. Instead what is experienced is a kind of holistic listening that can unite the therapist with the patient, yet allow the patient and therapist to remain fully separate in the healing process. It is in identification alone that we lose our objectivity and become destructively fused with the patient, as described earlier.

Thus, empathy is the intersubjective process that, among other things, empowers us to listen with the "third ear," to communicate humanistically and therapeutically with patients, thus contributing to helpful helping.

SETTING APPROPRIATE BOUNDARIES WITH PATIENTS/CLIENTS

The challenge, then, is for the health professional to be in therapeutic relationship with patients, yet maintain the helper-helpee relationship. It is imperative that this relationship remains functional, always serving the purpose of healing. How does the clinician reveal just enough about herself or himself to maintain the trust and collegiality without allowing the relationship to change into a more involved friendship or intimate relationship? Revealing too much might confuse the patient by seeming to convey that you are willing to give more than is appropriate for the helping process. Powell[3] describes 5 different levels of communication that one can use as guidelines for communicating effectively without revealing too much about oneself. These levels lie on a continuum from near indifference to extreme intimacy.

❖ *Level Five: Cliché Conversation.* No genuine human sharing takes place. "How are you?" "It's nice to see you." Protects people from each other and prevents the likelihood of meaningful communication.

❖ *Level Four: Reporting Facts.* Almost nothing personal is revealed. Some sharing takes place about information such as diagnostic data or the weather.

❖ *Level Three: Personal Ideas and Judgments.* Some information about oneself is shared, often in response to the patient's conversation. Topics talked about often relate to the patient's illness or the process the patient is going through, and if the patient looks bored or confused, conversation reverts back to Level Four.

❖ *Level Two: Feelings and Emotions.* A deep trust is required to share at this level, and if a person fears judgment, it will be impossible to relate at this level. True friendship and caring require this level of communication. Each person wants to be deeply known and accepted just as he or she is.

❖ *Level One: Peak Communication.* Mutual complete openness, honesty, respect, and love are required to communicate at this level. An all-encompassing intimacy is shared, often involving relating sexually. The minority of human interactions takes place at this level.

In therapeutic communication with patients, it is important for the professional to have a clear idea about appropriate boundaries that will facilitate healing. Once crossed over, interaction beyond this boundary will confuse patients, and the health professional will appear to be offering more of him- or herself to the relationship than is facilitative to the helper-helpee relationship. In most instances, interaction will take place at Levels Five, Four, and Three, with an occasional interchange at Level Two, but never at Level One.

New professionals often confuse the appropriate boundaries and find themselves caring too much, spending more time with one patient than is wise, or telling inappropriate stories or jokes in an attempt to make the patient feel at ease. The reverse often occurs when the patient feels compelled to help put the practitioner at ease. Patients don't need this added anxiety; they need to relax and trust that the health professional has his or her best interests at heart, and can manage the healing interaction free of awkwardness or threats to confidentiality and trust.

BELIEFS OF EFFECTIVE HELPERS

A.W. Combs[4] and colleagues at the University of Florida conducted research on the characteristics of effective helpers and concluded, "Good helpers are not born, nor are they made in the sense of being taught... Becoming a helper is a time-consuming process. It is not simply a matter of learning methods or of acquiring gadgets and gimmicks. It is a deeply personal process of exploration and discovery, the growth of unique individuals learning over a period of time how to use themselves effectively for helping other people."

Helpers were evaluated for their effectiveness, and the most effective responded to specific questions about their beliefs in 6 major categories. The results are summarized in Table 5-1.

These beliefs are all developed in a growth process that is very much influenced by the way the lenses we talked about in earlier chapters are set. The key to becoming an effective helper is to allow one's self to grow, to mature, to become more aware of feelings as well as thoughts, to be able to identify those beliefs that lead to behaviors that facilitate healing, and grow beyond defensive behaviors that result in negativity and fragmentation.

Professionals will act according to what they believe their purpose is. The purpose of the mature healing professional is to listen carefully with the "third ear," to evaluate, to assist, to support, to help problem solve alternatives that lead to healing, to apply therapeutic measures aimed at alleviating pain and dysfunction, to teach, to help others discover how to maneuver successfully in the world, and to solve their own problems that interfere with the highest and deepest functioning possible.

Carl Rogers[5] suggests 7 key questions that lead to a form of self-examination that will help us evaluate the quality of one's helping:

1. Can I behave in some way that will be perceived by the other person as trustworthy, as dependable, or consistent in some deep sense? Here congruence is the key factor. Whatever feeling or attitude is being experienced must be matched by an awareness of that attitude, and actions must match feelings.

2. Can I be expressive enough as a person that what I am will be communicated unambiguously? The difficulty here is to be fully aware of who one truly is. Rogers says this: "...if I can form a helping relationship to myself—if I can be sensitively aware of and acceptant toward

Table 5-1

SUMMARY OF THE BELIEFS OF "EFFECTIVE" HELPERS

Combs et al describe commonly held beliefs and perceptions of effective helpers in 6 categories.

1. Subject or Discipline

One is committed to knowing one's discipline well, but mere knowledge is not enough. Knowledge about one's discipline is so personally integrated and meaningful as to have the quality of belief. Effective helpers are committed to discovering the personal meaning of knowledge and converting it to belief.

2. Helper's Frame of Reference

Effective helpers tend to favor an internal frame of reference emphasizing the importance of people's attitudes, feelings, and values that are uniquely human over an external frame of reference that emphasizes facts, things, organization, money, etc.

3. Beliefs About People

Effective helpers believe that people are essentially:

- Able to understand and deal with their own problems given sufficient time and information.
- Basically friendly and well-intentioned.
- Worthy and have great value; they possess dignity and integrity that must be maintained.
- Essentially internally motivated, maturing from within and striving to grow and help themselves.
- A source of satisfaction in professional work rather than a source of suspicion and frustration.

4. Helper's Self-Concept

Effective helpers have a clear sense of self and their own personal boundaries before they enter into relationships with others. They feel basically fulfilled and adequate, so self-discipline is well practiced. Therapeutic presence for the other is made possible by a strong sense of self, of personal fulfillment, and of personal adequacy.

5. Helper's Purposes

Effective helpers believe that their purpose is to facilitate and assist rather than control people. They favor responding to the larger issues, the broader perspective rather than the minute details in life. They tend to be willing to be themselves, to be self-revealing. Their purpose includes honesty, acknowledging personal inadequacies, and need for growth. Another purpose is to be involved and committed to the helping process. They are process-oriented and committed to working out solutions rather than working toward preconceived goals or notions. They see themselves as altruistic, oriented toward assisting people rather than simply responding to selfish needs.

6. Beliefs About Appropriate Methods or Approaches to the Task

Effective helpers are more oriented toward people than toward rules and regulations or things. They are more concerned with people's perceptions than with the objective framework within which they practice. In helping people, the most effective approach is to discover how the world seems to that person. Self-concept is at the heart of the way one views the world, and so working with self-concept is imperative. Helpers have to be committed to gaining the trust of helpees so that self-control can be relearned in a positive way. The helping relationship makes this growth possible.

Adapted from Combs AW. *Florida studies in the helping professions*. Gainesville, Fla: University of Florida Press; 1969.

my own feelings—then the likelihood is great that I can form a helping relationship toward another."

3. Can I let myself experience positive attitudes toward this other person—attitudes of warmth, caring, liking, interest, or respect? This often engenders the fear that if we allow ourselves to openly express these feelings, the helpee might misinterpret our intentions, and the therapeutic distance might be blurred. The key here is to remain in our professional identities and yet still relate in a caring way to the other person.

4. Can I be strong enough as a person to be separate from the other? This question speaks to avoiding identification. I must be ever aware of my own feelings and express them as mine, totally separate from the feelings I may perceive that the helpee is experiencing. Likewise, I must be strong in my otherness to avoid becoming depressed when my patient is depressed, or fearful in the face of my patient's fear, or destroyed by his or her anger.

5. Can I let myself enter fully into the world of my patient's feelings and personal meanings and see these as he or she does? The key effort here is to avoid judging the patient's perspectives, but instead allow empathy to occur. In this way, once the world of the other is more fully experienced, the help that is offered can be based on this holistic level of knowing made possible by empathy. Meanings can be confronted with acceptance and modified to work toward healing. Judgment and criticism of meanings places a barrier between the helper and the helpee.

6. Can I act with sufficient sensitivity in the relationship that my behavior will not be perceived as a threat? A patient who feels free of external fear or threat feels free to examine behavior and change it. Patient care can be threatening in and of itself. Whatever we can do to lower anxiety will assist the effectiveness of our helping.

7. Can I meet this other individual as a person who is in the process of becoming, or will I be bound by his (or her) past and by my past? Martin Buber uses the phrase "confirming the other." This means accepting the whole potentiality of the other... the person he or she was created to become.[6] People will act the way we relate to them. The Pygmalion effect was described following the famous Broadway play in which a poor working girl showed that she could behave like a princess when she was treated like one and taught carefully.

The more one fully comprehends the importance of the nature of the helping interaction, the more one will become committed to the growth required for consistent therapeutic use of self. Yes, our professional knowledge and skill are critical to our effectiveness, but without the ability to interact in healing ways, we sabotage most efforts.

AWARENESS THROUGH ACTION

The exercises that follow are aimed at helping you discover your currently held ideas about the nature of helping, and why you are interested in becoming a health professional. Your beliefs about your self are explored, and you are given the opportunity to practice one of the major factors of effective helping: active listening. You'll be surprised how difficult it is to really hear what someone else is saying.

REFERENCES

1. Davis CM. *A phenomenological description of empathy as it occurs within physical therapists for their patients.* Boston University, Boston, Mass, 1982. Unpublished doctoral dissertation.
2. Stein E. *On the Problem of Empathy.* 2nd ed. The Hague: Martinus Nijhoff; 1970.
3. Powell J. *Why Am I Afraid to Tell you Who I Am?* Niles, Ill: Argus Communications; 1969.
4. Combs AW, Avila DL, Purkey WW. *Helping Relationships—Basic Concepts for the Health Professions.* 2nd ed. Boston, Mass: Allyn and Bacon; 1971.

5. Rogers C. The characteristics of a helping relationship. In Rogers C, ed. *On Becoming a Person.* Boston, Mass: Houghton, Mifflin; 1961.
6. Buber M, Rogers C. Transcription of dialogue held April 18, 1957, Ann Arbor, Mich. Unpublished manuscript.

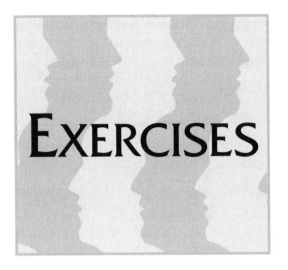

EXERCISES

EXERCISE 1: SELF-AWARENESS/ WHY DO I WANT TO HELP?

Respond to the following questions. Discuss with 2 or 3 others and then with the entire class. Note the variety of reasons why people are drawn to the helping professions, and note the responses most of you share in common.

1. Why do I want to be a helping professional?

2. Whom do I most want to help?

3. What specific rewards do I get from helping people?

4. How do I want to be perceived by those I intend to help?

5. Do I believe people are essentially lazy and will want to have me do all the work for them, or do I believe people most of the time want to help themselves? Is there a category of patients/clients who I believe are mostly lazy? How did I decide this?

6. I feel most anxious when I'm helping, whom?

7. Those who require the most help from others are who?

8. Answering these questions made me feel what?

Journal Reflections

As I reflect on my response to the above questions, what did I learn about myself?

EXERCISE 2: BELIEFS ABOUT SELF

Complete the following self-awareness continuum. Place a mark on the line that reflects your current belief about yourself. Discuss with a person in the class that you trust and can be open and honest with. Compare your responses to the beliefs of effective helpers as outlined in Table 5-1.

What I Believe About Myself Today

1. IDENTIFICATION

Feel apart from those I work with. Important to keep my distance, stay somewhat aloof.

Identify with others; I feel a part of those I work with, those I lead, those who are my patients.

2. ADEQUACY

Life is very complex, and I flounder a lot in trying to keep it together for myself. Hard to keep aware of all my choices in life.

Most of the time I'm capable of solving my own problems, at least dealing with them. Life situations usually offer several choices for me to make, and I usually do okay.

3. TRUST

The future of my health profession is somewhat shaky. I may not have a job; my curriculum is somewhat tenuous, dependent solely on the quality of various instructors that come and go. I may end up not being able to help much.

Basically, I feel I am a dependable, reliable person, capable of coping with the future of health care and of coping with my new growth no matter where it leads me.

4. DEGREE OF FEELING WANTED

Most days I feel pretty rejected and ignored. People on the whole don't act like they really want me around.

I may not be the most attractive person in the world, but mostly I feel I am essentially likable, attractive, and wanted.

5. WORTHINESS

My worthiness and integrity are often overlooked by most people, especially by those who really matter to me.

I feel I am a person of consequence, dignity, integrity, and worthy of respect.

(Adapted from Combs AW, Avila DL, Purkey WW. *Helping Relationships—Basic Concepts for the Health Professions.* 2nd ed. Boston, Mass: Allyn and Bacon; 1971)

EXERCISE 3: EFFECTIVE LISTENING

According to Rogers[5], good listening involves:

1. Not only hearing the words of the speaker, but hearing the feelings behind the words as well.

2. Putting oneself in the place of the other, or self-transposal; feeling the other's feelings and seeing the world through the speaker's eyes.

3. Suspending one's own value judgments so as to understand the speaker's thoughts and feelings as he or she experiences them.

Really listening is very difficult and takes practice, especially if you disagree with what is being said. Most normal conversations involve talking at one another rather than with one another.

Divide into groups of 3. One person serves as monitor, the other 2 as discussants. The monitor helps the discussants find a topic of mutual interest but one on which they fundamentally disagree. The first discussant states his or her position. In the typical discussion, we are so concerned with what we are going to say next, or so involved with planning our response, that we often tune out or miss the full meaning of what is being said. In this exercise, before any discussant offers a point of view, he or she must first summarize the essence of the previous speaker's statement, so that the previous speaker honestly feels his or her statement has been understood. It is the monitor's role to see that this process takes place with each exchange.

Discussion takes place for 10 minutes with the monitor assuming the responsibility of insuring that the procedure described above is followed. At the end of 10 minutes, discussants give each other feedback about how well they felt they had been heard, understood, and responded to.

The process is repeated with the monitor assuming the role of discussant and one of the discussants becoming monitor.

One more note: The role of monitor is critical to the success of this exercise. The monitor must insist that each person summarize the other's statement before speaking. This is difficult to do but essential to the success of the exercise. So, be insistent, and be brave!

EFFECTIVE COMMUNICATION:
Problem Identification and Helpful Responses

Carol M. Davis, PT, EdD, MS, FAPTA

OBJECTIVES

1. To teach communication strategies for interactions that are confused and/or emotion laden.
2. To define congruence and give the opportunity to examine one's own congruence or lack of it.
3. To emphasize the importance of both thoughts and feelings in communication.
4. To point out the risks and rewards of communicating clearly in the presence of intense feelings.

Very often the bulk of our communication throughout the day is quite superficial. Rarely do we communicate with the express purpose of trying to understand in order to be helpful. Even when we make a greater than usual attempt to listen carefully because we care and are concerned, it is rare that our interaction might be said to be truly helpful. Therapeutic communication requires learning a new skill, but more than that, it requires unlearning habitual, nonhelpful ways of interacting. This chapter is devoted to teaching you a new way of communicating with the express purpose of developing your abilities to use communication as an integral aspect of your therapeutic presence with patients. It might be helpful to begin with a case example.

> Jonathan was enjoying the seventh month of his first position as a physical therapist in a rehabilitation center. Each day he was experiencing more confidence in his skills in evaluation and treatment, especially using therapeutic exercise for patients with spinal cord and brain injury. One of his favorite patients was a young, 14-year-old high school cheerleader who had been referred to him 2 months ago while still in a coma in the intensive care unit. Diane had gone through the front windshield of her mother's car, a consequence of not having her seat belt fastened. Her mother escaped injury but was feeling tremendous guilt. She and Diane had been arguing at the time, and she mistakenly ran a stoplight that resulted in the accident.

> Just last week Diane began to respond to light and sound, and yesterday she opened her eyes and looked at Jonathan for the first time after he had transferred her to a chair at bedside. He was feeling elated, and was very hopeful that soon she would be responding to verbal commands.
>
> Diane's mother visited every day and often was present while Jonathan treated Diane. Today Mrs. Graham seemed particularly discouraged. Even though Diane was showing obvious signs of recovery from her coma, she was still unable to move. When Jonathan came to treat Diane, Mrs. Graham left the room but returned as he finished and told him she wanted to speak to him. As they walked out into the hallway, Mrs. Graham turned to Jonathan and shouted, "You're not helping her! No one is helping her recover. I asked around and found out you're a new therapist, and you can't know what you're doing or my daughter would have been well long before this! I want you to stop seeing her. I want a therapist with experience to treat my daughter. I never want you to set foot in her room again!"

The above is an example of an emotion-laden interaction similar to many that take place daily in hospitals and health care facilities. If you were Jonathan, how would you have responded? What would you have felt? Would you have quickly defended yourself? Would you have argued that Diane was showing remarkable signs of improvement? Would you have shouted, "Nobody speaks to me like that"?

When people are ill and injured, emotions run high both on the part of the ill and their families and on the part of those who are caring for them. Illness and injury stir up feelings of vulnerability and fear. People generally feel out of control and must give over control of their lives to strangers, often in institutions which seem like strange, impersonal, frightening cultures all their own.

At the root of every emotion-laden interaction is a problem. *What, exactly, is the problem in this situation, and whose problem is it?* Mrs. Graham would say that the problem is that her daughter is being treated by an inexperienced physical therapist and is not recovering because of it. Therefore, Jonathan and his inexperience are the problem. Jonathan might say that the problem was that Mrs. Graham was feeling helpless and responsible for her daughter's pain and injury and lashed out at him in her frustration. Another analysis might offer that the problem is that Diane did not have her seat belt on, and if she had, she would not even be in a coma.

This chapter focuses on identifying problems and clarifying problem ownership in interchanges that are characterized by intense emotions. In the midst of an interchange like the above, it is often difficult to sort out what is happening and what might be appropriate responses that would help resolve the situation. Different skills are required depending on the nature of the problem and who "owns" the problem.

The underlying theme in this chapter is this: **communicating in ways that help to solve problems, while at the same time respecting and honoring human beings, will facilitate the healing process**. Because we work with people who are ill and disabled, it is not enough simply to make the correct diagnosis and give the most appropriate treatment. Something more is expected of us. That "something more" includes helping the patient understand his or her illness or disability to the extent that he or she can make choices with regard to treatment and with regard to modifying lifestyles to prevent further problems and to live successfully with the problems that are not going to be resolved.

LEARNING NEW COMMUNICATION SKILLS

Each of us enters the helping professions having communicated all of our lives. It doesn't take much patient care experience to learn that the communication skills that served us quite adequately in our private lives often fall short of helping us to relate adequately to patients and colleagues in day-to-day patient care. As Dr. Eric Cassell writes in his book, *Talking with Patients*,[1] without effective communication we are unable to acquire objective and subjective information in order to make decisions that are in the best interests of the patient, and, more importantly, we are unable to utilize the relationship between practitioner and patient for therapeutic ends. This chapter focuses on sorting out emotion-laden communication in order to help patients identify and solve their own problems. Chapter 7 extends this theme in teaching you the skills of assertiveness, and Chapter 10 will instruct you in carrying out a helping interview.

EMOTION-LADEN INTERCHANGES

Communication connects us to the world. Humans are essentially social and need to feel a connection to others. Getting our basic needs met more often than not requires some form of communication.

Barriers to the effectiveness of communication might include the use of a foreign language (or the use of jargon), carelessness in choosing the words that convey exact meaning, and/or an inability or unwillingness to listen to each other carefully (hearing deficit, distraction by environmental "noise," unwillingness to concentrate, defensiveness). Many of us are rather unaware of how effective we are in day-to-day communication. It is difficult to come outside of ourselves and watch ourselves interact with others, reflecting on our feelings and the way in which we react to others. Others of us have been given direct feedback about our communication. Statements such as "I love the way you listen so intently to what I say, and wait until I'm finished before you respond" vs "I wish you'd hear me out instead of mentally practicing a quick comeback" give us clear information about how we're doing as we communicate in that moment.

The fundamentals of communication consist of a sender, a message, a receiver, and an environment. In an emotion-laden interchange, the message is obscured by the fact that someone is upset and unable to identify clearly what the heart of the problem is and how to best go about solving it. What is most important is that you realize that the luxury you experienced as a "private citizen," before you made a commitment to becoming a health professional, of simply reacting to others must now be replaced by a commitment to use emotion-laden communication, even when you feel personally attacked.

LESS THAN HELPFUL RESPONSES

The most unhelpful response is indifference. To fail to listen is indicative of an inability or unwillingness to be therapeutically present to the one in need of help. Other less than helpful techniques include the following:[2]

❖ *Offering reassurances.* Statements such as "Oh, it can't be all that bad" or "If you think you have it bad, you should just look around you" do little but signal an unwillingness to listen to patients' perceptions of their problems. At the heart of this reply is a practitioner who is not aware of his or her own feelings about the topic, or one who pretends to offer more time and attention than there is to give, and is trying to get away as rapidly as possible.

❖ *Offering judgmental responses.* Judgmental responses include several types. For example, those responses that convey approval or disapproval, either verbally or nonverbally, at an inappropriate moment; those that convey advice at a time when it is more important for the patient to make his or her own decision; and responses that are stereotypical: "Adults should know better than to act like children."

❖ *Defensiveness.* When we feel threat to the ego, we respond defensively. Defensiveness indicates a personalization and a refusal to listen carefully to what the patient is saying. A response such as "You're always late. I've got better things to do than wait for you, you know" may be true, but does little to solve the patient's tardiness problem.

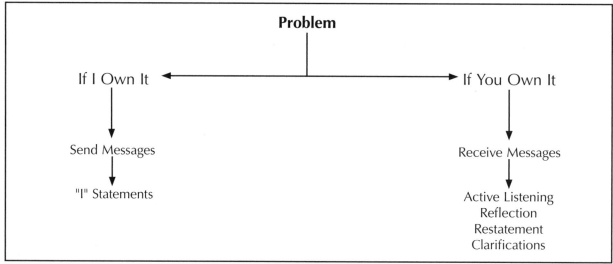

Figure 6-1. Identifying problem ownership.

VALUES THAT UNDERLIE THERAPEUTIC RESPONSES

Very often nonhelpful responses are impulsive and reactive and do not reflect value-based behavior. The values that underlie therapeutic responses are described in Chapter 3. Attitudes such as caring and warmth, respect, compassion, and empathy will help interrupt an immature, impulsive response to an emotion-laden communication.

Acceptance of the other person as doing the best he or she can in the moment, and acceptance of the responsibility to be therapeutic in the midst of a chaotic situation are signs of a mature healing professional. These responses emanate from the essential self, not the ego or persona.

Remember that the goal of rehabilitation is to help the patient regain control over his or her life such that independent function at the highest and deepest levels is restored. The role of the practitioner in emotion-laden communication is to ascertain, what is the problem, and whose problem is it?

IDENTIFYING PROBLEM OWNERSHIP

Learning to send clear messages and to receive accurate messages in intense situations requires identifying who "owns" the problem.[3] Different skills are required for each. For the sake of learning this skill, the rule that applies in every case is the person exhibiting the intense emotion is the owner of the problem, even if he or she is trying desperately to inform you that the problem is really yours.

For example, if the patient is upset with you for being late and shouts at you as you enter the clinic, "You're late!" you don't have a problem. You just walked into the clinic. The patient who is upset has a problem, even though he might be trying to convince you that you are his problem.

In identifying problem ownership, the person with the emotion "owns" the problem. The first step to resolving the issue is to realize the different skills required depending on who owns the problem. Figure 6-1 illustrates the 2 sets of skills required: active listening and "I" statements.

Emotion-laden exchanges are cluttered with intense feelings, derogatory remarks, apologies, illustrations, etc. In order to sort out the problem, special listening skills are needed to defuse the emotion and get at the problem. Critical to this method is the resistance of the desire of the unhelpful response to want to "fix" it right away to get rid of the anger or conflict. The alternative is to listen by resisting the quick advice, or the defensive reply.

ACTIVE LISTENING—
WHEN THE OTHER HAS THE PROBLEM

Active listening is a form of therapeutic listening that helps the agitated person with the problem hear clearly what he or she is trying to say. It involves paraphrasing the speaker's words rather than reacting to them in order to clarify if you have caught the intended meaning. You must suspend your thoughts and attend exclusively to the words of the other person. This is not easy and requires development as a new skill. In a sense, it requires self-transposal, where you work to put yourself in the other person's shoes, to understand rather than judge or defend against. For some, it will require great effort to resist responding with a suggestion of what to do, since the desire to fix it is so habitual.

Active listening is made up of 3 different processes:[3]

1. *Restatement*—Repeating the words of the speaker as you have heard them.

    Example: "I get so frustrated that I never have a day free from my back pain."

    Restatement: "You're frustrated because the back pain never leaves you?"

    Restatement can be annoying if not timed appropriately. Notice that the restatement is formed as a question. When done well, it assures the patient that you have, indeed, heard the content of what he or she is saying. The main purpose of restatement is to help the person continue speaking and should only be used in the initial phases of active listening. Once you have reassured the patient that you are hearing his or her words, reflection and clarification become more useful responses.

2. *Reflection*—Verbalizing both the content and the implied feelings of the sender.

    Example: "This pain has been going on for months. I just can't go on any longer."

    Reflection: "You're exhausted and feeling defeated from the constant pain?"

    The purpose of reflection is to express in words the *feelings and attitudes sensed behind the words of the sender*. This aspect of listening indicates you're hearing more than just the words, you're hearing the emotion behind them. Sometimes we guess incorrectly, but this gives the sender the chance to clarify for us and for him- or herself exactly what he or she is feeling. Awareness of feelings is critical to identifying the real problem. When the listener wants to help the sender to examine more extensively both thoughts and feelings, or to focus thoughts and feelings, clarification is used.

3. *Clarification*—Summarizing or simplifying the sender's thoughts and feelings and resolving confused verbalizations into clear, concise statements.

    Example: "When the doctor told me I needed physical therapy, I knew that you would be the person who would help me get rid of my pain. But it's been 2 weeks now, and the pain just keeps coming back. I am afraid that I'll have this pain forever. I'm not sure what it is that I'm supposed to do. Do I just have to live with this or will somebody please help me?"

    Clarification—"When you first came to physical therapy, you thought the pain would be relieved immediately. Now you realize that ridding yourself of the pain is going to take longer than you expected and is more than a matter of somebody just fixing it?"

    These skills take practice, as does resisting the answer that tends toward "fixing it." The exercises at the end of the chapter will give you an opportunity to practice.

CLEAR SENDING—USE OF "I" STATEMENTS WHEN I OWN THE PROBLEM

When I feel the emotion and want to communicate to another person that I am upset, clear communication is facilitated when I am congruent. That is, my words clearly match my feelings. I express my feelings with "I" messages rather than the commonly used editorial "they," "you," or "everyone." First let's look at congruence.

Congruence

Congruence is a term that indicates that the words and the music match. Congruence is present when *what I say matches what I do and what I feel.*[3] Incongruence appears ingenuine and dishonest, "not ringing true." How often we have been caught in incongruence when someone asks for a compliment: "Well, do you like my new haircut or not?" "Well yes, it's okay I guess." What was felt was less than okay but no one likes to appear rude. When a person is congruent, he or she appears open, honest, genuine, and authentic. Nonverbal cues and tone of voice are consistent with the words spoken.

Congruence requires reflection. Before speaking, you must realize both feelings and thoughts, and reconcile such pulls as wanting not to be hurtful, yet wanting to be honest. A congruent response to the requested compliment might be: "You know, I noticed you had a new haircut, but I believe I liked it better the old way." With this response, the person realizes that you value honesty and are willing to be honest and can avoid being rude. The message "rings true" and you feel better. More important, the person knows you will resist responses aimed at trying to please others.

Congruence is best conveyed when it is communicated with sensitivity and thought. It should never be used as a rationalization for insensitive and rude "honesty."

"I" Messages

"I" messages are necessary when you feel emotion, you own the problem, and you want to get the problem solved. Our tendency is to blame when we feel uncomfortable. An example might be: "You always leave the dirty dishes in the sink! I'm getting sick and tired of cleaning up after you." What is the problem, and whose problem is it?

Well, I'm upset, so the problem is mine, and it requires a clearer message than that if I want to get it solved in a helpful way. Using an "I" message, that is the way I would proceed: "I'm feeling very frustrated. This is the third night in a row that I've found dirty dishes in the sink, and I'm tired of doing them for you. Let's talk about this."

With "I" messages, I clearly own my frustration. Then it's up to the other person to respond, hopefully with concern, perhaps even with active listening. *Please note, however, that use of an "I" statement does not guarantee that the other person will respond in a helpful way.* What it does guarantee is that my feelings will be expressed, and I will take responsibility for my upset, rather than blaming someone else. Another person might never get upset over dirty dishes in the sink!

Using "I" statements involves taking a risk. I speak in the first person, I "own" my feelings rather than ignore, disclaim, or minimize them. It takes reflective thought to decide what it is that I'm feeling and how it is I can express that. Sending "I" messages tells the other person that you are owning your upset, and both you and he or she are worthy and capable of solving this problem with appropriate, clear, respectful discussion.

The exercises at the end of the chapter will help you practice this important skill as well.

CONCLUSION

Communication that is helpful resists the need to impulsively respond, or to offer quick advice or a quick solution to a problem. Instead, therapeutic communication strives to clarify the problem, and to assist the person with the problem to solve it for him- or herself. When we were children, we needed older adults to fix it for us, to put a bandage on our bruised knees or our bruised egos. As mature health practitioners, we must unlearn the natural tendency to help by giving advice. We must respect and value the communication process as one more tool in our repertoire of therapeutic responses where we help the other person help him- or herself.

Let's return to the case example at the beginning of the chapter. Jonathan and Mrs. Graham are standing in the hallway outside Diane's room, and Mrs. Graham has just let Jonathan have it. What is the problem and whose problem is it?

Clearly it is Mrs. Graham's problem. Jonathan has practiced his therapeutic communication skills, and instead of defending himself, he responds with, "You're obviously upset and frustrated at the apparent lack of progress on Diane's part, and you believe that is due to my inexperience."

Mrs. Graham says yes and goes on for another few minutes, while Jonathan keeps up with her with active listening responses. Soon she calms down, and, feeling really listened to, she looks at Jonathan and admits that the real problem is that she feels that this is all her fault, and she feels so helpless. Jonathan explores with her what he believes are her choices in dealing with the guilt she feels and then promises to include her in his therapy sessions to a greater extent tomorrow, so that she can provide minor aspects of treatment in the evenings. Mrs. Graham shakes his hand, thanks him, and agrees to see a counselor to work on her feelings of guilt.

Not all communications will end that amicably, but the majority will end far less amicably if the practitioner responds impulsively or simply reacts. Therapeutic communication is the most useful way to insure a helping response to emotion-laden communication.

REFERENCES

1. Cassell EJ. *Talking With Patients.* Vol 1. Cambridge, Mass: MIT Press; 1985:4.
2. Kozler B, Erb GL. *Fundamentals of Nursing. Concepts and Procedures.* Reading, Mass: Addison-Wesley; 1979.
3. Munson PJ, Johnson RB. *Humanizing Instruction or Helping Your Students Up the Up Staircase.* Chapel Hill, NC: Johnson Self Instructional Package; 1972.

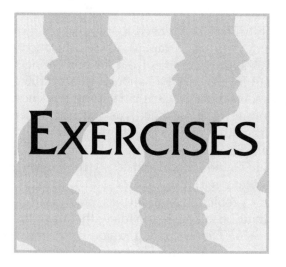

EXERCISE 1: CURRENT PATTERNS

1. Think of a recent situation in which you felt emotionally upset or frustrated. Briefly describe the situation on paper.

2. Whose problem was it? If you were upset, it was your problem. How did you communicate? Did you communicate at all, or did you swallow it and hope it would go away, or at least change so it was no longer a problem?

3. What did you communicate, exactly?

4. How would you change that now, using "I" statements or active listening? Do you think the outcome would have changed if you had used "I" messages or active listening?

5. Write an "I" statement designed to communicate upset.

EXERCISE 2: ACTIVE LISTENING

Active listening involves restatement (of the words of the sender), reflection (of the words and underlying feelings of the sender), and clarification (summarizes and focuses the sender's message). Practice writing all 3 types of responses as requested below.

Restatement

SENDER

I'm very worried about my shortness of breath.

I used to be able to jog for a whole hour, but now my joints start to ache.

I wish I could swim for 100 laps without getting so tired.

RESPONSE FROM YOU

You're worried about your shortness of breath?

Reflection

SENDER

This pain has been going on for months now. I just wish someone would fix it for me. I wish someone would help.

Yesterday was a good day, but today I feel the same old way.

It's hard remembering to do my exercises. I want to get better, but it's hard.

RESPONSE FROM YOU

Your pain just drags on and you wish to relieve it. Perhaps you're concerned that it will never go away?

Clarification

SENDER

I wish someone would tell me what's going on with my knees. When I get up in the morning they're fine, but by noon they're swollen and feel tired. I'm too young to be suffering with joint problems. Is this arthritis or what? Do I have to live with this forever?

So when the chiropractor told me I had a curved spine and I had to keep coming back for more adjustments every day I felt that surely there must be something I could do for myself. I got a little frustrated by having so little to do to help myself.

I almost didn't make it here. I got a horrible headache as I was driving here. The traffic is so stressful in this city. Will it ever end? There are new cars every day on the road. I don't know if I can keep up driving, with these headaches. Is there anything you can do for me?

RESPONSE FROM YOU

You're worried that your knee problem might be arthritis and that you'll never be rid of it?

Exercise 3: "I" Messages

Read each situation and the "you" message (blaming response), then write an "I" message in the third column of the following table.

Situation	*"You" Message*	*"I" Message*
The aide has neglected to clean the whirlpool for 3 days in a row.	What's the matter with you? Are you getting lazy or what?	I'm confused and frustrated. For 3 days the whirlpool hasn't been cleaned. What's the problem?
Your patient has arrived late and set your schedule back by a half-hour all day.	You're late again! Now I'm going to be a half-hour behind for the last 3 treatment sessions.	
The patient seems depressed and has been reluctant to speak up for several days.	You're so quiet lately. Did I do something to make you mad?	

Exercise 4: Patient/Practitioner Interactions

A series of vignettes follows. Divide up into groups of 3, where 1 person is the health professional, 1 person is the patient, and 1 person is the observer.

Role play the first vignette for 5 minutes or so, or until an appropriate place to stop occurs. The observer should have in hand a copy of the "Patient/Practitioner Interaction Checklist" which follows Vignette 4 on page 107. At the conclusion of the vignette, the observer asks the patient how he or she is feeling, then asks the practitioner the same question. The observer then gives the practitioner feedback as recorded on the checklist. At the end of the first round (approximately 15 minutes), remain in the same group of 3, but exchange roles and repeat the same vignette. After all 3 of you have role played the practitioner, discuss the experience among yourselves. Take a risk and give each other helpful feedback, negative and positive, about your communication skills. Journal about the experience focusing on what it felt like to be the therapist, to be the patient, and to be the observer giving negative feedback to a classmate or colleague.

Vignettes

Each person playing a role should see the description for that role only. Read the brief description and then act out the part as you would if it were happening to you. These vignettes are written for the role of physical therapist, but feel free to alter the descriptions to make them more applicable to the role that you are preparing for in your education if it is not physical therapy.

Vignette 1

Physical Therapist

You've been working with this patient who is wheelchair bound for 4 months. In the last 3 weeks, the 2 of you have focused on the patient's discharge home. The patient seems pleased to be returning home, but also anxious. You notice lately that the patient is short-tempered and cuts people off who try to help. You hate conflict and want to avoid it at all costs.

Patient

You are wheelchair bound and have been working in physical therapy for 4 months with the same therapist. In the last 3 weeks, the 2 of you have focused on your discharge home. You've begun to be very anxious about separating from the rehabilitation center and are experiencing intermittent episodes of chest pain. You're afraid to tell anyone about this, for you fear they will discount your symptoms and label you as overdependent, and actually you're afraid that they might be right. You're exhausted because you haven't slept more than 1 or 2 hours for the past 3 nights. You decide to confide your fears to your physical therapist, but you're feeling very exhausted and defensive. You decide to just blurt it all out and hope that your therapist will understand.

Vignette 2

Physical Therapist

You are the therapist for a cerebral palsy children's program. One mother brings her child 3 times a week to your center and stays and watches you treat her daughter along with the other children. This child is African American, and several races are represented at the center. You are Anglo American. This center is the only place where children with cerebral palsy can get treatment in this small town.

Patient's Mother

You are the mother of a child with cerebral palsy. You bring your child to physical therapy at the rehabilitation center in your small town 3 times each week and wait while she receives treatment. You notice that the physical therapist seems to spend less time with your daughter than she spends with 2 other children. You are African American and the others are Anglo American, as is the physical therapist. You've decided to confront the therapist with your suspicions. You're angry and hurt, but you fear that if you say the wrong thing, your daughter will be treated even less than before. This is the only center in town that offers treatment for your child. This is not the first time you've felt that you and your family were being discriminated against because of your race.

Vignette 3

Physical Therapist

Your 20-year-old patient had minor knee surgery a week ago and is still complaining of pain. He keeps his knee elevated with ice, hates to do exercises, screams with pain, and uses his crutches only with assistance to go to the bathroom. The surgeon is anxious to discharge the patient home, but you're convinced that he is not ready and will surely fall. He has 10 stairs to climb just to get from the sidewalk to the front door of his house. You're subconsciously afraid that your lack of experience in caring for patients with knee surgery has contributed to his poor recovery, so you're feeling guilty.

Patient

You have just had knee surgery 1 week ago and are experiencing a lot of postoperative pain. You're protecting your knee, keeping it very still so it will heal faster and hurt less. Your physical therapist seems to think you should have been discharged home days ago and is frustrated with your oversensitivity to the pain. You've never had surgery before, and no one really prepared you for this experience. You're afraid you'll be discharged tomorrow, and you feel very shaky with your crutches. You have no idea how you'll climb up the 10 steps to your front porch, let alone the 15 to your bedroom. You're upset with yourself for being afraid, you hurt, you're fearful of being thrown out in the cold with no help. You decide to talk to your therapist before physical therapy today. You feel angry at her for putting you in this position.

Vignette 4

Physical Therapist

You are with a private practice assigned to cover the patient care needs at a nursing home, and although you love the patients and enjoy the interaction with them, you realize that much of their functional activity has to be supervised by the nursing staff when you are not there. The nurses love the patients also, but they are short-staffed. They are constantly asking you to help them with nursing functions while you are doing therapy, and you cooperate but are becoming more and more frustrated. You decide to talk to the head nurse about this after you discuss one of your patients who needs to be ambulated 3 times a shift to build endurance. You approach the nurse as she is making out her daily census report.

Nurse

You are in charge of a unit of elderly patients and you are understaffed. The administrator has been criticizing you for inefficiency, and you feel she is being unrealistic in her demands on you. Secretly you fear that if one more thing goes wrong you are likely to lose your job. The physical therapist has asked to see you, and you are angry with her because she seems to make more work for your nurses so that their nursing tasks do not get completed. The physical therapist is always asking the nurses to dangle patients to help ambulate them; you think they should hire another therapist and let your nurses do nursing care.

Journaling

At the conclusion of the exercises, create a journal that details your feelings about this new form of communicating. How do you feel about its usefulness? Do you believe you will be able to develop skill in using "I" statements? Are you willing to practice at home? How about active listening skills? Make a commitment to practice using these skills at least once each day until you believe you have developed some skill, and remember that this form of communication is now a choice for you in any situation.

Patient/Practitioner Interaction Checklist

The observer in the triad responds to these questions during each role-play situation and then uses this information to give feedback to the practitioner about his or her therapeutic communication.

How well did the practitioner:

1. Attend to the patient's (or nurse's) emotional state and feelings?

2. Identify what the problem was and who had the problem?

3. Use reflection and clarifying responses during active listening? Use "I" statements when he or she owned the problem?

4. Use open-ended questions and statements to encourage the patient to talk more?

5. Remain silent when appropriate?

6. Respond to the patient with signs of sympathy and self-transposal?

7. Avoid judging, defensive, or blaming statements?

8. How could the therapist improve communication next time?

ASSERTIVENESS SKILLS AND CONFLICT RESOLUTION

Carol M. Davis, PT, EdD, MS, FAPTA

OBJECTIVES

1. To identify the importance of using assertive communication in healing interactions.
2. To distinguish between nonassertive, assertive, and aggressive communication.
3. To point out that there are situations in which each person tends to give up personal power.
4. To describe how to defuse a hostile, angry reaction.
5. To identify the rights we all share as human beings.
6. To offer the opportunity to contract for changing negative, reactive behavior to positive, assertive behavior.

ASSERTIVENESS TRAINING

In the previous chapter we learned a new way of communicating in intense or emotional moments. This chapter expands on the skills previously learned and teaches a way of communicating that will improve one's sense of personal power and self-esteem in situations where stress would have us give up that power. Let's begin with a case example.

> Sheila Lester, registered nurse, was standing at the nurses' station reading her patient's chart before going into the patient's room to give her treatment. The patient's physician came to the station and was searching for the chart. When he saw that Sheila was reading it, he turned to her and said, "Give me the chart, Honey; that's my patient and I have to see her now." Sheila felt as if she were being treated in a nonprofessional way, to say the least. She felt her heart begin to race, she knew she was blushing, and she realized that she felt degraded and humiliated. Before she could stop herself, she turned to the physician and shouted, "My name is not Honey, and this is my patient, as well!" The physician looked up with amusement and returned, "Well, well; what is your name then, Honey?" Sheila felt as if the battle were lost, and put the chart down and walked away in anger.

Assertiveness training has become well-known in the past decade and many people claim its benefits as a communication skill, but it also carries a negative connotation in some circles. Images of the "uppity" woman or the aggressive man come to view. These images result from our socialization, from the messages we heard from our parents as we grew up. As rambunctious children, many of us were taught that we should "know our place" and practice humility. As we grew older, we heard other messages and rules such as: "Children should be seen and not heard;" "Go to your room until you can come out with a smile on your face;" and "If you can't say something nice, don't say anything at all." Certainly the traditionalists, baby boomers, and families from strong ethnic cultural backgrounds heard, "Women belong in the supportive role to their husbands," while more recently we hear phrases such as, "Don't worry, be happy!" and "Don't sweat the small stuff."

The accumulative effect, especially on all those who suffer from low self-esteem, and on those who feel disempowered in the community, can result in communication that is not healthy or healing in nature. Following rules that do not encourage genuine and appropriate expression of feelings results in multiple unhealthy behaviors: the bottling up of genuine emotion; the repression of feelings over time that often results in stress-related illness; passive-aggressive silence or manipulation, and inappropriate outbursts of anger, rage, defensiveness, and frustration. At the extreme, we see the rampage of killings at high schools in the United States committed by adolescents who were enraged by "bullies" and felt powerless to communicate their feelings to others.

THE CHALLENGE IF COMMUNICATING WISELY IN HEALTH CARE

Health care calls for a great deal of practice when dealing with fellow practitioners who are often working under stress and when dealing with patients and their families who are feeling intensely vulnerable. Emotional communication, including anger, is very prevalent in the practice of health care. There are many situations that occur daily in which a person is stimulated to react either in anger or in giving up personal power and feeling helpless.

GENDER DIFFERENCES

Women predominate in all of the health professions except medicine and surgery, and medical school admissions data indicate they are fast catching up to balance male applicants. However, we live in an evolving society that has been, and continues to be, essentially male-dominated and patriarchal. The culture of the west has been slow to accept the balancing of the opposites, while the reality of the need for both is well established in all cultures. In spite of the fact that health care consists of much more than physician care, medicine was created by men to be practiced by men. Nurses, who are predominantly women, feel especially affected by this disparate power structure. In a study conducted by Friedman on nurse-physician relationships, nurses reported that they had to deal with:[1]

1. Condescending attitudes.
2. Lack of respect as either a person or a professional.
3. Public humiliation as physicians rant and rave in front of patients, families, or anyone who will listen.
4. Temper tantrums.
5. Scapegoating (nurses are blamed for everything that goes wrong).
6. Failure to read nurses' notes or listen to nurses' suggestions.
7. Refusal to share information about the patient.
8. Frequent public disparaging remarks.

The continuum of insensitive behavior issuing from people in power to those in less powerful positions can run from poor taste and bad manners to outright sexist abuse and harassment. The sources of verbal abuse to nurses described in the Friedman article were primarily physicians, then patients' families, and lastly, the nurse's supervisor.[1] So although it is true to point out that part of the power struggle in health care has to do with the difficulties in our culture of men and women relating equally with each other, it is not as simple as that.

As much as all children are alike, developmentalists have shown us that boys and girls are different in the way they are treated by adults, in their goals and ideals, in the way they see their place in the world, and in the way they make decisions about right and wrong. However, all people have a genderless essential self, a core identity that is good that underlies the public self or persona and the ego. All people have the natural desire to become more, to grow, to learn, to increase self-esteem, to have influence, and to feel capable and able to facilitate change for the better. People in health care, both men and women, for the most part, want to help others, to change conditions of illness and pain, or inability to function fully as a human being in the world. To help in healing ways, one must exercise personal and professional power for the good. The goal must be to mature beyond the need for the ego to defend itself and to reach down to the essential self, where we are confident of our personal rights and assured of our equality and from where we can communicate with empathy and understanding.

EXERCISING OUR PERSONAL POWER

In Section I, we learned that how we feel about ourselves has everything to do with how we view the world and how we view other people. How we feel about our own self-worth also is directly connected to how much personal power we feel we have, and how we use that power.

Webster defines power as a possession of control, authority, or influence over another; the ability to act or produce an effect; legal or official authority, capacity, or right; physical might; or political control or influence.[2] Notice that power is a neutral term, having neither positive nor negative value connotations. If we want to facilitate change and make the world better, we have to learn how to exercise power.

Women in our society have been taught to play a role secondary to or supportive of men. Men have been taught to seek out and expect the support of women, but we are all born equal. *We learn to give up our power.*

Some beliefs that we develop that result in a giving up of personal power include the following.

1. I am not as important as the other person (often the physician or supervisor).
2. I am lucky to be treated with respect by others (those in authority).
3. I have years of training and experience, but they still do not compare to medical school.
4. I must act in ways that indicate I know my place so that I can keep my job, keep referrals coming, keep peace for others' sake.
5. When criticized by a superior, I must not respond, but agree in order to save face and avoid further criticism.
6. My needs are not as important as others'.

Some situations seem inherently more apt to stimulate stress than others, thus we can predict that we might be tempted to give up power or respond defensively with anger when we find ourselves required to respond. Ten such situations that cause stress for some or all of us include:

1. Command—Someone orders us to do something.
2. Anger—Includes name-calling, using obscenities, and shouting.
3. Criticism—Someone judges us as being less than adequate.

4. Unresponsiveness—Indifference to us or to our request.
5. Depression—A feeling of gloom in another, extreme sadness.
6. Impulsivity—Someone flies off the handle, acts crazy.
7. Affection—Someone expresses love and affection, or asks us for it.
8. Making mistakes—Fear that you cannot make a mistake; feeling as if you must always have the right answer.
9. Sexual content—Someone makes an overt or covert sexual comment or sexual advance.
10. Pain—Feelings of wanting to flee in the face of pain.

PERSONAL RIGHTS

Thoughts or beliefs we developed even before we could talk lead to feelings (rational or not) which then lead to behavior or reactions. It is a universal right that every person is entitled to act assertively and to express honest thoughts, feelings, and beliefs.

Assertiveness training teaches us that we have a choice of communicating in a way that allows us to convey our thoughts and feelings with tact and respect for others and honor for ourselves. As human beings, each one of us has the right to:[3]

* ❖ Be treated with respect.
* ❖ Have needs and to have those needs be as important as other people's needs. We have the right to ask (not demand) that other people respond to our needs and to decide if we want to respond to others' needs.
* ❖ Have feelings and express those feelings in ways that do not violate the dignity of others.
* ❖ Change our minds.
* ❖ Determine our own priorities.
* ❖ Ask for what we want.
* ❖ Refuse without making excuses.
* ❖ Form our own opinions and express them, and to have no opinion at all on a certain topic.
* ❖ Give and receive information as fellow health professionals.
* ❖ Act in the best interests of the patient.

When we allow our rights to be overlooked, we assume a dependent role that lowers self-esteem and fosters nonassertive behavior. Recognizing that we have rights is the first step in the cognitive retraining that is essential to assertiveness.

ASSERTIVENESS

What exactly is assertiveness? The concept of assertive behavior can best be described in comparison to what it is not—nonassertive (passive) and aggressive behavior.

Nonassertive Behavior

* ❖ Failing to get your point across by remaining quiet or passive. Perceived by others to be weak, easily taken advantage of, or manipulated.
* ❖ *Key message conveyed*: I don't count; my feelings are not as important as yours.

Aggressive Behavior

* ❖ Getting your point across but perceived by others as hostile, angry, offensive, sarcastic, or humiliating.

❖ *Key message conveyed*: This is what is true. Any reasonable person would agree. You are stupid to disagree. What I want is most important; what you want, feel, or think does not matter.

Assertive Behavior

❖ Getting your point across without offending others using direct, congruent expression of thoughts, feelings, beliefs, and opinions in a nonoffensive way.

❖ *Key message conveyed*: This is how I view the situation. This is what I think and feel at this moment.

❖ Alberti and Emmons[4] list 10 key elements to assertive behavior:
1. Self-expressive.
2. Respectful of the rights of others.
3. Honest.
4. Direct and firm.
5. Equalizing; benefiting both self and relationship.
6. Verbally appropriate, including the content of the message (feelings, rights, facts, opinions, requests, limits).
7. Nonverbally appropriate, including the style of the message (eye contact, voice posture, facial expression, gestures, distance, timing, fluency, listening).
8. Appropriate for the person and the situation; not universal.
9. Socially responsible.
10. Learned, not inborn.

Examples of Assertive Responses

Many of us have found ourselves in the situation when, dining out, we order our meal and something happens to make it less acceptable than we had expected. We find ourselves in a situation where we feel it is necessary to speak up in order to enjoy the meal that we've requested. Let's say that the dinner is completely cold. What are our choices in this situation?

❖ Passive—Say nothing at all. When the waitress asks, "How's your dinner?" we respond, "Fine." However, the person we're dining with receives the brunt of our hostility all evening.

❖ Aggressive—Stand up, shout for the waitress or waiter, and say in a loud and angry voice, "This meal is ice cold. I'm willing to pay good money for a good dinner, but you have the nerve to bring me a meal that has been sitting around for half an hour, and I resent it. Take this meal back immediately and bring me some hot food."

❖ Assertive—Motion for the waiter, state calmly that your food has become cold and request that it be heated and brought back to you as quickly as possible.

Upon comparison, it's easy to value assertive communication as superior to the other 2 modes. Difficulty acting assertively in appropriate situations with any consistency stems from the real or perceived threat of rejection, anger, or disapproval. Often this reluctance to be assertive is based more on habit and subconscious fears that we learned long ago, and that now guide our responses in an automatic way. Assertiveness helps us realize that we have a real choice to stand up for ourselves and to hold on to our power in difficult situations. Why in the world would anyone sit and eat a cold dinner while not enjoying it, and be willing to pay for it? What is the fear behind speaking up to ask for your rights? For many of us it is simply a matter of over-learning the dictate, "Don't make waves, don't cause a fuss, don't do anything that will bring attention to yourself." Behind this admonition is the basic feeling that others' rights are more important than mine and that I don't count.

TYPES OF ASSERTIVE RESPONSES

There are 8 types of assertive responses that can benefit us in the practice of health care and in our day-to-day interactions:[4]

1. Being confrontational.
2. Saying no.
3. Making requests.
4. Expressing opinions.
5. Initiating conversation.
6. Disclosing self.
7. Expressing affection.
8. Entering a room of strangers, willing to get to know others, and allowing ourselves to be known.

The first 2 areas can be described as assertive responses that express what commonly appear to be negative emotions; the next 3 are emotionally neutral responses that are task specific, and the last 4 call for expressing positive emotions. In the exercises, you will be given the opportunity to draft assertive, passive, and aggressive responses to each situation.

ATTRIBUTION AND THE DESIRE TO ACT ASSERTIVELY

A person can be quite knowledgeable about assertiveness but will not think to use these skills for any number of reasons. For example, if one believes that no matter what is done, the attempt will end in failure, assertiveness does not seem important. This problematic way of thinking illustrates one aspect of behavior that can partially be explained by attribution theory.[5]

The exercise in Figure 7-1 will help you discover the nature of your attributions, or how your lenses are set today.[6] Now, chart your numbers in the grid at the bottom of the figure.

Note the differences in your perceptions of the causes of success and failure. If you are like most people, you tend to attribute success to causes that are different in nature than those to which we attribute failure.

Attribution theory provides a framework to understand the ways that a person's lenses are set. An attribution is what we feel or think caused an outcome we have experienced.[7] How we view outcomes, as successful or failing, is critical in determining our expectations and out future actions. The 3 dimensions of the causes to which we attribute success or failure are the *locus* (due to something inside or outside of me), *stability* (lasting or temporary), and *controllability* (to what extent I can control this) dimensions.

Attributions that we assign to outcomes have a great deal to do with how we think about ourselves, or relate directly to how our lenses are set with regard to self-esteem. If we have *good self-esteem*, we are likely to attribute the cause of our successes to something *inside of ourselves*, something that is *stable or controllable*. If we have low self-esteem, we are likely to see our successes as due to forces outside of ourselves that are unstable and uncontrollable like luck or the difficulty of the task. In contrast, with failure, a person who indicates a cause that is internal, unstable (changeable), and controllable, such as the amount of effort we expended or the strategy we chose, will be more likely to expect success in the future by increasing effort or changing the ineffective strategy.[5]

In other words, with high self-esteem, we choose to believe we are going to succeed directly because of our actions, and if we fail, it is not because of a fixed internal trait (we have low ability or a poor personality), but because of circumstances that can change if we apply a different, more successful strategy to the task. In summary, when failure is attributed to stable, external, and uncontrollable events, there is little we

Put yourself in a time when you've done a project that was highly praised. What did you do? Who praised you? How did you feel? How did this influence future activity? Write down one major cause of your success.

1. Is the cause due to something about you, or due to something outside of you?

| Internal (Inside you) | 1 | 2 | 3 | 4 | 5 | 6 | 7 | External (Other resources) |

2. Is the cause something that will remain stable or be only temporary?

| Lasting (Stable) (Constant {IQ}) | 1 | 2 | 3 | 4 | 5 | 6 | 7 | Temporary (Unstable) (Changing [weather]) |

3. Do you see this cause as something you can control or is this beyond your control?

| Controllable (Whether I study or not) | 1 | 2 | 3 | 4 | 5 | 6 | 7 | Uncontrollable (Other person's mood) |

4. How likely are you to experience the same outcome in the future?

| Highly likely | 1 | 2 | 3 | 4 | 5 | 6 | 7 | Unlikely |

Now, think of a time when you have experienced a failure, for example, given an important talk and the audience reacts negatively, or cooked a meal that no one liked. Write down one major cause.

5. Is the cause due to something about you or something outside of you?

| Internal | 1 | 2 | 3 | 4 | 5 | 6 | 7 | External |

6. Is the cause something that will remain stable or be only temporary or changing?

| Lasting (Stable) | 1 | 2 | 3 | 4 | 5 | 6 | 7 | Temporary (Unstable) |

7. Do you see this cause as something you can control or is this beyond your control?

| Controllable | 1 | 2 | 3 | 4 | 5 | 6 | 7 | Uncontrollable |

8. How likely are you to experience the same outcome in the future?

| Highly likely | 1 | 2 | 3 | 4 | 5 | 6 | 7 | Unlikely |

Now chart your numbers on this grid:

	Success	*Failure*
Internal/External		
Stable/Unstable		
Control/Uncontrol		

Figure 7-1. Attribution exercise.

can do to affect change and we are unlikely to use assertiveness or any other strategy to get the job done. This is a loser's or victim's "script."

It is important to describe the nature of success and failure in ways that allow success to be judged realistically and over the long term.[7] The most adaptive attributions, according to Curtis,[8] occur when success is defined in other than all-or-nothing terms; are realistic in the circumstances; and are attributed to one's personal ability, effort, or good judgement. In health care, many frustrating situations are unlikely to change, but we can change how we think about them and how we deal with them to experience success over the long term. If success is seen as having all patients be discharged from our care fully cured, or have Medicare pay for 100% of treatment in 100% of eligible cases, few practitioners would ever feel as if they succeeded. Compromise, realistic expectations, and acceptance of long-term strategies are necessary, along with avoiding dualistic right/wrong judgments.

In sum, we must change the way we define failure and think about the causes of failure in order for assertiveness to be useful and successful. If we believe failure is attributed to external events that are uncontrollable and stable, we will be unlikely to use assertiveness. However, if we reframe our thoughts, decide that our goal might have been a little too unrealistic, and decide to employ another strategy to work for success, assertiveness can be a useful tool to solve problems.

LEARNING TO ACT ASSERTIVELY

Assertive behavior is not inborn; it is a skill, and to develop it requires learning 5 new behaviors:[4]

1. **Recognize situations in which you are tempted to become passive or aggressive in your communication**. Develop the skill of observing yourself. Be conscious of situations where you automatically give up your power, have irrational thoughts that do not relate to the present moment, or feel the necessity to put the other person down.

2. **Recognize when you are tempted to attribute failure to forces that are uncontrollable and stable**, such as a powerful person's unpleasant personality traits or a medical system that fails to acknowledge patient needs. Challenge yourself to think of a strategy to replace feelings of hopelessness or negativity.

3. **Replace these old thought patterns with different, more positive and powerful thoughts**. Cognitively interrupt the old thought patterns of, "You're right, I'm no good," "How dare you attack me, you arrogant fool?" or "It's no use!" Alone, or with another trusted person:

   a. Discuss the nature of the situation that aroused the emotion.

   b. Confront the tendency to react passively or aggressively.

   c. Identify the belief that lies behind your reaction.

   d. Replace the erroneous belief with a counteracting right.

   e. Identify a more positive thought that will bring more confident feelings.

4. **Practice thinking new thoughts** as a first step in changing the feelings that go with the old thoughts, thus deflating the energy behind the old reaction. You will know you are on the right track when the new thoughts make you feel positive and hopeful.

5. **Practice the new behavior that goes along with the ownership of the right**. Be assertive. Count your blessings and feel good about your ability to make a positive difference in the world.

How might Sheila, the nurse in the example at the beginning of the chapter, communicate assertively? Well, Chapter 6 taught one aspect of assertive communication, the use of "I" statements. This mode of communicating transforms an aggressive, blaming, or accusatory response to an assertive, responsible, and clear expression of feeling, essentially telling the other person the effect that his or her behavior has on you. In many cases, an "I" statement alone is initially sufficient to get your assertive message across. The situation Sheila found herself in calls for a confrontive assertion. Sheila feels diminished, less than a colleague, more like a slave being asked to do the master's bidding. Her feeling response is anger at being treated so poorly, and her initial reaction is to be angry. When her anger does not get her what she wants, the messages in her head revert to: "See, you're just not as good as the physician. Your rights are not important here." She gives up and walks away in frustration. What she hoped for was a collegial relationship with the physician, as both of them carry out their clinical responsibilities with the patient. This calls for a confrontive response aimed at helping her avoid becoming aggressive in anger and also to avoid passively giving up her power by silently complying with the physician's rude request.

First, Sheila must be aware of her feelings in the situation, her tendency to react in anger and give up her power. She must be aware of to what causes she attributes the outcomes in this situation. Next she must pay attention to the messages she gives herself and challenge the negative thoughts with more affirming, positive thoughts that confirm her rights as a human being. Then she is ready to respond with an assertive reply aimed at exercising her right to express her honest thoughts, feelings, and beliefs around this situation. One format for an effective response is the DESC response.

DESC RESPONSE AS A FORMAT FOR ASSERTIVE COMMUNICATION

The DESC format described by Bower and Bower[9] incorporates "I" statements but expands them and is useful when a more detailed interaction is required to get the other person's attention to your point of view. DESC is an acronym for:

D: Describe the situation.
E: Express your feelings about the situation: "I feel _____."
S: Specify the change you want: "I'd like for you to _____."
C: Consequences. Identify the results that will occur: "In that way _____."

Let's compose a DESC response for Sheila in the situation outlined at the beginning of the chapter:

D: Yes, Dr. Dutton, I realize that this is your patient. She's my patient as well; I'm her nurse.
E: My name is Sheila Lester. When you call me "Honey" it demeans me and I don't appreciate it.
S: I'd like you to call me Sheila or Ms. Lester because I'd like to discuss this patient with you as a colleague would. I would like you to treat me as a colleague.
C: In that way, I feel the patient will receive better care because we are working together with her in a more respectful and collegial way.

Sheila took a big risk with this physician by speaking up to tell him how his behavior made her feel. She must have trusted that this was a risk worth taking. We would hope that the physician would respond in a mature way, and treat her request with respect. Assertive communication does not guarantee this, however, as we'll discuss in a moment.

Sometimes you know that the risk is not well-placed. An alternative to the DESC confrontation is the DISC confrontation, which is used when you are confronting a person who will not care what you feel, so you eliminate the expression of feeling and substitute I for Indicate, indicating the problem the behavior is causing. DESC and DISC are really just amplifications of the effective "I" statement, but using them in a practiced, disciplined way provides an opportunity to erase an old, ineffective way of responding by replacing it with an assertive response.

An illustration of the DISC response for a physical therapist would be:

A powerful physician refers a patient with low back pain to you, a physical therapist, and specifically orders:

❖ Evaluate and treat with heat and massage.
❖ No exercise, no mobilization.

Upon evaluation you realize that this back pain is the result of an acute muscle spasm that occurred recently and was facilitated by poor body mechanics and weak flexor and extensor muscles. Your professional knowledge requires that you treat with ice and teach exercises to relax the current problem and prevent recurrence.

Your DISC confrontation might go something like this:

D: I'd like to talk with you about Mr. Doughty's back problem.

I: Your physical therapy referral for heat and massage is a logical place to start for a chronic problem, but my examination reveals this to be an acute spasm that the literature indicates responds faster and more effectively to ice. Likewise, his back extensor and abdominal muscles are quite weak, and he needs gentle relaxation exercise to reduce the spasm and eventual instruction in proper body mechanics.

S: I'd like for you to approve my plan to treat with ice and massage, then follow with gentle pelvic tilt and bridging exercises to tolerance to release the spasm, and eventually teach him stretching and strengthening exercises and proper body mechanics to prevent recurrence.

C: That way perhaps we can help him recover and get him strong enough and wise enough to keep him from reinjuring himself.

Organizing your thoughts will be more difficult, at first, and so the exercises for this chapter will provide practice following this 4-step method by writing out your response to a past situation that was particularly difficult for you. The key to your success will be paying attention to the way you feel. When you feel negative feelings, reach for a more positive thought. Thoughts are very creative, and we have a built-in indicator of how well we are doing with moving in a positive and growing direction. Good thoughts feel good. It's as simple as that.

You're probably wondering how you'll learn to respond quickly and on the spot with such a detailed DISC or DESC format when an assertive response is indicated. At first you will not be so organized. The most you can hope for is to recognize your feelings, avoid giving up your power angrily or passively, and buy time before responding at all. Eventually, however, it will become second nature to speak up with an "I" statement or a DESC response.

Assertively Dealing With Anger

Every once in awhile you will have to deal with an angry, defensive person. Feeling trapped in another's lashing out usually stimulates a flight-or-fight response or either passive or aggressive behavior. The ego is stimulated into defending itself, or the ego caves in to fear and wants to run away. In the previous chapter we learned to use active listening when the other person has the emotional outburst; this continues to be the most effective response in an assertive mode. Using active listening skills to help the person defuse the energy behind the outburst, which is most often secondary to fear, allows you then to use "I" statements to offer your assertive response. In other words, be a Teflon sponge; absorb the emotion by using restatement, reflection, and clarification, and let it slide off of you.[10]

Hostility Curve

A hostile, angry person will use a predictable pattern when raging that looks somewhat like what is shown in Figure 7-2.[11]

When you argue or respond defensively with someone who is raging, this will only fuel their fire and produce another take-off, escalating the argument to higher levels. Likewise if you interrupt the hostile person and appeal to him or her to "be reasonable," a similar response will result. One person just keeps setting off the other, and no problem gets identified, let alone solved.

Skillful handling of a person who is raging involves the active listening skills we practiced in Chapter 6 (Figure 7-3). During the raging person's irrational phase, it is best to simply wait and listen carefully, but do not say anything. Wait for the moment when the angry person seems to run out of steam, and then demonstrate that you have been listening, and say something supportive, such as, "If the same thing had happened to me, no doubt I would be angry too," or "I know this has been a very difficult experience for you."

Being supportive does not require that you agree with the person, but simply that you hear him or her. This eventually will serve to defuse the increasing emotion, and he or she will begin to cool

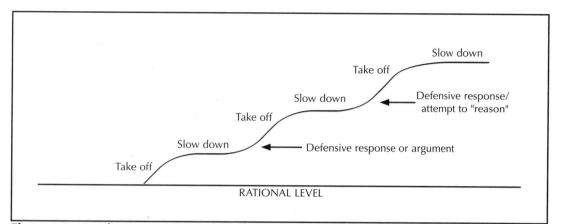

Figure 7-2. Hostility/rage pattern of escalation. (Adapted from American Hospital Association Pamphlet. *Teaching Patient Relations in Hospitals—The Hows and Whys*; 1983.)

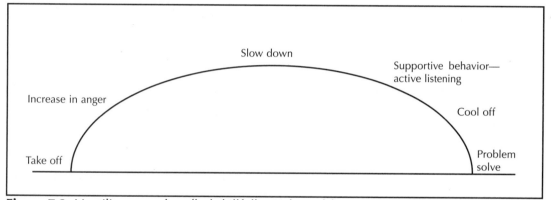

Figure 7-3. Hostility curve handled skillfully. (Adapted from American Hospital Association Pamphlet. *Teaching Patient Relations in Hospitals—The Hows and Whys*; 1983.)

off. Very often he or she will apologize for losing composure. At this point, it is important to help the angry person save face by leading him or her to a private area where you can sit down, and use your neurolinguistic psychology match, pace, and lead skills outlined in Chapter 8.

What people are most asking for is recognition and understanding. Active listening gives you the chance to stand still and offer a therapeutic response which will increase the chances for a positive outcome to the interchange. Once emotions have been dissipated, offer your assertive point of view and offer to work together to solve the problem.[9]

It is important that you vent your own feelings with a trusted friend after the incident is over. And keep in mind the words of Mother Theresa: "People are often unreasonable, irrational, and self-centered. Forgive them anyway. If you are kind, people may accuse you of selfish, ulterior motives. Be kind anyway... The good you do today will often be forgotten. Give your best anyway. In the final analysis, it is between you and God. It was never between you and them anyway."

BENEFITS OF ASSERTIVENESS

There are several benefits to using assertive behavior:
- ❖ It is our ethical and healing responsibility.
- ❖ It increases our self-respect.
- ❖ It increases our self-control.
- ❖ It improves self-confidence.

❖ It helps us develop more emotionally satisfying relationships with others.

❖ It increases the likelihood that everyone's needs will be met.

❖ It allows us to exercise our personal rights without denying the rights of others.

To exercise our personal rights relates to competency as a citizen; as a consumer; as a member of an organization or school or work group; or as a participant in public events to express opinions, to work for change, to respond to violations of one's own rights, or those of others.[4]

In the health professions, we must work side by side with colleagues, helping our patients regain their feelings of confidence and ability to function independently in the world. In order to make sure this happens, everyone's rights become important, and the exercise of those rights is critical to the healing process.

COMMON MYTHS ABOUT ASSERTIVENESS

As valuable as assertive communication is, there are some common myths that accompany this process:

1. **If I speak up with assertiveness, others will like what I say and do what I ask.** Using assertive communication is no guarantee for anything, except that you have expressed yourself with dignity, honesty, and with regard for others. How others respond to you is always a question and has much to do with the other person. Most important, you never have the right to violate another person's rights, even when you use assertiveness.

2. **All I have to do is say the assertive words and I will be perceived as being assertive.** Assertive words are critical to an assertive message, but assertive words spoken passively or aggressively destroy the basic message of assertiveness. The posture of assertiveness is an appropriate tone of voice, a steady voice, open posture, and good eye contact.

3. **Once I learn assertiveness skills, I must use them all the time in every situation that tends to make me feel powerless.** There are times when the best assertive response is to simply walk away and say nothing. One good example is deciding not to retaliate to an aggressive person. Then it is best to say nothing. Always remember, you are free to choose not to assert yourself in a situation.

   Ask yourself:

   a. How important is this situation to me?

   b. How am I likely to feel afterwards if I don't assert myself?

   c. What do I gain by being assertive? What do I lose?

   d. What do I gain by not being assertive? What do I lose?

4. **One assertive reply is all that's needed.** The first assertive response is the easiest. It's the "comeback" response that is more difficult. People will argue with your assertive response and try to get you to give up your power in spite of your effectiveness. For example, saying no when you mean no often takes several repeats of the no, and you may decide to end the conversation with, "Don't try to make me feel guilty. I told you I care about you, but I will not say yes this time. I said no; I mean no. End of discussion."

PRACTICE LEADS TO ACTION

The exercises begin with self-awareness about your own tendencies to respond passively or aggressively in certain situations. They proceed into opportunities for you to practice assertive communication with your classmates in role-playing situations. Don't forget to journal about the impact that the readings and exercises have on you. How does all of this make you feel? The exercises conclude with the opportunity for you to negotiate a personal contract for change—to truly change behavior that has been practiced for many years takes more than good intentions, it takes a promise. For some of you, at first your new behavior will feel awkward and ingenuine. My advice is, fake it until you make it. Rarely will I suggest ingenuineness, but many of us have overlearned the feelings that accompany low self-esteem and need to dramatically break up harmful, reactive behaviors to false beliefs. Ideally we could all experience the necessary inner transformations quickly and congruently. Life is a bit more complex than that. So, this time, start the process from outside-in rather than from inside-out. The goal is the same. The outer behavior, as inauthentic as it feels, for example, to be equal to a physician or experienced colleague, is still in everyone's best interest. Act as if you have every one of those rights listed above, and eventually you will accept it as the truth. Act as you believe someone you admire would act in this situation. Soon you will feel the inner confidence needed to ensure authentic, assertive, and kind behavior under the greatest of stress. Believe in yourself, imagine your success, and it will come quickly.

REFERENCES

1. Friedman FB. A nurse's guide to the care and handling of MDs. *RN.* 1982;March:39-43.
2. *Webster's Seventh New Collegiate Dictionary.* Springfield, Mass: G & C Merriam Co; 1963.
3. Chenevert M. *STAT—Special Techniques in Assertiveness Training for Women in Health Professions.* St. Louis, Mo: CV Mosby; 1978.
4. Alberti RE, Emmons ML. *Your Perfect Right.* 5th ed. San Luis Obispo: Impact Publishers; 1986:34.
5. Anderson C, Jennings DL. When experiences of failure promote expectations of success: the impact of attributing failure to ineffective strategies. *Journal of Personality.* 1980;48:393-407.
6. Curtis K. Personal communication.
7. Weiner B. Attribution theory and attributional therapy: some theoretical observations and suggestions. *Br J Clin Psychol.* 1988;27:93-104.
8. Curtis K. Altering beliefs about the importance of strategy: an attributional intervention. *J Appl Soc Psychol.* 1992;22:953-972.
9. Bower SA, Bower GH. *Asserting Yourself.* Reading, Mass: Addison-Wesley; 1976.
10. Silber M. Managing confrontations: once more into the breach. *Nursing Management.* 1984;15:54-58.
11. American Hospital Association Pamphlet. *Teaching Patient Relations in Hospitals—The Hows and Whys;* 1983.

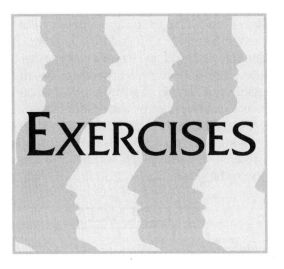

EXERCISES

EXERCISE 1: MY RIGHTS AS A PERSON

When we hear terrifying stories of people's inhumanity to each other, we're often moved to righteous indignation. For example, none of us can hear recountings from Holocaust victims without cringing with horror. Likewise, prisoner-of-war stories recently revealed from the Iraq war and Guantanamo Bay move us to anger and outrage. Human beings deserve to be treated in certain ways simply because we are human. What rights do all people have, as human beings? What does each human being deserve, simply by virtue of the fact that he or she is a person, alive on this earth? Make a list of the basic rights of all human beings.

Now reflect on that list in your journal. Do you act in ways that are consistent with your beliefs about your rights? Are there certain rights that you fail to claim for yourself? If so, why is that?

How does this list change when a human being becomes ill or disabled? Journal about the rights of people who are ill or in need of health care.

EXERCISE 2: SELF-AWARENESS— ASSERTIVENESS INVENTORY

Complete the Assertiveness Inventory (Table 7-1) from Alberti and Emmons' *Your Perfect Right*.[4] As directed at the bottom of the survey, circle the 3 statements that most often result in your giving up your power and becoming passive, or becoming so angry that you become aggressive.

Look at your responses to questions 1, 2, 4, 5, 6, 7, 9, 10, 11, 12, 14, 15, 16, 17, 18, 19, 21, 22, 24, 25, 27, 28, 30, and 35. These questions are oriented toward nonassertive behavior. Are you rarely speaking up for yourself? Or is there one situation that gives you more problems than the others? If so, journal about it starting with the earliest memories you have about that incident.

Look at your responses to questions 3, 8, 13, 20, 23, 26, 29, 31, 32, 33, and 34. These questions are oriented toward aggressive behavior. Are you pushing others around more than you realized? Does one question give you more trouble than the others? Again, journal about it, as above.

Few people are assertive all the time, aggressive all the time, or passive all the time. The situation often dictates the response. On rereading your total responses, do you see a pattern? Do you favor one way of responding over the others? Draw some conclusions about yourself from the inventory and journal about them. Which situations cause you most trouble? Which situations do you handle with no trouble at all? Why is that?

Can you identify obstacles that stand in the way of asserting yourself confidently? What beliefs do you hold about yourself and the world that make it difficult or easy to assert yourself? What is the worst thing that could happen? Journal about your learning.

Ask family members and trusted friends to give you honest and specific feedback about their observations of your behavior under stress. Do you show patterns of passivity or aggressiveness? Ask them to illustrate their points with examples. Resist the natural desire to defend yourself as they respond. Just listen, and take notes, then journal about what you learned and about your feelings.

Table 7-1

ASSERTIVENESS INVENTORY

The following questions will be helpful in assessing your assertiveness. Be honest in your responses. All you have to do is draw a circle around the number that describes you best. For some questions, the assertive end of the scale is at 0, for others at 4. Key: 0 means no or never; 1 means somewhat or sometimes; 2 means average, 3 means usually or a good deal; and 4 means practically always or entirely.

1. When a person is highly unfair, do you call it to his or her attention?................................ 0 1 2 3 4
2. Do you find it difficult to make decisions? 0 1 2 3 4
3. Are you openly critical of others' ideas, opinions, behavior?...0 1 2 3 4
4. Do you speak out in protest when someone takes your place in line? 0 1 2 3 4
5. Do you often avoid people or situations for fear of embarrassment? 0 1 2 3 4
6. Do you usually have confidence in your own judgment?..0 1 2 3 4
7. Do you insist that your spouse or roommate take on a fair share of household chores? 0 1 2 3 4
8. Are you prone to "fly off the handle?" 0 1 2 3 4
9. When a salesperson makes an effort, do you find it hard to say "no" even 0 1 2 3 4
    though the merchandise is not really what you want?
10. When a latecomer is waited on before you are, do you call attention to the situation?.........0 1 2 3 4
11. Are you reluctant to speak up in a discussion or debate?...0 1 2 3 4
12. If a person has borrowed money for a book, garment, (thing of value) and 0 1 2 3 4
    is overdue in returning it, do you mention it?
13. Do you continue to pursue an argument after the other person has had enough?................0 1 2 3 4
14. Do you generally express what you feel? 0 1 2 3 4
15. Are you disturbed if someone watches you at work? 0 1 2 3 4
16. If someone seems to be kicking or bumping your chair in a movie or a lecture, do.............0 1 2 3 4
    you ask the person to stop?
17. Do you find it difficult to keep eye contact when talking to another person?.......................0 1 2 3 4
18. In a good restaurant, when your meal is improperly prepared or served, do you.................0 1 2 3 4
    ask the waiter/waitress to correct the situation?
19. When you discover merchandise is faulty, do you return it for an adjustment? 0 1 2 3 4
20. Do you show your anger by name-calling or obscenities?..0 1 2 3 4
21. Do you try to be a wallflower or a piece of the furniture in social situations? 0 1 2 3 4
22. Do you insist that your landlord (mechanic, repairperson, etc.) make repairs,...................0 1 2 3 4
    adjustments, or replacements that are his or her responsibility?
23. Do you often step in and make decisions for others? 0 1 2 3 4
24. Are you able to openly express love and affection? 0 1 2 3 4
25. Are you able to ask your friends for small favors or help? 0 1 2 3 4
26. Do you think you always have the right answer?...0 1 2 3 4
27. When you differ with a person you respect, are you able to speak up for your 0 1 2 3 4
    own viewpoint?
28. Are you able to refuse unreasonable requests made by friends?......................................0 1 2 3 4
29. Do you have difficulty complimenting or praising others?..0 1 2 3 4
30. If you are disturbed by someone smoking near you, can you say so?................................0 1 2 3 4
31. Do you shout or use bullying tactics to get others to do as you wish?...............................0 1 2 3 4
32. Do you finish other people's sentences for them? 0 1 2 3 4
33. Do you get into physical fights with others, especially with strangers? 0 1 2 3 4
34. At family meals, do you control the conversation? 0 1 2 3 4
35. When you meet a stranger, are you the first to introduce yourself and begin 0 1 2 3 4
    a conversation?

Now go back and circle the 3 statements that most often result in you giving up your powers and becoming passive or that anger you so much you become aggressive.

EXERCISE 3: ASSERTIVE, AGGRESSIVE, AND PASSIVE RESPONSES

Practice making responses to the following situations. The first situation is done for you as an example.

Saying No

The head nurse stops you on the floor as you are just about to evaluate a new patient. "Mr. Johnson needs to be supervised in the use of his walker as he goes to the bathroom and none of us have time. I wonder if you'd mind walking with him right now."

1. Passive: Well, I'm very busy, but if he has to go right now, I suppose I can help.

2. Aggressive: Look, I taught him how to use that walker. It's your job to supervise him in bathroom activity. I've got a patient to evaluate, and I don't appreciate your inconsiderate views of the value of my time.

3. Assertive: No, I can't do that right now. Mrs. Adams is able to help him, as can his family members. I have a new evaluation that can't wait.

Making Requests

It's the end of the day and you have 3 more patients to evaluate before leaving. You're going to need some help or you'll be working very late. How do you ask for it?

1. Passive:

2. Aggressive:

3. Assertive:

Expressing Opinions

An edict comes down from above that all staff must treat at least 4 "units" of patient care per hour. You feel that this is unreasonable and that it interferes with establishing a therapeutic presence with your patients. How do you respond?

1. Passive:

2. Aggressive:

3. Assertive:

Initiating Conversation

You're attending a workshop and you've always wanted to talk with the speaker about a topic of great interest to you. You feel shy and somewhat intimidated by the speaker and his reputation.

1. Passive:

2. Aggressive:

3. Assertive:

Self-Disclosing

Your parents are in the midst of a year-long divorce battle that has brought great grief to your younger brother. Last night he called you and spoke of thoughts of suicide. They live far away, and you feel frightened and helpless. At work, you seem distracted and upset. A friend asks, "Is there anything wrong? You seem preoccupied today."

1. Passive:

2. Aggressive:

3. Assertive:

Expressing Affection

A patient that you have been working with is being discharged. You go to the room and his family is there packing to help him move back home. He asks to speak to you privately, takes your hand, and thanks you for everything you've done for him, and gives you a warm hug.

1. Passive:

2. Aggressive:

3. Assertive:

Entering a Room of Strangers

You've just moved to a new city to begin your first position after graduating. A new colleague invites you over for a party. You walk into the apartment and you realize you do not know one person in the room except the host. Everyone else seems to have known each other for years. No one is dressed the way you are.

1. Passive:

2. Aggressive:

3. Assertive:

Reflect in your journal which of these situations was easiest for you to envision handling assertively, and which was most difficult. Which responses were easiest to come up with? Do you find that how you might respond has very much to do with your perception of the stress inherent in the situation?

EXERCISE 4: ASSERTIVE COMMUNICATION

In this chapter, you learned about DISC and DESC communication. Now you have a chance to role play various assertive responses to the following vignettes. Before role-playing, however, you are asked to write the DISC or DESC response. The practitioner or student is in the assertive response position; the other person should use this opportunity to practice the *active listening skills* learned in the chapter just previous to this one. A third person serves as the observer, giving feedback at the end of the dialogue on the effectiveness of the communication. Use the Observer Response Sheet following Vignette 9 to jot down your observations as they occur. Each person should choose an appropriate "difficult" vignette, and write a DISC or DESC statement before breaking up into groups of 3.

Vignette 1

You are a student on your first of 2 final clinical assignments. The clinical facility is very high-powered with a superior reputation. You feel no matter what you do, you could never achieve the level that is expected of the staff. You truly feel that you're doing your best, but you are under constant stress to prove yourself. You are to be checked out on a knee evaluation, but you've forgotten some of the basic steps, and you've asked for help from the orthopedic star of the staff, who always says, "Yes, but I'm too busy. Catch me tomorrow." Your clinical instructor stops you as you are ready to go home and relax at the end of the day and says, "I've let you off the hook long enough. You should have that knee evaluation down by now. Come with me and let me check you out."

❖ Write a DESC response.
❖ Role play.

Vignette 2

You are a clinical instructor. You've observed your student for 3 weeks and feel he may be quite weak in evaluation skills, and you feel he or she is not taking the assignment seriously. When you suggest a checkoff session, your student always asks for more time. Yet all you hear is talk about lots of parties, after-hours fun, and you notice a real reluctance to read or show initiative in looking things up or asking for help. You think he might be trying to squeeze through without the appropriate amount of responsibility. You've decided to confront your student and ask for checkoff on a knee evaluation.

Vignette 3

You've just accepted a position at a health care facility that also has an active student program. The staff seems to ignore the dress regulations and everyone wears what he or she wishes, and so you also decide to wear what you wish, and come to work in comfortable clothes: hip huggers and a tunic top. Your supervisor tells you to go home and change your clothes and come back in the "regulation uniform." You decide to confront him or her.

Vignette 4

In the middle of a treatment, your patient, a young and rather seductive member of the opposite sex, grabs your arm and tells you that he or she has very strong sexual feelings for you and wonders if you might meet privately at the end of the day.

Vignette 5

You are a professional on the staff for over a year. You still lack skill in one treatment technique that an aide knows how to do flawlessly. In front of the patient, the aide comes up to you and chastises you for not knowing how to do even the simplest procedures. You are embarrassed, and decide to confront the aide.

Vignette 6

Your colleague who always takes advantage of others comes up to you in front of a patient and asks you to cover for her, as she has to make an important phone call. She disappears and does not return for 2 hours. When she returns you decide to confront her.

Vignette 7

You are instructing a 35-year-old woman in pelvic stabilization exercises, and the patient is having difficulty recruiting her lower abdominals and pelvic floor. All of a sudden the patient begins to cry, saying that her back hurts so much, and that she and her husband had not been able to be intimate for 6 months and she feels as if he no longer desires her. How do you respond? (Resist the common desire to "fix" patients' problems and remember active listening skills.)

Vignette 8

Your supervisor notices that you are taking longer with one of your patients who suffered a stroke than is common for a patient treatment. She suggests you delegate the care of this patient to an assistant. You believe the patient requires the attention of a professional. What do you say?

Vignette 9

Review your responses from the Assertiveness Inventory. Create a vignette that typifies a situation that is predictably problematic for you. Teach your partner how to act in a way that is sure to elicit passive or aggressive behavior from you. Then write a DISC or DESC response and role play.

Observer Response Sheet

As an observer, your role is to facilitate a dialogue that has an adequate assertive response. The dialogue may begin with the "aggressor" making the statement that requires the assertive response, or it may begin with time having elapsed since the incident, and the assertive response is occurring now. Keep track of time, and keep the interchange to 2 or 3 minutes. At the conclusion, *ask the assertive responder how he or she feels, then ask the other partner the same.* Then proceed to give feedback to both on these various aspects of their communication.

How well did the assertive communicator:

1. Communicate using the "I" statements, DISC, or DESC responses?

2. Stay nonaggressive, nonjudgmental, nonaccusatory?

3. Listen and respond in an assertive way to the other's response?

4. How well did the "aggressor" use active listening skills and still stay in character? How would you suggest each could improve his or her communication?

Chapter 8

COMMUNICATING TO ESTABLISH RAPPORT AND REDUCE NEGATIVITY USING NEUROLINGUISTIC PSYCHOLOGY

Helen L. Masin, PT, PhD

OBJECTIVES

1. To recognize the importance of developing rapport in effective communication.
2. To teach principles of neurolinguistic psychology (NLP) to assist practitioners in developing effective verbal and nonverbal communication skills.
3. To recognize primary representational systems in NLP and how they impact on effective communication skills.
4. To learn the problem-solving approach of MYOUR as used in NLP as a model for enhancing effective communication skills.

The importance of rapport has long been recognized in health care; it is commonly referred to as "bedside manner." Exactly what constitutes appropriate bedside manner? A patient can easily tell you when it is present and when it is not present, although the patient may not be able to describe specifically what it is. If the physician has good rapport, the patient may perceive the doctor as warm and caring. However, if the physician has poor rapport, the patient may perceive the doctor as cold and distant. The purpose of this chapter is to help you to recognize rapport and to develop skills in utilizing rapport to enhance your therapeutic presence.

Stop now and think of a time when you went into a physician's office for the initial visit. In your mind's eye, envision this experience from beginning to end before proceeding with the reading of this chapter.

If you felt comfortable with the physician, you may have decided to utilize his or her services again. If you did not feel comfortable, you probably decided to find another physician. Take a moment to list the factors that made your experience very comfortable or not very comfortable. Specifically, what were some of the physician's behaviors that you identified? What were some of your responses to those behaviors? Finally, focus on what role verbal and nonverbal communication played in your interpretation of the behaviors.

Table 8-1

GENERIC ABILITIES

Generic abilities are attributes, characteristics, or behaviors that are not explicitly part of the profession's core of knowledge and technical skills but are nevertheless required for success in the profession. Ten generic abilities were identified through a study conducted at University of Wisconsin-Madison, 1991-1992. The 10 abilities and definitions are:

Generic Ability	Definition
1. Commitment to Learning	The ability to self-assess, self-correct, and self-direct; to identify needs and sources of learning; and to continually seek new knowledge and understanding.
2. Interpersonal Skills	The ability to interact effectively with patients, families, colleagues, other health care professionals, and the community; and to deal effectively with cultural and ethnic diversity issues.
3. Communication Skills	The ability to communicate effectively (ie, speaking, body language, reading, writing, listening) for varied audiences and purposes.
4. Effective Use of Time and Resources	The ability to obtain the maximum benefit from a minimum investment of time and resources.
5. Use of Constructive Feedback	The ability to identify sources of and seek out feedback, and to effectively use and provide feedback for improving personal interaction.
6. Problem Solving	The ability to recognize and define problems, analyze data, develop and implement solutions, and evaluate outcomes.
7. Professionalism	The ability to exhibit appropriate professional conduct and to represent the profession effectively.
8. Responsibility	The ability to fulfill commitments and to be accountable for actions and outcomes.
9. Critical Thinking	The ability to question logically; to identify, generate, and evaluate elements of logical argument; to recognize and differentiate facts, illusions, assumptions, and hidden assumptions; and to distinguish the relevant from the irrelevant.
10. Stress Management	The ability to identify sources of stress and to develop effective coping behaviors.

Adapted from May W, Morgan B, Lemke J, et al. Model for ability-based assessment in physical therapy education. *J Phys Ther Ed.* 1995;9:1.

To be effective, health care requires interaction with people who often are not functioning at top levels. Increasingly, health care professionals are bombarded with information regarding the importance of effective communication skills. In 1995, May[1] identified 10 generic abilities that clinicians determined were essential for success as a physical therapy professional (Table 8-1). Three of the 10 generic abilities were directly related to communication skills. One was *communication skills*, which includes the ability to communicate effectively (speaking, body language, reading, writing, listening) for varied audiences and purposes. A second was *interpersonal skills*, which included the ability to interact effectively with patients, families, colleagues, other health professionals and the community, and to deal effectively with cultural and ethnic diversity issues. A third was use of *constructive feedback*, which involves the ability to identify sources of feedback, seek out feedback, and to effectively use and provide feedback for improving personal interactions. In addition, Schmoll[2] states that "Increasingly, our professional role will encompass that of an educator. If I treat you, it's for today. If I teach you, it's for a lifetime." Burcham[3] contends that an essential component for success in the managed care environment is to listen to the customer (patient). He claims that by listening carefully to your customers (patients), you will find that the things that satisfy them are not the costly things that you do. Be sure that what you are doing has demonstrated value to your customer (patient). All of these interactive processes are critical to the rendering of effective health care.

As discussed in Chapter 5, The Nature of Effective Helping, professional knowledge and skill are critical to health care providers, but we also need the ability to interact in healing ways. Indeed, Davis states "How we approach patients, speak to them, touch them, and listen to them has as much or more of an impact on healing than do knowledge and skills of our professional preparation."[4] For the health care practitioner, the ability to communicate with patients is a critical component to being successful in our therapy with patients. To be successful in these therapeutic processes, we must understand the nature of communication, the nature of therapeutic relationships and the context in which this communication takes place (see Chapter 9, Communicating With Cultural Sensitivity).

COMMUNICATION FROM A QUANTUM PERSPECTIVE

Current research in quantum physics supports a view that acknowledges the importance of relationships. In the quantum world, relationships are not just interesting. To many physicists, relationships are *all* there is to reality.[5] The physics of our universe is revealing the primacy of relationships. As we let go of our Cartesian, linear, and mechanistic models of the world, we begin to step back and see ourselves in new ways, to appreciate our wholeness.[5] We are observing in ourselves, as well as in all living entities, boundaries that both preserve us from, and connect us to, the infinite complexity of the outside world. Indeed, Jantch states that "in life, the issue is not control but dynamic interconnectedness."[6] None of us exists independent of our relationships with others.[5] If this is true, then all of us need to develop better skills in communicating in all of our relationships.

The developments in quantum physics present us with a dramatic paradigm shift regarding what we perceive as real. Newtonian physics taught us that the basic elements of nature were small, solid, indestructible objects. However, quantum physics teaches us that atoms, the building blocks of all matter, actually consist of vast regions of space in which very small particles move. Depending on how these small particles are observed or considered, they may behave as particles or as waves. Given this quantum interpretation, solid objects are no longer perceived as solid. Even though our 5 senses tell us that we are made up of solid matter, we are probably more like a mass of energy set in constant motion. This energy is constantly breaking itself down and building itself back up. The current research in psychoneuroimmunology addresses this "energy flow" as a force which responds to our own inner chemistry. Mind and body are united in a whole nurtured by the flow of vital energy, or chi.[7] This paradigm shift is important for health care practitioners to understand in facilitating the healing process. Many complementary and alternative health care procedures such as reflexology, craniosacral therapy, and acupuncture address this concept of "energy flow" in the therapeutic process.[7]

In quantum physics, relational holism demonstrates how whole systems are created among subatomic particles. Through this interaction of particles, parts of the whole are changed, drawn together by a process of internal connectedness. Electrons are drawn into intimate relations as their wave aspects interfere with one another, overlapping and merging; their own qualities of mass, charge, spin, position, and momentum become indistinguishable from one another. According to Zohar,[8] it is no longer meaningful to talk of the constituent electrons' individual properties, as these continually change to meet the requirements of the whole. If we apply this microcosmic model from quantum physics to the macrocosmic model of human communication, then we have a dynamic paradigm for communication that reflects the interactive processes that occur with each communication encounter. Remember from Chapter 5, that the process of empathy as described by Stein[9] and Davis[10] includes self-transposal followed by a "crossing over" or shared moment of meaning, followed by sympathy. This unique form of intersubjectivity illustrates the dynamic interactive aspect of communication.

Another fascinating finding from the research in quantum physics indicates that a very small change may have an impact far beyond what could have been predicted. Until recently, observations from empirical research that fell outside the predicted, linear, hierarchical model were generally discounted or explained away. For example, we were trained to believe that small differences averaged out, that slight variances converged toward a point, and that approximations would give us a fairly accurate picture of what could happen. However, the research in chaos theory has changed these beliefs because when we view the world as a dynamic, changing system, the slightest variation can have explosive results.[5] If we were to create a difference in 2 values as small as rounding them off to the 31st decimal place, after 100 iterations or repetitions of the values, the whole calculation would be skewed. Indeed, scientists now find that the very small differences at the beginning of a system's evolution may make prediction impossible. They call this "sensitive dependence on initial conditions."[5] Iteration or repetition creates powerful and unpredictable effects in nonlinear systems. For example, in the first 6 months of human pregnancy, the embryo may experience a change that will significantly modify the outcome of the newborn infant, such as a cleft lip or palate. In complex ways that we do not understand, the system feeds back on itself, enfolding all that has happened, magnifying slight variances, and encoding it in the system's memory. In this way, prediction is prohibited. If we apply this concept to communications models, slight variations in communication patterns may produce dynamic changes in communicative interactions.

As stated in Chapter 6, Effective Communication, therapeutic communication requires learning new skills as well as unlearning habitual, nonhelpful ways of interacting. The purpose of using effective communication is to improve one's therapeutic presence with patients. By communicating in ways which help to solve problems, while at the same time respecting and honoring the human being, practitioners can actually facilitate the healing process. In sum, practitioners can utilize the patient-practitioner relationship itself, so important in the nonlinear quantum model, for therapeutic intervention.

Neurolinguistic Psychology

The utilization of neurolinguistic psychology (NLP) has been reported to enhance communication effectiveness in health care settings.[11-13] Laborde[14] defines NLP as a discipline based on the idea that neurology, language, and behavior are interrelated and can be changed by specific interventions. The theoretical basis for NLP emerged from studies of the work of masters in several fields.[14] O'Connor and Seymour[15] define NLP as the art and science of excellence, derived from studying how top people in different fields obtained their outstanding results. They describe NLP as practical. It is a set of models, skills, and techniques for thinking and acting effectively in the world.

NLP first evolved in the 1970s from the work of John Grinder, an assistant professor of linguistics, and Richard Bandler,[16] a psychology student at the University of California, Santa Cruz. Bandler and Grinder believed that by identifying excellence one could analyze it, model it, and use it.

Their initial work studied 3 outstanding communicators: Fritz Perls,[17] founder of gestalt therapy; Virginia Satir,[18] founder of family therapy; and Milton Erickson,[19] psychiatrist and hypnotherapist. Grinder and Bandler were also strongly influenced by the work of Gregory Bateson,[20] a British anthropologist who wrote on communication and systems theory.

The basic framework for NLP comes from the awareness that our neurological processes are sensory based, and that we use linguistics or language to order thought and behavior and to communicate with others. In our roles as health care providers, we are constantly challenged to communicate effectively with our patients, their families, our colleagues, and our support staff. NLP gives us the tools and skills to assist us in enhancing our verbal as well as our nonverbal skills.

In NLP terms, the *meaning of communication is based on the response that you get.* As health care professionals, this puts a great deal of responsibility on the provider to use forms of communication to which the patient can respond. Research conducted by Mehrabian[21] using the word "maybe" has shown that communication has multiple aspects. In Mehrabian's study, asking the listener how he or she interpreted what the communicator meant by "maybe," the interpretation by the listener was 55% from body language (including posture, gesture, and eye contact), 38% from tone of voice, and 7% from the verbal content of the message. Since Mehrabian's study only used one word, it is difficult to generalize his findings to multiple word communications. However, the study does indicate that the process of our communication may be even more important to the message than the content of our communication.

RAPPORT

In order to effectively communicate, we must first establish rapport with our client, establishing an atmosphere of trust and confidence. Rapport also helps to solidify the participation within which people can respond freely. Think back to your opening visualization at the beginning of this chapter. What were the behaviors that you identified in the scenario with the physician that helped establish rapport? What were the behaviors that broke rapport? When 2 people in conversation are in rapport, communication seems to flow. Body language and voice tonality flow together; bodies as well as words match each other. What is *said* can create or break rapport, but remember that verbal communication is only part of the total communication. People in rapport tend to match each others' posture, gestures, and eye contact. When rapport is established, people mirror each other and their body language is complementary.[15] At its best, rapport flows into a focus of concentration that takes on a life of its own, and for a few moments, time is forgotten.

Rosenzweig[11] states that rapport implies a working relationship between 2 people. Patient and practitioner recognize each others' needs, share information, and set common goals. Rapport implies mutuality, collaboration, and respect. However, rapport results from more than just good intentions. Words and actions must be carefully and sensitively chosen.

Studies have shown that the presence of rapport treats illness, enhances satisfaction and compliance, and *prevents* malpractice litigation.[11] Egbert and colleagues[22] describe a special therapeutic rapport that was established with an experimental group of patients undergoing elective laparotomy. These patients received "extra" reassurance and information. As you might expect postoperatively, these patients needed only half as many analgesics and were discharged home almost 3 days earlier than controls. Another study by Inui and colleagues[23] found that enhanced communication skills of physicians resulted in clinically significant improvement in blood pressure control in their patients. Studies of mothers' compliance with physicians' recommendations were studied by Korsch and Francis.[24] They found that mothers' satisfaction and compliance with treatment depended on whether the doctor was perceived as friendly and on how well the physician conveyed information. Finally, malpractice specialists report that poor rapport between physician and patient might be the single most common cause of malpractice suits. The risk of litigation increases when patients experience the physicians as uncaring, when they fail to discuss or disclose, or when patients are left with unrealistic expectations.[11]

NLP AND RAPPORT

NLP provides a framework that may assist professionals in establishing rapport with their clients. The 3 key steps in establishing rapport are *matching, pacing,* and *leading.*[15] Matching a person's body language with sensitivity and respect helps to build a bridge between the practitioner and the patient's model of the world. The premise is based on the idea that when people are like each other in body language, they will be more easily connected and in sync. In a sense, the practitioner is matching the patient's "explanatory model" as described by Kleinman[25] through matching the patient's body language (see Chapter 9, Communicating With Cultural Sensitivity).

Matching

Matching is very different from mimicry. Matching involves the subtle modeling of others' movements by small hand movements, body movements, and head movements. It also involves matching distribution of body weight and basic posture. Matching breathing and voice matching are other ways to develop rapport. Matching can occur with voice tonality, speed, volume, and rhythm of speech. Vocabulary and voice matching can be used in telephone conversations as well as in face-to-face encounters.[15]

> Tim and Chris were trying to decide whether to spend the evening by going to a movie or studying for an exam they both had coming up the next week. Chris really wanted to go to the movie and was angry with Tim for "never wanting to have any fun." Chris was disappointed that Tim was not interested in going to the movie with her. However, she decided to "see" the situation from Tim's perspective. She matched his posture and his tone of voice, and suddenly she remembered that he had barely passed the last exam and was worried that he might not pass this course. As she matched his voice and posture, she felt his fear and vulnerability, and suggested that they both study alone for awhile and then quiz each other later. Tim breathed a sigh of relief, and suggested that if they got enough accomplished, they might go out for a while later on.

For some people, matching another initially may feel uncomfortable or unnatural. For others, it may happen naturally. Notice your reactions when you are matching or when you are being matched. If you want to establish rapport, and the person has fidgety movements, you may want to cross match by subtly swaying your body or moving subtly without actually fidgeting yourself. It is not necessary to *like* the person to establish rapport. You are using this skill to better understand the person, and thus develop a working relationship with him or her.[15] Try it with someone you have difficulty understanding. Matching their body posture and movements may help you grasp the other person's point of view. In some situations, by matching the other person's body language, you may experience what they are feeling in your own body and thus better appreciate the client's nonverbal communication with you.

In some cases, you may choose not to establish rapport. For example, in a situation in which the other person appears hostile, you may choose to break rapport. You can break rapport by mismatching body language, tonality, speed, volume, or rhythm of speech. If you are seated, you may stand up to indicate nonverbally that the interaction is over. If you need to continue the communication at a later time, you can suggest another time to meet once the person has had some time to calm down. You might ask the person to write down his or her concerns to bring to your subsequent meeting. By writing down his or her concerns, he or she may release some of the tension that caused you to end the initial meeting. If you sense that you are still unable to resolve the issue at your rescheduled meeting, you may wish to ask another colleague to be present for your meeting.

A good example of a time when you would want to break rapport would be when a patient was acting inappropriately in a sexual way.

> Judy, a physical therapist, was treating a man with cervical disc herniation with massage while he lay supine on the treatment table. She was seated at his head and was gently mobilizing his very tense neck muscles when he asked her out of the blue, "Are you turned on when you do this?" She responded, directly but not unkindly, that she was thinking about his neck pathology and that sexuality was not at all a part of what she was concerned with. Besides that, she was happily married, and wanted to keep the relationship with her patients on a strictly professional level. Not to be put off, her patient replied, "Well, does your husband make you happy in bed?"
>
> At that point, Judy knew she had to break rapport. She stood up, looked at her patient in the eye and said firmly, "This treatment is over. As I said, it is very important that we keep a professional relationship between us. If you cannot do that, I will have to refer you to another therapist. Please make a follow-up appointment for next week, but recognize that I will not see you if you continue to be inappropriate with me, and I will have to refer you to a male colleague."

Pacing and Leading

Once you have established rapport with someone, you can change your behavior and he or she is likely to follow you. This is referred to in NLP as *pacing* and *leading*. Pacing and leading, basic concepts in NLP, involve the use of rapport and developing respect for the other person's worldview, and they assume a positive intention. To pace and lead successfully, one must pay attention to the other person and be flexible enough in one's own behavior to respond to what one sees, hears, and feels.[15] Superior teachers do this intuitively. First, they establish rapport with their student, enter the student's world, and then pace the student to move into the subject or skill that is being taught. Pacing or matching behavior creates the bridge through rapport and respect. When leading, you change your behavior so that the other person can follow. However, one must have rapport *before* one can pace and lead. When the teacher is pacing the student, the teacher matches the student's posture, verbal tonality, and speed of speaking to establish rapport. When the teacher recognizes that she has matched the student's pace and that he or she has rapport with the student, he or she introduces a change in posture, verbal tonality, and speed of speaking, and the student then follows the teacher's lead. This only occurs once the teacher has established rapport with the student by first matching and pacing the student on several levels of communication (eg, posture, tonality, speed).

Rapport is a critical skill in intercultural communication, as discussed in Chapter 9. Without rapport, intercultural communication may be doomed from the outset. Since much of communication is perceived nonverbally, there is a chance to establish rapport even though there are language differences. Nonverbal communication is the language of culture. Through the development of rapport, the practitioner matches the patient's body language, tonality, speed, volume, and rhythm of speech.[15] If the dialogue is between a low context (individualistic) and a high context (collectivistic) individual, the practitioner can take nonverbal cues from the patient that will assist in establishing rapport even if the practitioner does not speak the language of the patient. The person from a low context (individualistic) culture will generally rely heavily on the spoken word and demonstrate little gesturing or touching in the communication interaction. The person from the high context (collectivistic) culture will generally rely less on the spoken words but will use more gesturing or touch in the communication interaction.

Pacing is especially helpful in dealing with intense emotions in communications. If someone is angry, you must first match his or her anger at lower intensity. This will keep the anger from escalating. Once you have matched, you gradually reduce the intensity of your own behavior to lead the person to a calmer state. If someone approaches you with a sense of urgency, you can match him or her by speaking a little louder and quicker than usual and then pace the person to a softer and slower speed.[15]

PREFERRED REPRESENTATIONAL SYSTEMS—PREDICATES

As human beings, we are all capable of thinking. However, we tend to think about what we are thinking *about,* rather than *how* we think. Because of this, we often believe that other people think in the same manner we do. This often causes difficulty in communications with people who have different *ways* of thinking. In NLP, these patterns or ways of thinking are called *representational systems*. They are another tool in NLP that may assist practitioners in communicating with patients. Representational systems are the ways in which we take in, store, and code information in our minds, through seeing, hearing, feeling, taste, and smell. Thought patterns have direct physical effects on the mind and body. For example, think about eating your favorite food. Although the food may by imaginary, your production of saliva is measurable. This Pavlovian conditioned reflex is a good example of the influence of the mind on the body. We use the same neurological paths to envision or represent experience inwardly as we do to experience it outwardly or directly. These same neurons generate electrochemical charges that can be measured by EMG readings. We use our sensory systems (sight, touch, hearing, smell, taste) to perceive the world and then we inwardly "re-present" the world in our minds.[15]

According to O'Connor and Seymour,[15] **visual (V), auditory (A), and kinesthetic (K) systems are the primary representational systems in Western cultures. In NLP, the senses of taste and smell are often included with the kinesthetic sense.** People from Western cultures generally use all 3 of these primary systems all the time, but they are not equally aware of them. They tend to favor some over the others. The visual system has external (E) representations when one is looking at the outside world (VE), and internal (I) representations when one is mentally visualizing (VI). The auditory system is divided into hearing external sounds (AE) and internal sounds (AI). The auditory system of internal sounds includes the internal voices and dialogue of the individual.[15] For example, the therapist may be hearing the client say "good morning" in the external environment of the clinic, and at the same time, she may be having an internal dialogue about why she got a speeding ticket on the way to work. Remember from Chapter 2 that the way we view ourselves and the world is directly influenced by the internal sounds of the voices of our parents that we've introjected or incorporated, usually not on purpose.

The kinesthetic system includes the feelings that accompany tactile sensations like touch, temperature, and moisture (KE); internal feelings (KI) of remembered sensations; emotions; and inner feelings of balance, body awareness, and proprioception. Human behavior is based on a mixture of these internal and external sensory experiences. **If a person uses one internal sense habitually, it is called his or her** *preferred representational system* (PRS). The words that a person uses in conversation will indicate his or her PRS and thus yield important clues for establishing rapport.[15] For example, we all know some people who constantly respond, "Oh, I see" and others who reply, "I hear you."

According to Jepson,[26] the visual PRS is found in about 60% of the population. People who are organized, appearance-oriented, and observant tend to fall into this category. They are good spellers and memorize in their "mind's eye." They are distracted by noise, but often have difficulty following verbal instructions. They prefer reading for themselves rather than being read to. They become distracted if they are given too much verbal information.[12] Stop and think—are you a person who will read the written instructions first, before attempting to put a new purchase together out of the box?

People with auditory PRS account for about 30% of the population. They are experts at matching pitch, accents, timbre, and tones. When reading silently, they may move their lips. They may have a tendency to talk out loud to themselves. They are good listeners and can follow verbal instructions easily.[12] Stop and think—would you rather have someone verbally teach you a new theory than read about it?

The remaining 10% of people have a kinesthetic PRS. They enjoy "hands on" experiences and prefer to learn by doing. They are generally physically oriented and physically demonstrative. They may tend to appear restless. They may live in a disorganized environment.[12] Stop and think—do you want to put that new purchase together from the box without reading the directions first?

Remember that to build rapport, the listener matches the speaker. As a practitioner, one can listen for the language that a person uses to find out whether someone's PRS is visual, auditory, or kinesthetic. Since language communicates our thoughts, words will reflect the PRS which we prefer using. For example, 3 people with different PRSs may read the same book. The visual individual might say that he or she saw eye to eye with the author's premise. The auditory person might say that the author's message sounded clear as a bell to her. Someone who is primarily kinesthetic might say that she had a solid grasp of the author's premise. Although all 3 read the same book, they all responded differently. One was thinking in pictures, one in sounds, and one in feelings. **In NLP terms, these sensory-based words (verbs, adjectives, and adverbs) are called** *predicates.* **Understanding the use of predicates enables a practitioner to match predicates with the patient as another means of gaining rapport.** When working with a patient who is nonverbal, it is a good idea to use a mixture of visual, auditory, and kinesthetic predicates to optimize the communication because the person's PRS cannot be elicited verbally. It is also important to use a mix of predicates when addressing a large group of people to engage all 3 PRS styles.[15]

WATCHING EYE MOVEMENTS TO ASCERTAIN PREFERRED REPRESENTATIONAL SYSTEMS

Another important tool in NLP is the observation of what is termed "eye accessing." Dilts[27] discovered visible behavioral changes that signaled neurophysiological outputs that were clues to preferred representational systems. These clues include eye movements made during accessing of memory, breathing changes, skin color changes, and body postural changes. Neurological studies have shown that eye movement laterally and vertically appears to be associated with activation of different parts of the brain. So it becomes useful to observe eye movements in someone to better understand that person's experience as we are communicating with him or her.

There appears to be some common neurological connection between eye movements and PRS because the same patterns are found worldwide (except for the Basque region of Spain).[15] When patients visualize from the past, they tend to move their eyes up, and to the left. When they construct a picture or imagine something they have never seen, they tend to move their eyes up and to the right. Defocusing the eyes or looking straight ahead is another way to know if the speaker is using visualization. The speaker will appear to be looking beyond the listener as if watching an imaginary movie picture in front of them. The eyes tend to move to the left for remembered sounds and across to the right for constructed sounds. When the eyes go down and to the right, the patient is usually accessing feelings. When the patient talks to him or herself, the observer will see the eyes go down to the left[15] (Figure 8-1).

Eye accessing cues occur quickly, so the observer needs to watch the patient closely. In some cases, the eye accessing directions may be reversed. The person observing needs to ask several questions to determine if the patient may have a reverse eye accessing pattern. This is sometimes seen in individuals who are left-handed, but it may occur in anyone.

Figure 8-1. This illustration shows what you see when looking at another person.

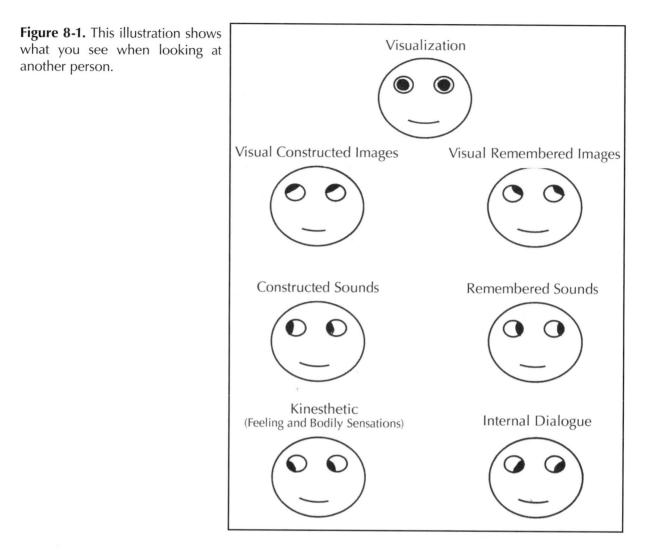

Visualization

Visual Constructed Images   Visual Remembered Images

Constructed Sounds   Remembered Sounds

Kinesthetic
(Feeling and Bodily Sensations)   Internal Dialogue

POSITIVE DESCRIPTIVE STATEMENTS

The NLP tool of using positive descriptive statements is a very useful tool in communicating with patients. A positive descriptive statement is a statement describing the behavior that you want the patient to do, rather than the behavior that you don't want. For example, if you tell a child, "don't spill the milk," he or she first has to visualize spilling the milk in order to "not" spill it. If I tell an adult, "don't cross your legs" as a hip precaution, he or she first has to visualize crossing his or her legs in order to "not" cross them. The health care practitioner might want to say "keep your legs parallel" or "keep your feet pointing straight ahead" so that the person can visualize only the outcome that you are recommending.

When working with children, elderly patients, or patients who are easily confused, the use of positive descriptive statements can make a big difference in the patient's understanding of your directions. When writing home programs for patients, using positive descriptive statements can be extremely helpful in assisting the patient to understand the exercise you want him or her to practice.

The Map vs the Territory Described by the Map

Another concept in NLP is that the map is not the territory it describes. The map is a symbol for the territory but it is not the territory itself. Chapter 2 describes how each individual has a perception of the world from his or her point of view. The perceptual filter is our bias by which we experience the world around us. Conflicts may occur between us because we have different maps of reality. Each of us has personal models of the world (explanatory models as described in Chapter 9) with our own sets of filters that may include visual, auditory, or kinesthetic PRS, as well as ways of sorting or categorizing stimuli in the environment. For example, one individual may observe a glass as half full and another individual may observe the same glass as half empty. The glass is exactly the same, but each individual perceives it according to his or her own sorting style. Different sorting styles also act as filters for how the individual perceives a situation in the environment. Another example might be a patient who perceives exercise as an unpleasant requirement in his or her recovery process, while another patient might perceive it as a blessing in his or her recovery process.[15]

If we choose to be successful in our communications with our patients, families, colleagues, and support staff, we must recognize that each person has a different map (or explanatory model) and different filters for the territory in which we all find ourselves. Through the use of NLP, we can learn to respect and appreciate the different maps and filters. LaBorde[14] suggests utilizing the acronym MYOUR as a way to remember and summarize the communication skills in NLP. MY is what I want, YOUR is what you want, and OUR is making sure everyone gets it. Once we appreciate the different maps and filters that we all have, we are in a better position to work together toward common goals in health care, education, intercultural communication, and ultimately world peace.

Conclusion

It's very important to remember that NLP provides us with tools for helping us to connect with our patients, their families, and our colleagues. We must be willing to be sensitive and flexible to match and pace for the benefit of others. Whether our patient prefers visual, auditory, or kinesthetic cues, there is no right or wrong way. The health care practitioner who is able to understand and adapt to the client's way of thinking will have better results. Our task is to make the therapeutic relationships as smooth, as helpful, and as free from conflict as possible. Practicing these basic NLP principles and techniques will assist you greatly in building rapport and calming negative interactions. The exercises that follow will give you a start in this process.

References

1. May W, Morgan B, Lemke J, et al. Model for ability-based assessment in physical therapy education. *J Phys Ther Ed.* 1995;9:1.
2. Schmoll B. Physical therapy today and in the twenty-first century. In: Scully, Barnes. *Physical Therapy.* Philadelphia, Pa: Lippincott Raven; 1989.
3. Ketter P. Understanding driving forces behind managed care is crucial for survival. *PT Bulletin.* 1997;12(29):6-7
4. Davis CM. *Patient Practitioner Interaction. Instructor's Manual.* Thorofare, NJ: SLACK Incorporated; 1994:17.
5. Wheatley MJ. *Leadership and the New Science.* San Francisco, Calif: Berrett-Koehler Publishers; 1994.
6. Jantch E. The self organizing universe. In: MJ Wheatley, ed. *Leadership and the New Science.* San Francisco, Calif: Berrett-Koehler Publishers, Inc; 1994:126.
7. Davis C. *Complementary Therapies in Rehabilitation: Holistic Approaches for Prevention and Wellness.* Thorofare, NJ: SLACK Incorporated; 1996.

8. Zohar D. The quantum self: human nature and consciousness defined by the new physics. In: MJ Wheatley, ed. *Leadership and the New Science*. San Francisco, Calif: Berrett-Koehler; 1994:118-119.

9. Stein E. *On the Problem of Empathy*. 2nd ed. The Hague: Martinus Nijhoff; 1970.

10. Davis CM. *A Phenomenological Description of Empathy as it Occurs Within Physical Therapists for Their Patients*. Boston University, Mass, 1982. Doctoral dissertation.

11. Rosenzweig S. Emergency rapport. *J Emerg Med*. 1993;11:775-776.

12. Jepson C. Neurolinguistic programming in dentistry. *CDA Journal*. 1992;20(3):28-32.

13. Konefal J. *Chronic Disease and Stress Management*. Denver, Colo: NLP Comprehensive International Conference; 1992.

14. Laborde G. *Fine Tune Your Brain*. Palo Alto, Calif: Syntony; 1988.

15. O'Connor S. *Introducing NLP*. San Francisco, Calif: Aquarian; 1990.

16. Bandler R. Grinder J. *The Structure of Magic*. Palo Alto, Calif: Science and Behavior Books; 1975.

17. Perls FS. *Gestalt Therapy Verbatim*. Moab, Utah: Real People Press; 1969.

18. Satir V. *Peoplemaking*. Palo Alto, Calif: Science and Behavior Books; 1972.

19. Gordon D, Anderson M. *Phoenix: Therapeutic Patterns of Milton H. Erickson*. Cupertino, Calif: Meta Publications; 1981.

20. Bateson G. *Steps to an Ecology of Mind*. New York, NY: Ballantine Books; 1972.

21. Mehrabian A, Ferris S. Decoding of inconsistent communications. *J Pers Soc Psychol*. 1967;6(1): 109-114.

22. Egbert L, Battit G, Welch C. et al. 1964. In: Rosenzweig S, ed. Emergency rapport. *J Emerg Med*. 1993; 11:775-776.

23. Inui T, Yourtee E, Williamson J, et al. 1976. In: Rosenzweig S, ed. Emergency rapport. *J Emerg Med*. 1993;11:775-776.

24. Korsch V, Gozzi E, Francis V, et al. 1968. In: Rosenzweig S, ed. Emergency rapport. *J Emerg Med*. 1993; 11:775-776.

25. Kleinman A. Concepts and a model for the comparison of medical systems as cultural systems. *Soc Sci Med*. 1976;12:85-93.

26. Jepson C. Neurolinguistic programming in dentistry. *CDA Journal*. 1992;20(3):30-31.

27. Dilts R. Roots of neuro-linguistic programming part II (the experiment). 1983. In: Jepson C. Neurolinguistic programming in dentistry. *CDA Journal*. 1992;20(3):30.

EXERCISES

EXERCISE 1: CLINICAL ENCOUNTERS

1. Sit across from someone in your class. One person will role play the therapist and one person the client. Role play a situation which you remember from a patient therapist interaction that you have observed. Talk to the patient as you normally would without paying any special attention to matching or mirroring.

   a. What do you experience as the therapist?

   b. What do you experience as the patient?

   c. Do you experience rapport with each other? Why or why not?

2. Sit across from another person in your class. Again, one person is the therapist and one person the client. Role play the same situation that you recall from a patient therapist interaction that you have observed. This time, the therapist will subtly match the body posture, gesture, hand movements, and breathing of the patient.

   a. What do you experience as the therapist?

b. What do you experience as the patient?

c. Do you experience rapport with each other? Why or why not?

EXERCISE 2: UNDERSTANDING PREFERRED REPRESENTATIONAL SYSTEMS—PREDICATES

1. Sit across from another person in your class. One person tells a story about his or her favorite vacation. The other person listens to the story and responds as he or she normally would.

   a. What do you experience as the storyteller?

   b. What do you experience as the listener?

   c. Did you experience rapport? Why or why not?

2. Sit across from another person in your class. One person tells a story about a favorite vacation. The other person listens to the story and pays close attention to predicates—the use of visual, auditory, or kinesthetic words and phrases. The listener responds by matching the personal representational system (PRS) of the storyteller.

   a. What is the PRS of the storyteller? How do you know?

   b. What is the PRS of the listener? How do you know?

   c. Did you experience rapport? Why or why not?

   d. Describe a clinical situation where use of predicates may be helpful to establish rapport.

EXERCISE 3: EYE ACCESSING ACTIVITY

1. Get together with someone in your class. Ask that person the following questions and record his or her eye movements below. The person responding to the questions can have the eye motion chart on their lap facing the person asking the questions so that the person asking the questions can more readily identify what each eye accessing movement indicates. The thought process and the eye accessing are what you want to understand in this exercise. The verbal responses are not important.

   a. What color is the couch in your living room?

   b. What did you see on your way to class?

   c. What would your ideal house look like?

   d. What would you look like with "pink" hair?

   e. What is the sound of a busy signal on the telephone?

   f. How would your voice sound underwater?

   g. Recite a nursery rhyme in your head.

   h. How does silk feel next to your skin?

2. What did you discover about eye accessing with your partner?

3. How might you use eye accessing in a clinical situation to enhance rapport?

EXERCISE 4: CLINICAL DILEMMA

1. You are a physical therapist working with a patient who accesses information in the visual PRS. How would you communicate with this person? What type of home program would you give him or her?

2. You are a practitioner working with a patient who accesses information in the auditory PRS. How would you communicate with this person? What type of home program would you give him or her?

3. You are a practitioner working with a patient who accesses information in the kinesthetic PRS. How would you communicate with this person? What type of home program would you give him or her?

COMMUNICATING WITH CULTURAL SENSITIVITY

Helen L. Masin, PT, PhD

OBJECTIVES

1. To examine the impact of culture on delivery of health care services.
2. To examine research in intercultural communication.
3. To explore and appreciate one's own cultural heritage.
4. To explore and appreciate the cultural heritage of others.
5. To recognize that intergenerational communication difficulties represent cultural differences, and learn how to communicate effectively with people of various ages.
6. To learn a problem-solving approach that assists practitioners to enhance their intercultural communication skills.

Have you ever experienced "culture shock"? How did you know?

With the ever increasing options for travel and information exchange via the Internet and other technology, people who come from different cultures are meeting through work, play, travel, and shared interests. Because of the increasing exposure to different cultures, it has become extremely important to develop an appreciation of, and respect for, people whose culture differs from one's own. In order to prepare for the 21st century, health care professionals must learn to communicate with cultural sensitivity to work effectively with patients, families, colleagues, staff, and support personnel.

CULTURE SHOCK—WHAT IS IT?

Culture shock has been defined as the stress experienced when individuals cannot meet their everyday needs as they would in their own culture. They may have difficulty communicating, making themselves understood, or figuring out why the "locals" are behaving in a certain way. In response to this stress, they may feel a sense of loss and a sense of shock that others behave so differently and seem to have such a different worldview.[1]

When culture shock occurs, familiar ways of behaving that you learn through socialization in your own culture do not work in the new culture. Culture shock may occur when you visit another country, when you move from one type of climate to another, when you talk with people who are members of a different generation from yours, when you meet people who have a different sexual orientation from yours, when you meet people who have a disability, or when you meet people who have a different race, religion, or political view from yours. Culture has the broadest connotation when viewed in this way.

If these differences pose challenges to communication among people in daily life, you can imagine the impact of these differences in patient care.

As professionals, we are committed to putting the needs of our patients first. In order to do this effectively, the professional must be aware of and appreciate the cultural mores and expectations of the individual from the world view of that person. Once the other person's world view is understood, it may be easier to establish a therapeutic relationship. The goal of this chapter is to introduce you to intercultural communication in health care in order to assist you in developing awareness and skills to work effectively in our increasingly diverse communities.

A Personal Experience

One of my first challenges as a new therapist working in an early intervention program for infants and toddlers with disabilities in Miami, Florida was to develop a feeding and eating program. I had been involved with a feeding and eating program in the public school system in Maryland where I had worked prior to moving to Miami. The program had been quite successful in Maryland, and I was delighted to share my experiences with my colleagues in my new setting in Miami. I suggested that the classroom teachers begin the feeding program with a "food play" activity. The therapeutic objective was to encourage the children to "play" with the food on their tray. Through play, it has been shown that children will eventually want to bring the food to their mouths to explore it. This would lay the foundation for the hand to mouth feeding behavior which is essential for self-feeding.

Based on my previous success with this approach in Maryland, I enthusiastically asked the nutritionist at the program to give me several jars of baby food to use for the food play activity. Many of the children in the program were former premature infants who were generally extremely tactile defensive around their mouths and often were resistant to eating food other than in a bottle.

The nutritionist gave me the food, and I poured out the jar on the tray of the corner chair of one of the toddlers. The child enthusiastically placed both hands into the food and smeared it all over the tray, all over himself, and eventually brought his hands to his mouth to taste it. Of course, I felt extremely pleased that he had been so engaged in the activity and that he had indeed brought his hands to his mouth and tasted the food as I'd hoped. Because this child had a history of tactile defensiveness, this was an excellent response, a real success. The next day I hoped to use the food play activity with several of the other children in the program.

When I went to work the following day, I suggested that the preschool teachers might want to join me to help introduce the food play activity with several of the other children with tactile defensiveness. As the teachers politely declined one by one, I wondered why they were not very enthusiastic about my suggestion. I proceeded to work with another child, and was delighted to see that the food play also helped him develop the hand to mouth skill.

After several more successful days with the food play activity, I was hopeful that the preschool teachers would finally join in. Since they still politely declined, I decided to ask them if they had any concerns about the food play activity. They all said it made them feel extremely uncomfortable. When I asked them what caused them to feel uncomfortable with the activity, they responded that you are viewed as a bad mother in their culture (Cuban) if you have a messy child. This activity was simply too threatening to them, for it challenged their cultural norms about what was acceptable behavior for good mothers with their children.

Once I understood the cultural origins of the issue, I had a much better understanding of the teachers' and parents' concerns. I politely explained to the teachers that my intention had not been to offend them or the mothers, and I asked if there might be an alternative way that we could address the problem. After talking with them, we decided to implement a solution that addressed my concerns, as well as the mothers' concerns. We decided that we would have the children in diapers for the food play activity. That way, we could bathe them after the activity and then put their clean clothes back on them. Thus, the children had the benefit of the food play without the messiness. The teachers, parents, children, and myself were all pleased. If we had not taken the time to understand the cultural norms involved in this situation, the teachers and families might have been labeled as "noncompliant" and the children would not have had the benefit of the food play learning experience which was so valuable for the development of their independent feeding skills.

As a new therapist in Miami, I quickly realized that I wanted to learn as much as I could about the cultures of the children and families with whom I was working. I began a pilot study to investigate maternal perceptions and knowledge about physical therapy in an early intervention in Miami.[2] Through my reading and research in this area, I learned a great deal, which enabled me to provide more culturally competent care to my patients and their families.

CULTURAL DIVERSITY IN THE UNITED STATES

In order to understand the need for culturally competent care, one must first recognize the increasing diversity that is developing in the United States. According to the 1990 census, the population distribution was as follows[3]:

❖ 75% Anglo-European American

❖ 12% African American

❖ 9% Hispanic American

❖ 3% Asian American

The 1996 predictions from the US Department of Commerce for the year 2050 project the population distribution in the United States to be as follows:

❖ 53% Anglo-European American

❖ 15% African American

❖ 24% Hispanic American

❖ 9% Asian American

In 1992, Christensen's research with clinical professionals indicated that the ability to work effectively with culturally diverse families requires professionals to acknowledge their own cultural background and to develop a general understanding of specific cultures. She stated that cultural background can be a powerful force in the relationship between professionals and the families they serve.[4] As we have learned in most of the chapters in this text, relationship is critical to the therapeutic use of oneself in health care, or therapeutic presence.

According to Wheatley,[5] the quantum physics of our universe is revealing the primacy of relationships. In other words, each aspect of the universe is affected by its relationship to every other aspect of the universe. In quantum physics, nothing exists independent of its relationship with something else. This challenges our traditional Cartesian model of a linear, quantifiable universe. For example, in organizations, we may ask which is most important—the system or the individual. The quantum physicist will answer, "it depends." It is not an either/or question. It is not important to decide between the 2, but rather to recognize the *relationship* that exists between the person and the setting. That relationship will always be different and will generate different responses depending on the person at that moment in time. People, like quantum particles, are "fuzzy." They may go from being predictable to being surprising, just as wave packets of matter include potentialities for both forms—particles and waves. If we can appreciate the "wave-ness" and the "particle-ness" in ourselves as well as others, we have a better chance of developing the potential in all of us. The potential for being a wave or a particle depends on the environment/culture/context. If we can understand our own environment/culture/context and that of our clients, we have a better chance of developing the therapeutic relationship. Given this quantum physics paradigm of the primacy of relationships and their "fuzziness," we have more appreciation for our own culture and the cultures of our clients. With this perspective, we have better chances of developing effective therapeutic relationships.

The importance of understanding one's cultural worldview was emphasized when the US government mandated that care for children is delivered in a culturally competent manner. Indeed, the federal legislation that began with P.L. 94-142 in 1975 required that public school education be provided for all children from 6 to 21 years of age, regardless of handicapping condition. This law was modified as P.L. 94-457 (Education of the Handicapped Act of 1986) to include public school education for all children from 3 to 21, regardless of handicapping condition. It also specified that ancillary health services including physical therapy and occupational therapy (among others) are provided for all children in a "culturally competent" manner. These 2 laws were subsequently reauthorized as P.L. 101-119 (Individuals with Disabilities Education Act of 1991),[6] which also specified that these services be delivered in a "culturally competent" way.

CULTURAL COMPETENCE

What constitutes cultural competence? Cross, Bazron, Dennis, and Isaacs[7] define it as "the set of congruent behaviors, attitudes, and policies that come together in a system, agency, or among professionals to work effectively in cross-cultural situations." This type of service recognizes and incorporates the importance of culture, assessment of cross-cultural relations, understanding dynamics of cultural differences, expanses of cultural knowledge, and modification of services to meet culturally unique needs.

The concept of cultural competence is also referred to as "cultural sensitivity" or "intercultural communication." The term cross-cultural refers to comparative studies in multiple cultures. The study of people from different cultures interacting together is called intercultural communication. This chapter highlights results of research in both cross-cultural and intercultural communication as it relates to enhancing one's therapeutic effectiveness.

IMPACT OF CULTURE ON THERAPEUTIC EFFECTIVENESS

Given the increase in diversity of the population of the United States predicted in the 21st century, the ability to successfully communicate in culturally diverse settings will be essential for all health care providers. Research has shown that training in cross-cultural communication enhances the effectiveness of therapists working with clients whose cultures differ from their own.[8] In order to appreciate the importance of developing skill in intercultural encounters, one must first understand the nature of culture itself.

Anderson and Fenichel defined culture as the specific framework of meanings within which a population, individually and as a group, shares its lifeways.[9] Margaret Mead defined culture as "abstractions from the body of learned behavior which a group of people who share the same traditions transmit to their children and, in part, to adult immigrants who become members of the society. It covers not only the arts and sciences, religion and philosophies to which the world culture has historically applied, but also the system of technology, the political practices, the small intimate habits of daily life, such as the way of preparing or eating food, or of hushing a child to sleep, as well as the method of electing a prime minister or changing the constitution."[10]

Given these definitions, you can begin to grasp how culture is a critical element in understanding how someone responds to illness or disability. According to Brislin,[11] cross-cultural research shows that complex concepts *do not* have the same meaning in all cultures. For example, good health to someone in the United States may mean an absence of bacteria or viruses. To someone in China, good health may mean harmony between yin and yang. Therefore, health care practitioners must understand both general and specific components of complex health concepts.

Culture general concepts are concepts that are applicable across all cultures. Culture specific concepts are concepts that are unique to a particular group. People learn to express symptoms of distress in ways that are acceptable to others in the same culture. For example, in India, stress-related disorders are often suspected when the patient is suffering from an upset stomach. In the United States, stress-related disorders are often associated with headaches. This difference is apparent from the widespread advertising for painkillers in the United States for relief of headaches.[11] As part of the socialization in one's own culture, one learns that certain complaints about distress are acceptable and elicit understanding whereas other complaints are unacceptable. Understanding the cultural basis for the client's symptoms becomes more critical to accurate evaluation of the presenting problem leading to an accurate clinical diagnosis.

The majority of all health professionals are white. To examine one profession more closely, currently 93% of physical therapy professionals come from Anglo-European roots. Among physical therapy students, only 5.6% are minorities.[12] As the populations served by physical therapists become increasingly diverse, it is essential that therapists become skilled in communicating with clients and families who come from cultures different from their own. Indeed, the American Physical Therapy Association (APTA) has a Minority/International Affairs Division that is dedicated to increasing the presence of minorities in the profession, as well as educating the current membership regarding intercultural issues. Similar divisions exist in medicine, nursing, occupational therapy, and speech language pathology.

CULTURE AND BELIEF SYSTEMS

In order to understand the ramifications of culture in health care, one must also understand the relationship among beliefs, attitudes, and behavior. According to Dillman,[13] *beliefs* are what people think is true, *attitudes* are how people feel about something, and *behavior* is what people do. Since culture impacts all 3 of these areas, health care professionals must be sensitive to clients' beliefs, attitudes, and behaviors regarding their illness, injury, or disability. Researchers have found that when the professional understands what the client is experiencing, the client is more likely to feel that he or she can be helped. Belief in the possibility of positive outcomes is central to the delivery of and acceptance of health services.[14]

In order for health care practitioners to understand the belief systems of their clients, they must first understand the "explanatory model" of the client. Kleinman[15] first described the explanatory model as the explanations that are offered for the etiology, onset of symptoms, pathophysiology, course of sickness, and treatment for the particular problem being addressed. On the cultural level, there may be differences between the explanatory model of the family and the explanatory model of the health care professional. These differences can hamper effective delivery of health care. However, by respecting the explanatory model of the client, the patient/professional communication can be enhanced. For optimal healing to occur, there must be a "fit" between the expectations, beliefs, behaviors, and evaluation of the outcome between the client and the professional.

RESEARCH IN INTERCULTURAL COMMUNICATION

Transcultural studies in medicine and nursing have shown that understanding cultural variables is critical to working effectively with different ethnic groups.[16,17] Jackson[18] found that the amount of time spent with the client affected patient satisfaction with medical care in the African American population receiving treatment for hypertension. DeSantis[16] found increased compliance regarding nursing interventions with Hispanic and Haitian mothers when the clients' belief systems were explored and respected by the professional. Harwood[17] stated that ethnic differences appeared to be important determinants of observed differences in health behavior. He found that ethnicity was shown to be particularly relevant to what an individual believes and how he or she behaves with regard to various health practices.

CULTURE AND HEALTH CARE

Cultural differences in relation to health care are reflected in many facets of daily life. Some of the critical care issues that we'll examine which may assist health care practitioners to better understand their clients include understanding the characteristics of both *collectivistic (high context)* cultures and *individualistic (low context)* cultures; Eastern and Western perceptions of *locus of control* and how they differ; the concept of *"face"* heard so often in discussions of Asian and Oriental cultures; *nonverbal intercultural communication patterns*; *personalismo*, a concept critical to understanding expectations of Hispanic culture; and finally, *somatization*.

In addition to exploring these differences, health care practitioners must also understand differences related to disability, racism, ageism, sexism, sexual orientation, and intergenerational expectations. Finally, it is important to recognize that environmental conditions such as poverty, homelessness, and minimal formal education are variables that transcend all cultures.

HIGH CONTEXT AND LOW CONTEXT CULTURES

First, let's examine the difference between high context and low context cultures. Cultures that are usually associated with individualism (low context) include: North America (the United States is considered the most individualistic), Western Europe, Australia, and New Zealand. Cultures that are usually associated with collectivism (high context) include: Asia, Africa, Central and South America, and Pacific Island societies.[11]

In order for health care professionals to understand the meaning of the cultural distinctions listed above, they must first be cognizant of their own culture. Saunders[19] identified numerous characteristics of the Anglo-European culture and/or Western medical culture that may impact the patient-practitioner relationship. Since the majority of health care professionals currently are from Anglo-European roots, it is helpful to understand those values that impact health care, which include: the need for personal control over the environment, need for change, time dominance, human equality, individualism, privacy, self-help, competition, future orientation, action/goal/work, openness/honesty, practicality/efficiency, and materialism.[20] These values may conflict with other cultures which may espouse collectivistic beliefs, attitudes, and behaviors as described below.

Collectivistic cultures differ from individualistic cultures in some very critical ways. Collectivism refers to the tendencies of a system that emphasizes the importance of the *we* identity over the *I* identity, group rights over individual rights, and in-group oriented needs over individual wants and desires. Individualism refers to the tendencies of a system in emphasizing the importance of individual needs over group needs. The Western Cartesian (individualistic) tradition tends to perceive the self in opposing dualistic terms, whereas the Eastern (collectivistic) tradition tends to perceive the self in a complementary, relational, whole perspective.[21] These differences in world view create very different perceptions for the people who are members of these cultures.

In cross-cultural interactions, low context and high context cultures will also reveal marked differences. Graham and Miller[22] state that low-context cultures, such as most North American and Northern European societies, place emphasis on individualism and individual goals, facts, the management of time, nonverbal communication, privacy, and compartmentalization. Essentially task-oriented, they focus on data to provide the answers to living well. Progress is measured in acquiring tangibles or material goods; goals are action-oriented and geared to produce short-term material profits. The driving force of low context cultures is work. The usual place in which a person is honored is at work. Low context societies are structured to honor individuals who are financially successful. Emotions may be considered inappropriate in most social and work settings. Low context individuals, such as the CEOs of major corporations in America, are highly individualistic, directive, and dominating. They tend to be results-oriented, independent, strong-willed, and quick to make decisions. They may also be impatient, time-conscious, solution-oriented, and self-contained. They often have a high need to be recognized for performance. When working in groups, low context individuals need less time to develop relationships in the group, so new and progressive programs can be changed easily and quickly. However, these individuals may create less cohesion and stability in the group and are less committed to group agreements or planned actions. Individualists find that clearing their plans with others may interfere too much with their desire "to do their own thing."[22]

In contrast, Tirandis[23] states that collectivistic or high context cultures and peoples place emphasis on relationships, group goals, the process and surrounding circumstances, time as a natural progression, verbal communication, communal space, and interrelationships. The high context norms are primarily group-oriented. They place the relationships of the cultural group before that of an "out-group" such as a university, company, or country. The ties to family and community are strong. In general, feelings and emotions are valued, and expression of feelings is encouraged. Religious and spiritual beliefs are highly valued. Behavior is perceived in a complex way. Nuances of meaning are important in nonverbal communication cues, and the status of others is viewed in context. In general, to repeat, Asian cultural norms are considered to be high context. The personal characteristics that are valued are being indirect, highly affiliative, team-oriented, systematic, steady, and quiet. The person is expected to be patient, loyal, dependable, sharing, and respectful; generally slow in making decisions; and a good listener. For these people, a longer amount of time is needed for individuals to become acquainted with and trusting of each other, but once the trust is established, the communication is fast. In general, the culture has strong links to the past and is slow to change. The society is highly stable and works as a unified group. The group members feel comfortable with the constant psychological presence of a group. The members are loyal to the group. They demonstrate cooperation, contribution to the group without the expectation of immediate reciprocity, and show public modesty about individual abilities.[23] Individuals are more committed to group agreements and planned actions.

The critical importance of understanding the cultural beliefs and norms of clients became apparent to me while providing physical therapy at a preschool for a 2-year-old boy with cerebral palsy and a history of grand mal seizures. His family had recently immigrated to Miami from Haiti. All the professional staff was extremely concerned about him because he was having grand mal seizures at the preschool. The staff contacted the mother to determine whether or not she was giving him the phenobarbital that had been prescribed by the neurologist. She assured the staff that she was giving her son the medication. When the seizures continued, the staff called the mother again and had a Creole translator speak with her about the phenobarbital. However, the boy still continued to have the seizures at school. We were all extremely concerned about him, so we invited his mother to school and asked her to show us how she was administering the phenobarbital. This turned out to be the critical question that we had not initially asked.

His mother showed us that she administered the phenobarbital to him by bathing him in it. We were all *stunned*! We had not even considered that the medicine would be given in any way other than by mouth. We had made an assumption based on our Western medical model of oral administration of the medication. Fortunately, we were able to explain that the medicine had to be administered by mouth to be effective. Once his mother understood this, she followed through with the oral administration. She explained that in the part of Haiti where she had lived, medicine was administered by bathing in it. The practice of oral administration was as strange to her as bathing was to us. According to Brislin,[11] whenever people have experiences during which they have to make adjustments, they learn that culture is much *more* than an abstraction!

Whenever a client is not responding in the way one would have anticipated, it is important to ask if cultural differences might be causing the difficulty. Professionals may ask "which of these symptoms is familiar to me, given my own cultural background, and which seem strange?" The symptoms will seem strange if the professional has not encountered them in his or her own socialization.

According to Turner,[24] there are 3 questions that a health care professional should ask when working with clients to avoid potential biases:

1. How is this client like all human beings?
2. How is this client like some human beings?
3. How is this client like no other human being?

By asking these 3 questions, the health care professional can avoid stereotypes and generalizations and move toward the person's unique problems, needs, and resources.

THE CONCEPT OF FACE

The concept of "face," regarded as a universal construct, refers to the sense of self-respect or self-esteem that people demonstrate in communicating with each other. The management of face differs from one culture to the next. According to Ting-Toomey,[21] managing face involves maintaining a claimed sense of self-dignity, or regulating a claimed sense of self-humility in interaction. Three possible issues related to face communication include: dignity-humility, respect-deference, and imposition-nonimposition. As anyone who has ever done business in the Orient will tell you, if one wishes to be successful in keeping face, one must understand the cultural background of face work issues, as well as the norms and boundaries inherent in face work negotiation.[21]

According to Haglund,[25] the issue of face dialectics proved to be critical to one hospital's retention of Asian nurses. In reviewing the employment records of the Asian nurses, the administration learned that the Asian nurses were leaving after only 90 days of employment. The hospital policy required that all employees receive performance evaluations after 90 days of employment. The Asian nurses were not accustomed to receiving negative feedback face-to-face, which is a Western norm. As a result, the nurses would immediately quit their jobs after the performance evaluation rather than "lose face." Such misunderstandings are likely to occur more frequently with increasing diversity in the health care workforce unless education in intercultural communication becomes a part of pre-service and in-service training for all health care providers and support staff.

What ideas can you think of that might solve this problem to avoid the loss of face yet still provide adequate feedback to the Asian nurses?

In general, one can predict that in individualistic cultures, individual pride is more likely to be overtly expressed, whereas individual shame is more likely to be demonstrated through other ego-based emotional reactions such as anger, frustration, or guilt. In contrast, in collectivistic cultures, relational shame or face loss, such as face embarrassment or face humiliation, is more likely to be experienced, while individual based pride is more likely to be suppressed. Overall, the individualistic cultures stress ego-based emotional expressions and individual self-esteem while collectivistic cultures values other focused emotions management and protection of collective self-esteem.

These differences have a profound impact on the ethical perceptions between the 2 systems as well. Gilligan's gender-based research studies indicated that Euro-American males tend to engage in the "morality of justice," whereas the Euro-American females tended to engage in the "morality of caring."[26] The ego-based emotions are associated with "morality of justice," whereas the other focused emotions are associated with the "morality of caring". In other words, in a moral dilemma between doing the right thing vs doing the caring thing, people from individualistic cultures will choose the "right" action over the "caring" action. Doing the caring action is more reflective of the high context or collectivistic worldview.

Numerous scholars[27] note that individualists in Western cultures tend to perceive emotion, cognition, and motivation as located in the mind, whereas collectivists in Eastern cultures tend to perceive these 3 constructs as stemming primarily from the heart. Western vocabularies tend to emphasize the relationship between self-conception and cognition, whereas Eastern vocabularies and metaphors tend to emphasize self-conception and emotional harmony issues.[27]

CULTURAL ISSUES OF TIME AND SPACE

Hall identifies time and space as factors of "context"[28] which are universal in all cultures. Hall distinguishes between "monochronic" time and "polychronic" time. In low context cultures, monochronic time is utilized. The individual pays attention to time and does only one thing at a time. Time is used to compartmentalize events, functions, people, communication, and information flow. In high context cultures, polychronic time is utilized. In this paradigm, many things may happen or get attention at the same time. There is more involvement with people and events. People take precedence over time and schedules. Emphasis is placed on completing human interactions.

In low context perception of monochronic time, information flow and communication are restricted. Meetings and communication in low context cultures are used to pass on information and/or determine information in order to evaluate and make decisions. In the high context perception of polychronic time, information flows freely among all participants. Because the information is available to everyone, it is expected that people will use intuition and understand automatically. In high context cultures, meetings are held to reach consensus about what is already known.

Each person has invisible boundaries of personal space or territory, which often infers ownership or power when linked to physical location. Spatial changes influence and give meaning to human interaction, even more so than the spoken word. Spatial cues such as distance between the speaker and listener are perceived by all the senses. Cultures may vary as to which senses are most attuned to spatial cues. For example, appropriate distance between speaker and listener in Anglo cultures is about 2.5 to 3 feet. In Middle Eastern cultures, it is about 2 to 2.5 feet. A popular example of this norm in North American culture is expressed when the speaker expresses annoyance that someone is "in their face". On the other hand, the Middle Eastern speaker may be confused as to why the North American listener keeps moving away from him or her in conversation.

In some cultures, spatial cues may be primarily perceived by vision, in some by hearing, and in some by touch or kinesthetic prompts. Vision, hearing, and kinesthetic cues as part of communication are described in Chapter 8.

For low context, monochronic societies and individuals, personal space is perceived as private, controlled, and often large. For high context, polychronic societies or individuals, space is frequently shared with subordinates and centralized or shared in an information network. Time and space are closely linked because access to individuals is often determined by both location and timing.[22]

HIDDEN DIMENSIONS OR IMPLICIT MEANINGS IN CULTURE

In order to understand the complete or true meanings in intercultural communication, one must understand the multiple hidden dimensions of "unconscious" culture. Hall[28] states that context will largely determine the message that the person receives. In collectivistic, high context communication, the vast majority of the information is already understood, either internalized in the individual or in the physical context of the situation. Only a small amount of the meaning is in the explicit transmission or coding of the message. For example, in high context cultures, the mere presence of an official representative at a meeting, regardless of whether or not something is said by the official, indicates that the meeting is understood to be important by all those present. In contrast, in low context, individualistic communication, the majority of information is in the explicit coding of the message rather than within the individual or the situation (context).

According to Hall,[28] it is up to each person to perform the critical function of correcting for distortions or omissions in the messages they receive. In order to be truly effective in intercultural communication, one must know the degree of information or context that has to be supplied in order to correctly interpret another individual's verbal and nonverbal behavior. The context or the information surrounding the event that gives it meaning will vary from culture to culture, and it is often the critical factor in determining whether individuals from different cultures will communicate effectively with one another. For the Anglo-American health care practitioner working with Native American clients, understanding the context of the situation is critical to effective intercultural communication. For example, Brislin[11] describes the very different cultural interpretations of silence in Native American communication as compared to Anglo-American communication. For the Native American, silence is a culturally acceptable response to ambiguity. For the Anglo-American, small talk is a culturally acceptable response to ambiguity. For the Anglo-American health care provider who does not understand the Native American context of silence, the client's silence may be perceived as disinterest or noncompliance with the health care provider's recommendations.

NONVERBAL COMMUNICATION

Nonverbal communication refers to information exchange (or difficulties in such exchanges) that does not require oral or written forms of language. These include gestures, positioning of the body, and tenseness of the facial expressions (see Chapter 8 on rapport using Neurolinguistic Psychology). Unfortunately, there are few cultural universals except the recognition that all cultures use both verbal and nonverbal means and that people should *avoid drawing any conclusions regarding nonverbal behaviors* without a great deal of knowledge.

Such knowledge involves developing understanding of specific gestures, expressions, and uses of the body, as well as a full grasp of the context of the communication. For example, the distance that people keep from each other is a potent means of nonverbal communication. In the United States, when a man and woman meet each other for the first time, they usually stand about 2.5 to 3 feet apart. If they stand closer, it may be interpreted as a sign of more than casual interest in each other. However, in Latin America, the typical distance people stand from each other while conversing is about 2 feet. This distance does not convey a special message of "desire for more interaction in the future."[28] For health care practitioners working with clients from Latin America, this information is critical to understanding the context of the intercultural communication.

PERSONALISMO

As a new therapist working in Miami, I was initially very surprised to receive invitations to attend celebrations at the homes of the children whom I treated. I was also confused when the parents of the children whom I treated asked me questions regarding my parents, marital status, and my siblings. Fortunately, I was able to ask my colleagues at the preschool, who served as my cultural informants, why the families were so interested in my personal life. They politely informed me that the families wanted to get to know me as a person as well as a professional. I later learned through my research that this is the concept of *personalismo* in the Hispanic culture, and that it is very important in establishing rapport with the families. Once I understood the cultural context of the communication, I felt much more at ease.

SOMATIZATION

Somatization, a behavior more common among Asians, Africans, and Latin Americans than in North Americans, refers to the tendency to report physical symptoms when a person is experiencing psychological distress. The patient does not present any identifiable organic causes for the problem, but experiences symptoms that are real and troublesome. Somatization is seen more frequently in cultures where complaints about anxiety, worries, and depression are perceived as signs of weakness. In many cultures, people have much less tolerance for mental illness than for physical illness. Therefore, the context of the communication must be understood by the professional in order to have effective intercultural communication. For non-Hispanic health professionals, the concepts of "nervios" and "ataques de nervios" may present with symptoms of heart palpitations, sleep disorders and generalized body pains. These somatic symptoms may reflect chronic feelings of stress related to various life challenges.

INTERGENERATIONAL ISSUES

Intergenerational expectations have recently been recognized as impacting communication across the generations. Generational differences have been found between *Traditionalists* (born prior to 1946), *Baby boomers* (born from 1946 to 1964), *Generation X* (born 1965 to 1981), and *Millenials* (born from 1982 to 2000). Each generation has traits that may not be understood by other generations. *Traditionalists* have traits that include loyalty, patriotism, faith in institutions, and fiscal conservatism. They survived the Great Depression, World War II, the Cold War, and the atomic bomb. *Baby boomers* have traits that include questioning authority, competitiveness, and a desire to put their own stamp on things. They witnessed the Vietnam war, Watergate, and human rights movements. They are often caught between raising teenagers and caring for elderly parents and are referred to as the "sandwiched" generation. Those from *Generation X* have traits that include self-reliance, resourcefulness, skepticism, adaptability, and eclectic interests. They were raised with personal computers, AIDS, and MTV. *Millenials* have traits including cyber literacy, realism, environmental consciousness, and global concerns. They witnessed the fall of the Berlin Wall, technological and media expansion, and natural disasters and violence.[29] When working with clients and colleagues from diverse generations, the clinician can recognize the diverse backgrounds and expectations of each generation, and modify his or her communication style to promote optimal intergenerational communication.

SIX UNIVERSAL ASPECTS OF HEALTH CARE IN ALL CULTURES

Scholars[11] have examined interactions between health care professionals and people seeking help in different parts of the world. Professionals include people with advanced degrees in highly industrialized nations as well as native healers, shamans, and herbalists in less industrialized nations. Six universal concepts in the delivery of health care were identified:

1. The health care specialist applies a name to a problem.

2. The qualities of the health care professional are important.[14] The professionals must be perceived by clients to be caring, competent, approachable, and concerned with identifying and finding solutions to the problem. (With minority groups in the United States, professionals must communicate a sense of credibility that they can be of help. In addition, they should be able to offer benefits of some kind as soon as possible. If they do not, the client is not likely to return for an appointment.)

3. The health care specialist must establish credibility through the use of symbols and trappings of status that are familiar in the culture.

4. The health care practitioner places the client's problems in a familiar framework (this implies recognition of the client's explanatory model by the practitioner).

5. The health care practitioner applies a set of techniques meant to bring relief (this implies recognition of the client's explanatory model).

6. Interactions between the clients and the practitioners occur at a special time and place (this implies recognition of the client's explanatory model).

In order to achieve these 6 universal requirements in the intercultural environment, health care professionals must be educated about their own culture as well as the cultures of the clients, families, colleagues, and support staff with whom they work. Many researchers recommend training in cultural sensitivity in order to provide optimal care through application of knowledge of culture and cultural differences. Research has indicated that counselors trained in cultural sensitivity were rated higher in the dimensions of expertise, trustworthiness, ability to show positive regard, and empathy as compared to counselors not trained in cultural sensitivity.[11] There is a difference between the pseudotolerance that results from "putting the lid on" one's intolerance and the genuine tolerance that stems from developing an open, courageous, and loving heart. Intolerance comes from fear. Knowledge and sensitivity training go a long way to quell the fear of what is different to yield true tolerance for and enjoyment of the differences among us. The professional must demonstrate willingness to bring knowledge to interactions with different clients and have the ability to take culture into account when discussing important topics related to alleviating pain and stress.

The 21st century offers health care providers both challenges and opportunities. Ethnocentrism, the belief that one's own culture is the best, will be challenged and people will need to expand their thinking to become tolerant of differences and tolerant of ambiguity. Intercultural researchers will be challenged to provide practical applications from their findings. Researchers will be challenged to develop the best culturally appropriate intervention programs in the areas of health, education, and worker productivity, while addressing ways to reduce stressors related to intercultural interactions. Basic information regarding the benefits and pitfalls of intercultural interactions will be widely discussed just as preventive health behaviors are discussed today.[11]

Opportunities will abound as discussions regarding tolerance, understanding, and mutual enrichment evolve and are disseminated. Women will have increasing choices in their lives and people will analyze the role that culture and cultural differences play in their lives and in the policies of their societies. If health care practitioners put time and effort into understanding cultural influences on their own behavior and the behavior of others, no doubt they will enjoy the challenges and the stimulation that intercultural interactions can bring.[11]

If we adopt the quantum physics paradigm regarding the primacy of relationships and their "fuzziness," we have a new model to assist us in appreciating and valuing our diversity. With our new awareness of, and appreciation for, our relationships to one another, we can introduce unconditional compassion, or love, into our organizations. According to Wheatley,[5] Chopra,[30] and many very wise people from the beginning of time, love in the broadest sense is the most potent source of power that we have available to us. Love, including respect and caring, is most thwarted when we emphasize how different we are from one another. Knowledge and sensitivity to cultural differences will facilitate our therapeutic presence and our sense of oneness with those fellow human beings that are our patients, their families and caregivers, and our health care colleagues. A few exercises follow to help you on your way to greater self-awareness and cultural sensitivity.

REFERENCES

1. Solomon, Greenberg, Pyszczynski. In: Brislin RW, ed. *Understanding Culture's Influence on Bbehavior.* Fort Worth: Harcourt Brace; 1993.
2. Masin HL. *Parental Attitudes Toward Physical Therapy Services at the Debbie School Early Intervention Program.* University of Miami, Department of Pediatrics, Fla, 1991. Unpublished manuscript.
3. Kellogg JB. Forces of change. *Phi Delta Kappan.* 1988;Nov:200-204.
4. Christensen C. Multicultural competencies in early intervention: training professionals for pluralistic society. *Infants and Young Children.* 1992;4(3):49-63.
5. Wheatley MJ. *Leadership and the New Science.* San Francisco, Calif: Berrett-Koehler Publishers; 1994.
6. *Individuals with Disabilities Education Act Amendments of 1991.* Public Law No. 101-119, 105 Statute 587, 1991.
7. Cross T, Bazron B, Dennis K, Isaacs M. *Toward a Culturally Competent System of Care.* Available from CAASP Technical Assistance Center, Georgetown University Child Development Center, 3800 Reservoir Road, NW, Washington DC, 20007, 1989.
8. Sue. In: Brislin RW, ed. *Understanding Culture's Influence on Behavior.* Fort Worth: Harcourt Brace; 1993:359.
9. Anderson P, Fenichel E. *Serving Culturally Diverse Families of Infants and Toddlers With Disabilities.* Available from National Center for Clinical Infant Programs, 733 15th St. NW, Suite 912, Washington, DC, 20005, 1989.
10. Mead M. Cultural problems and technical change in United Nations Educations Scientific and Cultural Organization, Paris, (pp9-10). In: Saunders L, ed. *Cultural Differences and Medical Care.* 1954: 247-248.
11. Brislin RW. *Understanding Culture's Influence on Behavior.* Fort Worth: Harcourt Brace; 1993.
12. APTA. *1994 PT Professional Education Program Fact Sheet.* Available from the Education Division, APTA, 1111 North Fairfax Street, Alexandria, VA, 22314.
13. Dillman DA. *Mail and Telephone Surveys. The Total Design Method.* New York, NY: Wiley Interscience Publication; 1978.
14. Sue, Zane, Draguns. In: Brislin RW, ed. *Understanding Culture's Influence on Behavior.* Fort Worth: Harcourt Brace; 1993:334.
15. Kleinman A. Concepts and a model for the comparison of medical systems as cultural systems. *Soc Sci Med.* 1976;12:85-93.
16. DeSantis L. Health care orientations of Cuban and Haitian immigrant mothers: implications for health care professionals. *Med Anthropol.* 1989;12:69-89.
17. Harwood A, ed. *Ethnicity and Medical Care.* Cambridge: Harvard University Press; 1982.
18. Jackson J. Urban black Americans. In: Harwood A, ed. *Ethnicity and Medical Care.* Cambridge: Harvard University Press; 1982:36-129.
19. Saunders L. *Cultural Differences and Medical Care.* New York, NY: Russell Sage Foundation; 1954.
20. Shilling B, Branan E. *Cross Cultural Counseling: A Guide for Nutrition and Health Counselors.* Available from United States Department of Agriculture and United States Department of Health and Human Services, 1989.
21. Ting-Toomey S. In: Wiesman RL, Koester J, eds. *Intercultural Communication Competence.* Newbury Park, Calif: Sage Publication; 1993.
22. Graham M, Miller D. *The 1995 Annual: Volume 1, Training.* San Diego, Calif: Pfeiffer and Co; 1995.
23. Tirandis HC. In: Graham M, Miller D, eds. *The 1995 Annual: Volume 1, Training.* San Diego, Calif: Pfeiffer and Co; 1995.
24. Turner. In: Brislin RW, ed. *Understanding Culture's Influence on Behavior.* Fort Worth, Tex: Harcourt Brace; 1993:325.
25. Haglund M. New waves—hospitals struggle to meet the challenge of multiculturalism now—and in the next generation. *Hospital.* 1993;May 20.
26. Belenky M, Clinchy B, Goldberg N, Tarul J. 1986. Gilligan, 1982. In: Gilligan, Ward, and Taylor, *Intercultural Communication Competence.* Newbury Park, Calif: Sage Publication; 1993.

27. Wiesman R, Koester J, eds. *Intercultural Communication Competence.* Newbury Park, Calif: Sage Publication; 1993:99.
28. Hall, Hall, & Hall. In: Graham M, Miller D, eds. *The 1995 Annual: Volume 1, training.* San Diego, Calif: Pfeiffer and Co; 1995.
29. Lancaster L, Stillman D. *Bridging generations in today's workplace.* Presented at: Combined Sections Meeting, APTA, Tampa, FL; February 2004.
31. Chopra D. *The Path to Love.* New York: Random House; 1997.

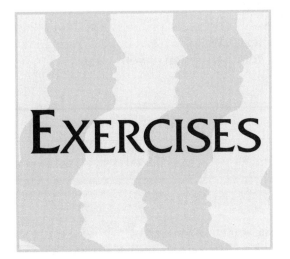

EXERCISES

EXERCISE 1: CULTURE SHOCK ACTIVITY

1. Have you personally experienced culture shock? Write a brief description of what you experienced. What did you see, hear, and feel? What was the context of the situation that shocked you?

2. Ask someone you know and admire if they have ever experienced culture shock. Write a brief description of what they experienced.

3. List similarities and differences in what you and your colleague or friend described.

4. What are the implications of culture shock for individuals of non-North American cultures when they immigrate to your state? What provisions does your state make for immigrants requiring government support?

EXERCISE 2: WHAT IS YOUR CULTURE/ETHNICITY?

1. Would you describe your culture as primarily individualistic (low context) or primarily collectivistic (high context)? Write out 2 examples from your daily life that indicate which context best describes your perception of your culture.

    a.

    b.

2. Describe the culture of someone you know whose culture is different from yours. Write out 2 examples from your observations of that person that validate your perception of that individual's culture as high or low context.

    a.

    b.

3. What did you learn from this activity? What did you take for granted before that has become more apparent through this activity?

4. What implications does this have for your clinical practice? What do you expect will be the nature of your patients' cultural background?

EXERCISE 3: CLINICAL DILEMMA

1. You are a therapist from an Anglo-European background working in an outpatient clinic which serves a primarily Hispanic patient population. You notice that your clients are frequently late for their appointments. Based on your knowledge of high and low context cultural differences, what might be the possible reasons for the lateness?

2. What strategies can you utilize to address these differences?

a. What is the worst thing you can do? Why?

b. What is the wisest thing you can do? Why?

3. What challenges and opportunities are presented to you personally in this situation?

EXERCISE 4: INTERGENERATIONAL DILEMMA

1. You are a physical therapist from the Millenial generation. You are working with a retired male accountant with a sports related injury from the Traditionalist generation. Based on your knowledge of generational expectations, what strategies can you use to increase your therapeutic effectiveness when working with this individual?

   a. How will you address this patient? Will you use formal or informal terms and names?

   b. How will you provide patient education for this patient? Will you suggest Web sites or provide written home programs?

   c. What challenges might you face in communicating effectively with this patient? How will you address those challenges?

2. How would this all change if you were a therapist from Generation X communicating with a person from the Millennial generation?

THE HELPING INTERVIEW

Carol M. Davis, PT, EdD, MS, FAPTA

OBJECTIVES

1. To emphasize the importance of communicating well in the initial stages of the relationship with the patient.
2. To describe the characteristics of a helping interview as compared to a nonhelping interview.
3. To teach the essentials of the helping interview.
4. To learn key points necessary to the successful interview of the adolescent and the patient in their 80s, 90s, or older.
5. To portray the qualities of a helpful interviewer.
6. To provide the opportunity to begin developing and practicing your interviewing skills.
7. To offer the opportunity to practice self-critique and to critique others.

In this chapter we focus on another specific application of communication skill: the art of establishing the relationship with our patients and gleaning from them the information we need to be of most help. First impressions very often count, and the importance of obtaining the patient's trust from the outset of our interaction together is invaluable to the healing process.

Interviewing is much more than obtaining a patient history. The interview serves as the cornerstone for the structure of care we give. Patients come to us worried and often in pain. They feel vulnerable and in need of our help and understanding. They want, often desperately, to put this problem behind them and get on with their lives, and they know they can't do it themselves. They come to us hoping that we will listen carefully, that we will know something about their problem, and that we will be able to help alleviate their worries. They sincerely want to trust that they have made a wise decision in coming to us. Not only do they want physical and psychological comfort, they want another human being to resonate with their distress.[1] All of this emotion, in varying degrees of intensity depending on the patient and the problem, is presented to us upon our initial contact with the patient. Most people will utilize maximum coping skills, however, and few will fully reveal the extent of their feelings about their problem. Most adults will convey varying degrees of ability to remain in control in an environment that appears, at the least, strange and at the worst, hostile.

As health professionals, the burden is on us to recognize that the patient feels at a distinct disadvantage and to reassure and support even those who convey a remarkable sense of confidence and comfort. At this initial meeting, interest, genuineness, acceptance, and positive regard are critical to establishing a healing relationship. And, as we have said before many times, the nature of the relationship we have with our patients is critical to the helping process.

HELPFUL ATTITUDE AND SKILLFUL QUESTIONING

Not only is it important to convey a healing attitude for our patients at the outset in the interview, it is imperative that the patient feel listened to and understood so that all of the information can surface that will lead to the most adequate and complete description of the problem. Thus, pragmatically, effective clinical decision-making depends on skillful interviewing, and skillful interviewing begins with a healing attitude and proceeds with artful questioning. Let's take a closer look at both.

THE HEALING ATTITUDE OF THE INTERVIEW

A good interview depends on appropriate attitude, good timing, and artful phrasing.[2] The nature of the questions and the process of the interview session will flow out of the beliefs that the questioner holds about such things as one's self-esteem, the appropriate nature of one's role in healing, and what patients are like as people. Let's take a look at some ideas, beliefs, and attitudes that facilitate a healing interview.

Positive self-esteem helps one assume a stance of "I'm OK and so are you. Neither of us is perfect, but each of us, I choose to believe, is doing the best we can to move forward in this world, and I want to help you get back to the business of life as soon as possible." This attitude fosters a healthy collegial relationship with the patient and keeps the locus of control within the patient. Likewise, it hinders any tendency on the practitioner's part to lay blame on the patient for behavior that might have contributed to the problem he or she comes to us with.

A helpful belief of the nature of one's role in healing is to assist the person needing help to identify and cope with his or her problems quickly and return to a felling of being in control of one's life as soon as possible.

Patients are simply people who have a problem that they would solve by themselves, if they could, but they need our professional help to identify, clarify the nature and cause of the problem, and to help them solve their problem and get on with living.

Obstacles to Conveying a Healing Attitude

People who have an attitude that facilitates healing are able to accept their patients just as they are without judging them. These practitioners will often have identified and dealt with biases and prejudices about certain behaviors such as alcohol abuse, laziness, smoking, use of profanity, and obesity. They will have reconciled their abhorrence of some behaviors such as rape and murder and are willing to be therapeutically present to people accused of such behaviors. As much as possible, they will be aware of and willing to underplay and/or eliminate deeply held prejudices about race, culture, gender, age, or sexual orientation.

How does all this happen? Obviously not overnight. The paragraph above describes a mature person whose ego is not bound by the fear that emanates from immature judgemental and dualistic thinking. Behavior that is accepting is nonjudgmental or nonblaming in nature. As much as we might abhor a person's behavior, it is helpful to believe that the person would have acted differently if he had more information and had been less impulsive.

Remember from Chapter 2 that many of the immature judgements and prejudices we continue to carry as adults stem from fear that we developed as children from the messages we heard from adults around us. As adults, we must confront the inappropriateness and negativity of these judgements and work to establish more whole, accepting, self-affirming beliefs.

One of the purposes of this text is to assist you in this maturation process by helping you to identify harmful attitudes and behaviors that would interfere with the healing nature of the interview. Practicing our active listening skills and assertiveness skills helps in an interview. True active listening and speaking out of an awareness of your own rights helps one to diminish a tendency to project one's own weaknesses and to minimize a judgmental attitude.

INTERVIEWING ADOLESCENTS

Over 2 million teenagers in the United States have chronic illnesses and disabilities. This is a diverse group, but at this developmental stage, they share some behavioral similarities that are important to understand and be sensitive to during the interview and during treatment.[3] Teenagers are preoccupied with their bodies and with peer acceptance and may be embarrassed by certain questions or feel some questions are trivial or none of the business of the health care provider. "The willingness of a teenager to share personal or intimate information depends on the perceived receptiveness of the provider... It is usually not difficult for patients and providers to discuss routine chronic medical conditions such as diabetes and asthma. Control of these conditions in some teenagers, however, may be related more to dietary indiscretions and marijuana or cigarette consumption, respectively, than to insulin or inhaler use. Such health-compromising behaviors must be identified before they can be dealt with; comments, facial expressions, or body language indicating disapproval can undermine the patient's willingness to disclose confidential behavior."[3] Remember that in Chapter 8, practicing the principles of neurolinguistic psychology will assist you in matching, leading, and pacing the patient to help solidify trust. A nonjudgemental and supportive attitude toward gay, lesbian, bisexual, and transgendered youth can help cushion the stigma they may perceive from family and peers.

Likewise teenagers who are depressed usually suffer from fear of exposure and the stigma of having a "mental illness" and need the support of the provider. Sleep disturbance, decreased appetite, hopelessness, lethargy, continual thoughts about suicide, illogical thoughts, or hallucinations are signs that the patient has an undiagnosed depression and should be referred for medical follow-up immediately, with the support of the parents or guardians. These symptoms, however, with questioning in the interview may be determined to be contextual—that is, there is no energy to do homework, exercise, or house chores, but unlimited energy to attend rock concerts, go to the mall with friends, and party. Likewise, these symptoms may also be secondary to an undiagnosed substance abuse problem, and further follow-up is required.

Reassure adolescents that the information that they provide will be kept confidential unless the threat of harm to the patient or others is revealed. Discussions about sex, their bodies or use of substances should always take place in a private area. If the patient is accompanied by an adult, first solicit appropriate information from the adult, but then request that the adult leave the room for the remainder of the interview.

With regard to compliance with a treatment plan, recognition of a parental problem is important. Teenagers need the support of parents to meet goals set in therapy. Adolescence is a time of testing boundaries. Chronically ill teenagers are often nonadherent with their therapy secondary to a need to be in control and test limits. The struggle for independence clashes with the need to follow a routine to improve or maintain health.[3] Local peer support groups can help, as well as an open and trusting communication with the provider. Emphasize the positive outcomes of adherence to quality of life, and have patients actively participate in developing a realistic treatment program.[3]

Interviewing Older Patients

Patients in their 80s, 90s, and older (the "old-old"—in contrast to the "young-old") are products of a traditional upbringing and respond most positively to certain respectful behaviors that may seem trivial to younger clinicians (see Chapter 9). Often they respond best if the practitioner calls them by their last names, shakes hands warmly, establishes good eye contact, walks with them to the treatment area, and makes "small talk" about family and the weather before starting the interview. Many old-old patients are concerned that any new thing "wrong" with them may spell the initiation of a downward slope toward death, and so they will be looking for reassurance and information about the nature of the illness or disability that is limiting them and will want a realistic perspective about a return to their previous level of function.

Often they suffer from hearing loss but do not appreciate being shouted at or patronized as if they are "stupid." Taking the time to get a thorough interview at the outset will pay off in the long run. Careful questioning about previous illnesses, medications they are currently taking, and comorbid conditions is critical in making an accurate diagnosis and planning an effective treatment. Likewise, a good understanding about support at home is critical to planning an effective treatment.

In sum, interviewing old-old patients simply takes longer, but a thorough interview that establishes trust and rapport is absolutely necessary for a successful treatment and recovery. Some older patients will be very difficult to communicate with, if they have held the identity of victim all their lives, and want you to fix their problems for them. They can be quite demanding, and it is important to set clear limits of what is possible in treatment and what you are willing to do, but also what the patient must do for a successful recovery. Perhaps you will find a certain deep pleasure in getting to know other older patients, for many enjoy a wisdom and humor that can be the high point of your day.

The Interview

Good Timing

With regard to timing, an effective interviewer avoids interruption (which often reveals an underlying harmful attitude of "this person is not very important to me") and listens carefully, effectively using silence. Those who are comfortable with silence will miss much of what a person will say when given a chance to pause and reflect. Time is positively manipulated to indicate a seriousness of attention and level of involvement. A specific amount of time is set to spend, uninterrupted, listening to the patient carefully as he or she tells you the story of the problem.

Artful Phrasing

Artful phrasing, a skill that is learned over time, involves using the right kind of question (open vs closed, direct vs indirect) at the right time; avoiding jargon, slang, and dialect; and tuning one's words and gestures to reassure the patient that he or she is being attended to at a serious and thoughtful level.[2]

Stages of the Interview

There are 3 stages in the interview: initiation, or statement of the purpose of the interview, development or exploration, and closure.

1. The **initiation** of the interview takes place as you, the interviewer, explain who you are, why you are here, and the purpose of the interview.

2. The **body** of the interview is the development or exploration stage. In it the interviewer leads an exploration on the part of the patient, perhaps beginning with the open-ended question, "What brought you here today?" A good interviewer will guide the patient down a meaningful path, assisting the patient to explore his or her problem but not allowing the patient to go too far afield from the problem. Active listening helps the patient to clarify and to zero in on the unique aspects of his or her situation. The interviewer listens carefully and sorts the information, jotting down significant revelations as he or she prepares for the clinical examination. The body of the interview unfolds in a unique story that the patient is invited and encouraged to tell. And the helpful interviewer confirms to the patient that he or she is being carefully and humanely listened to by a skilled and caring practitioner. When moving from one topic to another, it is helpful to use a transition statement. An example would be: "I think I understand the nature of your headaches; is it okay with you to shift now to the pain in your lower back?"

3. The **closing** of the interview takes place at a time that has been predetermined by the interviewer. If it becomes obvious that the interview is not complete, the interviewer doesn't just let the session drop, but says, for example, "We're beginning to run out of time for this session and I realize you haven't yet finished. What needs to be covered yet?" Then a second session is scheduled. Or the interviewer may begin the physical examination and continue discussing the problem with the patient during the exam. I offer a note of caution here, however. To begin the physical examination before allowing the patient to tell as complete a personal story as time allows is a mistake. As an interviewer, you cannot expect to establish a relationship and obtain meaningful information while engaging in palpation and physical evaluation methods. Your brain will attend to what you see and feel before it will attend to what it hears.

BODY OF THE INTERVIEW—INFORMATION GATHERED

The key questions that form the structure of the body of the interview and that set the boundaries for a meaningful story from the patient include the following:

1. What is the patient's reason for seeking health care? Why did she or he come today?

2. What is the patient's perception of the problem? What is it? Why did it begin? What are the consequences of the problem?

3. What impact, if any, does the problem have on the patient's life? How does he or she feel about it? Does it affect work, relationships, and quality of everyday life?

4. What are the characteristics of the problem? When did it begin? Precipitating factors? Where is it located? What is its quality and severity? What alleviates the problem? What makes it worse? What factors are associated with it?

5. What does the patient expect from this visit? What does he or she hope that you will do?

NONVERBAL COMMUNICATION

The nonverbal communication by the interviewer can either facilitate or hinder the quality of the interview. Revisiting Chapter 8 on Neurolinguistic Psychology and Chapter 9 on Cultural Sensitivity, and reviewing nonverbal communication in more depth, will help you develop your use of this important communication skill.

Key nonverbal elements of a helping interview include wise use of space (posture toward each other and at the same eye level, eliminating barriers), time (uninterrupted level of involvement), appropriate posture (leaning in, avoiding rigid posture or slouch or defiant gestures), voice inflection (appropriate speed and volume, warmth, and genuine curiosity conveyed vs flatness or excessive use of "you knows"), elimination of distracting body movements (twitching, shaking foot, tapping pencil), and good eye contact.

THE INTERVIEW—A UNIQUE FORM OF COMMUNICATION

Thus the interview represents a different form of communicating than we've learned growing up in our families and with our friends. The interview is the very first opportunity to convey a professional healing attitude, and it must be learned and practiced in order to develop skill. And behind every word needs to be an attitude of willingness and awareness that will result in congruence. The words and the inner attitude must be in harmony in order for the interview to be therapeutic. The interviewer must feel confident, peaceful, at one with self, and genuinely willing to establish a healing relationship.

MORE ON THE INTERVIEW ATTITUDE—WHAT WE ARE

Alfred Benjamin[4] says:

When interviewing, we are left with what we are. We have no books then, no classroom lessons, and no supporting person at our elbow. We are alone with the individual who has come to seek our help. How can we assist him (or her)? The same basic issues will confront us afresh whenever we face an interviewee for the first time. In summary they are:

1. *Shall we allow ourselves to emerge as genuine human beings, or shall we hide behind our role, position, and authority?*
2. *Shall we really try to listen with all our senses to the interviewee?*
3. *Shall we try to understand with him empathetically and acceptingly?*
4. *Shall we interpret her behavior to her in terms of her frame of reference, our own, or society's?*
5. *Shall we evaluate his thoughts, feelings, and actions and if so, in terms of whose values: his, society's, or ours?*
6. *Shall we support, encourage, urge her on, so that by leaning on us, hopefully she may be able to rely on her own strength one day?*
7. *Shall we question and probe, push and prod, causing him to feel that we are in command and that once all our queries have been answered, we shall provide the solutions he is seeking?*
8. *Shall we guide her in the direction we feel certain is the best for her?*
9. *Shall we reject his... thoughts and feelings, and insist that he become like us, or at least conform to our perception of what he should become?*

These are the central attitudinal questions that underlie every helping interview, and the response to each quite obviously reveals the values that form our attitudes. When you read the above questions carefully, you will see that Benjamin phrases a few to encourage a negative response, as if to have us examine our attitudes very carefully in order to be clear about our helping intentions. The humanistic values (and their subsequent actions) we discussed in previous chapters will lead to developing a healing attitude. Once that attitude is established, skillful and artful questions will become second nature, and the interview will become one more important tool in the practitioner's repertoire of healing behaviors. Automatically you will assume an active listening stance and convey a warm and genuine interest in your patient. Once this practiced routine becomes second nature, less stress will be attached to it, and you will experience great pleasure listening to most of your patients tell their story.

THE NONHELPFUL INTERVIEW

What would a nonhelpful interview look and sound like? Sometimes it is useful for us to explore a concept by describing its opposite. One interpretation of the opposite of a healing interview might go like this:

The clinician enters the treatment area where the patient has been waiting for quite a while. Without looking up from the patient record, or acknowledging the patient in any way, the clinician begins to read the chart, and mumbles, "Mr. Zuck?"

The patient replies, "Yes," and the clinician continues to read.

Clinician: "So, what's wrong with you?"

Patient: "I'm not sure. I hurt my back. I can't work."

Clinician: No response but thinks to herself, "Oh no, another back. This is the third malingerer I have seen today."

Clinician: "Well, take off your shirt and climb up on the table."

She leaves the area and returns 10 minutes later and, without speaking, begins the physical examination.

This, as you can see, is not really an interview at all. No rapport has been established, no active listening done, no meaningful information is gathered. The practitioner values only the information she will get from her physical examination. The patient is reduced to a "thing," another "low back" in a parade of "low backs."

How would you feel if you were the patient? Would you, as many patients do, make excuses for the poor, overworked therapist whom you are grateful has made the time to see you? Or have you decided already that here is a person without manners who will treat you only as a thing, another event in a long and uninteresting day? Would you throw up your hands in frustration and bury your disappointment even one more time, further convinced that no one really cares about your pain, and that you must endure this alone, without the understanding help of another person?

Whatever "treatment" gets accomplished in the above example, it will be of far less quality than it could be had the clinician used helping interview skills.

CONCLUSION

If you have ever been fortunate enough to have observed a master clinician at work, you have seen a person who truly values the interview and devotes the kind of attention to it described in this chapter. The greatest obstacles to consistent use of the helping interview are overwork and burnout. The more we feel over-extended in our day, and the more we feel that we are repeatedly facing unresolvable problems, the more difficult it will be to come outside of ourselves with a therapeutic presence for the interview. Therefore, the very foundation of the helping interview is a commitment to the discipline required to keep a balance in our lives so that we're rested and have good energy to give to our work. Also, we are required to keep a rein on the extent we commit ourselves to the work that must be done, avoiding giving up the right to keep a reasonable pace. People who feel consistently overworked are avoiding the responsibility they have to keep control of the workload and to fight for that right. Each patient we see ideally deserves 200% of our professional ability. It is our responsibility to make sure we have as much of ourselves to give as we can. Chapter 15 will expand on burnout and help you learn to balance your lives so that this ideal is more reachable.

The exercises for this chapter, again, are critical to effective learning. Conducting a useful interview requires maturation, experience, and practice. One of the most efficient ways to correct mistakes and improve style is to review videotapes of yourself interviewing in a role-play and, if possible, with a patient. Maturation and experience lead to quiet self-confidence and relaxation wherein the "third ear" automatically is engaged. Practice in interviewing will help you value and develop the artful balance of scientific discovery with compassionate intuition.

Don't forget to journal about this experience. What did you learn about yourself as an interviewer? What feelings did you have as you received feedback and/or watched yourself on videotape? Does a videotaping experience help you identify with patients even more than simply role-playing? Again, have fun as you learn and grow and mature into the role of the healing professional.

REFERENCES

1. Perlman HH. *Relationship: The Heart of Helping People.* Chicago, Ill: University of Chicago Press; 1974.

2. Enelow AJ, Swisher SN. *Interviewing and Patient Care.* New York, NY: Oxford University Press; 1972.

3. Friedman LS. Adolescents. In Feldman MD, Christensen JF, eds. *Behavioral Medicine in Primary Care.* 2nd ed. New York, NY: Lange Medical Books/McGraw Hill; 2003:88.

4. Benjamin A. *The Helping Interview.* 2nd ed. Boston, Mass: Houghton Mifflin; 1969.

5. Westberg J, Schachner T. *Material From Interviewing Course in Health and Human Values.* Miami, Fla: University of Miami School of Medicine; 1982-1988.

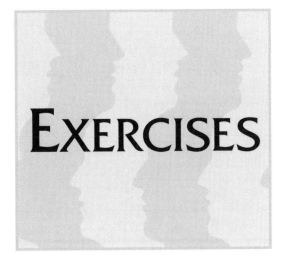

EXERCISES

EXERCISE 1: RESPONDING TO SITUATIONS

Below are situations in which you might likely find yourself as you interact with patients in the clinical setting. These situations are posed to help you explore in advance what you might feel in the situation, what may be underlying concerns in the situation, and what are some specific things you might say or do in a situation like this.

1. You are scheduled to interview Dr. Reynolds and report your findings to your clinical supervisor. Dr. Reynolds has been waiting for you for over an hour, pacing up and down in the waiting area. When you go out to introduce yourself to her, she turns to you angrily and says, "You clinicians don't give a damn about other people's time. Do you realize how long I've been waiting out here?" How might you feel at this moment?

   What might the patient's underlying concerns include?

   What are some specific things you might say or do at this point to try to salvage the interview?

2. You walk into the patient's room, and he is watching television. You introduce yourself, and the patient never even takes his eyes off the TV. He acts as if you are not present in the room. How might you feel?

What might the patient's situation be?

What are some specific things you might say or do in this situation?

3. The person you are interviewing is a street person who has not bathed in a long time. She has a severe body odor and an open sore on her leg that is infested with maggots. As she begins to speak to you, she asks for something to spit her tobacco into. What might you feel?

What might be underlying the patient's behavior?

What might you say and do to insure a helping interview?

4. You begin an interview with Mr. Selker who is 89 years old, with a good, open-ended question, but soon after you begin he begins talking abut his favorite football team. As you try to keep him on track about his problem, he consistently digresses to the topic of football. He is hard of hearing and seems to not understand what you are saying to him. How might you feel?

What may be underlying this patient's behavior?

What might you do to salvage the interview in the given amount of time allotted?

5. You are trying to conduct an interview with a patient, but each time you ask her a question, she looks to her husband and he answers it for her. What might you feel?

What might be underlying this situation?

What are some things you might say or do to get more information from the patient herself?

6. You are interviewing a teenager who has a sports injury. She has had Type 1 diabetes since childhood and indicates she is very tired of having to have insulin injections each day. She feels like an outsider with her friends. She loves playing sports, but it interferes with her insulin regimen and she is feeling pretty hopeless that she will never be accepted as a normal person. She tells you she wants to die. What might you feel?

What might be underlying this situation?

What might you say or do at this point to maintain a helping quality to the interview? (Practice your active listening skills of reflection and clarification. How serious is this wish to die, and has it been followed up by others?)

7. You are interviewing a patient and the patient suddenly leans forward, grabs your arm and says, "You are so attractive. I'd like to see you, you know, have a date with you. How about it?" How might you feel?

What might be underlying the patient's behavior?

What might you say or do to get the interview back on track?

8. You are interviewing an elderly patient who is sitting in a wheelchair. You believe he is able to understand you, but his responses are quite slow and labored. Suddenly you notice a stream of urine running down his leg and onto the floor. He seems not to pay attention to this. What might you feel?

    What decision must you make at this point of the interview?

    What might you say or do to insure that the interview remains helpful in nature? Practice self-transposal. What would you want someone to say to you? To do?

9. You are asked to interview a patient who only speaks Spanish. You cannot elicit meaningful information using rudimentary sign language. No one is close by who could translate for you. What might you feel?

    What decision must you make at this point?

    How can you solicit accurate information and informed consent? Be creative. (Sign language alone is not legally adequate.)

    Can you ethically or legally proceed without informed consent?

EXERCISE 2: VIDEOTAPING AN INTERVIEW

This exercise is offered to help you develop skill in conducting the helping interview and in critiquing your skills and the skills of your classmates. It consists of a role-play of an interview that, ideally, should be videotaped. Divide the class into several small groups, each small group serving as an observation and feedback unit.

The exercise begins with each class member receiving a description of the patient he or she is to portray. This description should include all pertinent personal and illness (symptom) information so that the actor/actress can carry out the role completely. Completion of the *Patient Information Form* is important to this process. Students are to be invited to submit patient descriptions from their experiences, or simply make up a description of a patient's situation. Each student should complete a *Patient Information Form*.

Class members number off, but first divide the class in half. If there are 50 students, number off 1 through 25, then start over and number 1 through 25 again. The two number 1's will interview each other. Each will role-play his or her own patient described on the *Patient Information Form*.

Some rearranging may take place (for example, a female student may prefer to interview another woman, or a man, whichever she feels she needs most practice with), but it is unwise to do much shifting around once the roles with numbers have been drawn.

When videotaping is done in small groups, an instructor should be with each group. The group should meet for as many sessions as it takes for each person to interview for 5 to 8 minutes. At that time the interview may not be over, but the instructor will call for an end.

During the interview, many thoughts and feelings are taking place. During the videotape play-back, the interviewer has control of the pause button and should stop the tape at any point he or she wishes to discuss the action and to review the various options that are available at that moment. The patient is invited to ask for the film to be stopped as well, but the interviewer is in charge of the playback. Once the tape is stopped, the interviewer and the patient are invited to discuss thoughts and feelings, and classmates may feel free to question, emphasizing a noncritical curious attitude.

During the interview, observers are asked to complete the *Reviewer Assessment Form*. After the interview, the patient is asked to complete the *Patient Assessment Form*. During the discussion of the interview, reviewers may add comments on their assessment form. At the end of the entire process, the interviewer completes the *Interviewer's Self-Critique Form*.

The total time for each interview session should take 20 to 30 minutes.

An Alternate Plan

Time and resource constraints may require that the patient and clinician meet outside class and arrange to have their interview videotaped, and then simply bring the tape to class for discussion and feedback. Classmates (reviewers) should have a summary description of the patient before viewing the tape, but, again, the class completes the *Reviewer Assessment Form* as they are watching the tape the first time.

Remember that the most important learning for this exercise grows out of the class discussion, not out of the tape itself. Feedback is best received when it is specific and given with kindness. Insights that contribute to learning are most effective when they are stimulated in a supportive and nonpunitive atmosphere.

You are reminded to journal about the experience. What was it like to play the role of an interviewer in front of a video camera and your classmates? What did you learn about yourself? What behaviors do you intend to develop?

Patient Information Form

Please answer the following questions about the situation, which you will be representing in your role as a simulated patient. This exercise will be most useful if you answer each item as accurately, completely, and authentically as a patient would who actually has the problem.

1. What is your reason for seeking care?

2. Why are you coming in to see the clinician *now*?

3. What other complaints or concerns have you had?

4. What do you think or fear the problem might be?

5. What do you think the consequences of the problem might be?

6. What are your past experiences with this problem?

7. How have your activities of daily living been modified as a result of this problem?

8. What other impact has this problem had on your life?

9. What has been the chronology of events in the development of this problem?

10. What is (are) the location(s) of the symptom(s)?

11. What is (are) quality(ies) of the symptom(s)?

12. What is (are) the quantity(ies) of the symptom(s) (eg, frequency, duration)?

13. What factors have you noted aggravate or alleviate the problem?

14. In what setting does the problem seem to occur (ie, what have you noted seems to precipitate the problem)?

15. What other manifestations or symptoms have you noted that seem to be associated with the problem?

16. What are your expectations of this visit to the therapist?

17. Describe your personal situation and characteristics.

18. What is the state of your underlying health?

19. What has been your past personal and medical history?

(Adapted from Course in Health and Human Values; University of Miami School of Medicine, 1982-1985.)

Reviewer Assessment Form

Circle the appropriate letters. KEY: Y = Yes; N = No; NA = Not Applicable
Note: Where indicated, use space under items to describe and give specific examples of what the Interviewer did.

Your Name:_____

Interviewer's Name:_____

BEGINNING OF THE INTERVIEW

Did he or she:

1. Greet the patient in a friendly, attentive, respectful manner?............................ Y N NA
2. Attend to introductions of himself or herself and the patient, ... Y N NA
   using the patient's name and his or her own name?
3. Define the purpose of the interview?... Y N NA
4. Help the patient get physically comfortable? .... Y N NA

EXPLORING THE PATIENT'S CONCERNS: GATHERING INFORMATION

Did he or she:

5. Use questions appropriately?

   a. Use a "general open-ended approach" to help establish .... Y N NA
      the reason(s) for the patient's visit?

   b. Use a "topic oriented approach" to explore new topics, ... Y N NA
      using specific questions only as needed?
      Give example:

   c. Avoid premature closed questions, which can be answered........................ Y N NA
      "yes" or "no"?

   d. Ask one question at a time? .... Y N NA

   e. Refrain from using leading questions? .... Y N NA
      If used, give example:

6. Nonverbally communicate attentiveness and openness?

   a. With a relaxed, open posture.. Y N NA

   b. With facilitating gestures, like head nodding .... Y N NA

   c. With natural, varied eye contact.. Y N NA
      Describe:

7. Verbally communicate attentiveness and openness?

   a. Using encouraging phrases, like "Please, go on?" .... Y N NA

   b. Repeating key words or feelings? .... Y N NA

   c. "Paraphrasing," reflecting back the essence of what .... Y N NA
      the patient is saying and/or feeling?
      Describe:

8. Remain silent where appropriate?
    a. Give patient an adequate opportunity to ask questions? .... Y N NA
    b. Didn't interrupt patient? .... Y N NA
    Describe:

9. Respond to patient in a warm and sympathetic manner? .... Y N NA
    Describe:

10. Organize interview in orderly fashion?
    a. Proceed from the general to the specific? .... Y N NA
    b. Proceed from the less personal to the more personal? .... Y N NA
    c. In history taking, proceed from present to past history? .... Y N NA
    d. When changing topics, make transitional statements? .... Y N NA
       Describe:

11. Speak clearly, using appropriate language without jargon? .... Y N NA

CLOSING THE INTERVIEW (COMPLETE ONLY IF INTERVIEWER GOT THIS FAR)

Did he or she:

12. Summarize what was said? .... Y N NA

13. Check if there were any further concerns or questions? .... Y N NA

14. Let patient know what will happen next? .... Y N NA

15. Other strategies Interviewer used that facilitated the interview.

16. Other strategies Interviewer used that blocked the interview.

(Adapted from Course in Health and Human Values; University of Miami School of Medicine, 1982-
    1985)

Patient Assessment Form

Name of Patient _____

Name of Interviewer _____

In response to the following, please be as specific as possible.

Behavior that facilitated my ability to communicate (eg, your use of silence which gave me a chance to collect my thoughts).

Behaviors that blocked my ability to communicate (eg, your use of leading questions, like "You don't have a sore throat, do you?").

Information and feelings, if any, that I was unable to share with you.

What I wished you had done or asked me.

(Adapted from Course on Health and Human Values; University of Miami School of Medicine, 1982-1985.)

Interviewer's Self-Critique Form

Circle the appropriate letters. KEY: Y =Yes; N = No; NA = Not Applicable
Note: Where indicated, use space under items and on back of document to describe and give specific examples of what you did.

Name:_____ Date:_____

BEGINNING OF THE INTERVIEW

Did I:
1. Greet the patient in a friendly, attentive, respectful manner?........................... Y N NA
2. Attend to introductions of myself and the patient, using.................................. Y N NA
   the patient's name and my own name?
3. Define the purpose of the interview?... Y N NA
4. Identify and reflect on my initial impressions of the patient? .... Y N NA

EXPLORING THE PATIENT'S CONCERNS: GATHERING INFORMATION

Did I:
5. Use questions appropriately?
   a. Use a "general open-ended approach" to help establish the.......................... Y N NA
      reason(s) for the patient's visit?
   b. Use a "topic oriented approach" to explore new topics, ... Y N NA
      using specific questions only as needed?
   c. Avoid premature closed questions which, can be answered.......................... Y N NA
      "yes" or "no"?
   d. Ask one question at a time? .... Y N NA
   e. Refrain from using leading questions? .... Y N NA
      If used, give example of leading questions to avoid in future:

6. *Nonverbally* communicate attentiveness and openness?
   a. With a relaxed, open posture? .... Y N NA
   b. With facilitating gestures, like nodding my head?...................................... Y N NA
   c. With natural, varied eye contact?... Y N NA
      Describe how use of nonverbals felt during interview:

7. *Verbally* communicate attentiveness and openness?... Y N NA
8. Remain silent, where appropriate?
   a. Give patient an adequate opportunity to respond to questions..................... Y N NA
   b. Didn't interrupt patient... Y N NA
      Describe positives and negatives of verbal communication:

9. Reflect on my own feelings and attitudes toward the patient?........................... Y N NA
   Describe:

10. Organize interview in an orderly fashion?
    a. Proceed from the general to the specific? .... Y N NA
    b. Proceed from the less personal to the more personal? .... Y N NA
    c. In history taking, proceed from present to past history? .... Y N NA
    d. When changing topics, make transitional statements? .... Y N NA
       Describe:

11. Speak clearly, using appropriate language without jargon? .... Y N NA

CLOSING THE INTERVIEW (COMPLETE ONLY IF YOU GOT THIS FAR)

Did I:

12. Summarize what was said? .... Y N NA

13. Check if there were any further concerns or questions? .... Y N NA

14. Let patient know what will happen next? .... Y N NA

15. Other strategies I used that *facilitated* the interview.

16. Other strategies that *blocked* the interview.

(Adapted from Course on Health and Human Values; University of Miami School of Medicine, 1982-1985.)

HEALTH BEHAVIOR AND EFFECTIVE PATIENT EDUCATION

Kathleen A. Curtis, PT, PhD

OBJECTIVES

1. To define health behavior and health literacy.
2. To illustrate how the concept of responsibility makes its way into the messages we give patients by way of examining Brickman's 4 models of helping and coping.
3. To present various health behavior theories so that we can better understand why patients sometimes act in ways that go against preserving their health.
4. To examine the influence of language and culture on health-related communications.
5. To teach principles of effective patient education.
6. To offer instructional planning guidelines when preparing patient and family education materials.
7. To teach instructional tips when working with groups.

The health care provider entered a note in the patient's medical record. An excerpt:

> The patient returns for follow-up today with essentially no change in his condition... questionable compliance with the prescribed treatment program. Plan: Review importance of continuing *daily medication.*

What happened?

The patient forgot, didn't have time, didn't have the money, didn't want to? It was too much trouble, too complicated, didn't meet his or her needs, couldn't fit it in with his lifestyle, didn't understand, doesn't speak English, has too many children, lost the instructions, felt it was just not that important!

Most health professionals would find one of these reasons to explain the patient's noncompliance with the treatment program. The reasons may be valid, but the patient's inability or choice not to follow through with the provider's instructions may result in serious illness, disability, or even death. If practitioners really want to influence patient behavior, they must understand health behavior and health literacy.

WHAT IS HEALTH BEHAVIOR?

Health behavior is a series of actions we take to maintain, promote, or improve our well-being. This might include getting immunizations, making regular dental visits, having an annual mammogram or Pap smear, using condoms during sexual activity, or starting a regular exercise program.

What health behaviors do you practice regularly? List at least one in each of the following categories:

❖ Screening examinations
❖ Health promotion activities
❖ Treatment of acute or chronic illnesses

WHAT IS HEALTH LITERACY?

Millions of adults have difficulty following self-care instructions due to limited health vocabulary and poor understanding of information and concepts. *Health literacy* is the patient's ability to read and understand all types of health-related materials. One of the first studies in this field documented that 1 in 3 English-speaking and 1 in 2 Spanish-speaking patients at public hospitals had marginal health literacy.[1] Individuals with health literacy problems lack sufficient health background knowledge and often have difficulty reading and understanding labels, appointment slips, and instructions for taking medications. In an era where cost containment has reduced the availability of follow-up services, this presents an ever-present danger to this population and raises the question of responsibility for one's well-being, the patient, or the provider.

WHO'S RESPONSIBLE... IN SICKNESS AND IN HEALTH?

If you are like most people, you are very likely to seek a physician's assistance when you have a painful problem. Imagine yourself visiting your physician for diagnosis and treatment of a minor but very irritating and painful skin infection. Your skin is cultured and you are given a prescription medication to put on your skin every day and an oral medication to take by mouth for 10 days. After 4 or 5 days, the lesion clears up and you discontinue your oral medication. A resistant strain of the same organism then shows up in the same location 2 weeks later. Your physician tells you that you will now have to undergo a complicated, prolonged course of treatment that is riskier to you and those around you. In addition, you will not be allowed to work at your job in the hospital due to the possibility of spreading this infection to immune-compromised patients.

WHO IS RESPONSIBLE NOW?

If the patient doesn't do what he or she is told to do, is it the provider's fault? Most providers would say NO! Do you believe the patient is responsible for the above situation? How would you feel as the patient in the above case?

Our beliefs about the patient's responsibility influence how willing we are to help our patients. Brickman's 4 models of helping and coping provide a framework for understanding how the concept of responsibility ties into the messages we give to patients in many patient education situations[2] (Table 11-1).

Table 11-1

BRICKMAN'S MODELS OF HELPING AND COPING APPLIED TO PATIENT EDUCATION

Provider's Perceptions of Patient Responsibility	*Responsible for Causing Problem*	*Not Responsible for Causing Problem*
Reponsible for Solution	**Moral Model** Patient admonished for causing problem. Patient education of high value but probably less likely to provide it.	**Compensatory Model** Provider has sympathy for patient's problems. Patient education highly valued. Provider highly motivated to provide it.
Not Responsible for Solution	**Enlightenment Model** Patient education of less value. Patient likely to be problem. Provider will be responsible for solution which minimizes need for patient education.	**Medical Model** Patient education of less value. Provider has been admonished for causing sympathy for patient. Provider will be responsible for solution, which minimizes need for patient education.

Adapted from Kahan M. *Physician assistants' models of helping behavior and their relationship to perceived responsibility, attributions and patient education.* University of California Los Angeles, Unpublished manuscript, 1988.

These 4 models vary in provider perceptions of the patient's responsibility for causing the problem and for taking action to solve the problem. Here are the rules:

1. If providers believe that patients are **not** responsible for *causing* their problems, they are *more willing to help* (Medical and Compensatory Models).

2. If providers believe that the patients **are** responsible for *causing* their problems, they are *less willing to help* (Enlightenment and Moral Models). If patients see themselves as **not** responsible for their problem and providers sees them **as** responsible for the problems, conflict may result. Patients may be angry and resentful of the providers' assigning blame to them.

3. If providers see patients as **not** responsible *for the solutions* to their problems (such as the treatment), they are likely to take most of the responsibility for patients and therefore do less patient education (Medical and Enlightenment Models).

4. If providers see patients **as** responsible *for the solutions* to their problems, they are likely to involve the patient in solving the problem and then hold the patient responsible (Compensatory and Moral Models).

Put yourself in the provider's shoes. What are your feelings about your patient's problems in this case? Who is responsible? If your provider holds you responsible for the solution, he or she may consider you unreliable and feel that his or her efforts have been wasted and are likely unappreciated, even though he or she may feel some sense of obligation to provide further treatment.

Table 11-1 may help to explain the relationship of the provider's perceptions of responsibility to their willingness to help. As you can see, only one set of conditions (Compensatory Model) exists where the provider is highly motivated to help and the patient is seen as responsible for participating in the solution to the problem.[3]

Some of you who are reading have already begun worrying about your health. Consider your perceptions about your own illnesses or problems. Then consider, would most patients see themselves as *causing* their obesity, their hypertension, their HIV infection? Do you think your health care providers hold the same perceptions of your responsibility for these health problems? It would be interesting to find out because the answer to this question has everything to do with the way patients are treated and cared for.

In designing effective patient education approaches, it is essential that we understand what influences health behavior. Researchers have published widely on this area for the past 50 years and still there are many questions. There are, however, several key schools of thought that can help health care practitioners to feel more informed about how to proceed with their patients.

HEALTH BEHAVIOR THEORIES

Health Belief Model

Perhaps the most influential theory of health behavior is the health belief model. This model explains why people fail to participate in programs or behaviors that prevent or detect disease.[4] For example, when the evidence is clear that smoking is harmful to one's health, why would a young person begin to smoke? Why would a health professional, fully aware of the risks and diseases associated with smoking, continue to smoke?

The health belief model proposes that the likelihood of an individual doing something to protect against a health threat is related to their perceptions in four areas:

- ❖ *Susceptibility to the health threat?* (ie, How likely is it that I will have this problem?)
- ❖ *Severity of the health threat?* (ie, How serious is this problem?)
- ❖ *Benefits of the recommended behavior?* (ie, What will I gain by doing this?)
- ❖ *Barriers or costs of the recommended behavior?* (ie, What are the obstacles that stand in my way or the costs to me of taking this action?)

Essentially, what this model proposes is that a person's action has little to do with the types of messages received or the validity of the information communicated and received. Thus, a person could simultaneously hold the belief that smoking is a potentially harmful behavior and because of conflicting beliefs, such as "My grandfather smoked for 55 years and died when he was 80," or "I will gain weight if I attempt to quit," this person will not take the essential action to reduce the health threat he or she may cognitively recognize.

Locus of Control

Another widely accepted theoretical approach uses the concept of *locus of control*, which refers to our perceptions that the outcomes and rewards we experience are either under our control or out of our control.[5] Remember that we first confronted this theory in Chapter 7 on Assertiveness. Individuals with an *internal locus of control* generally believe that their personal actions and choices have a direct bearing on the outcomes they experience. In contrast, individuals with an *external locus of control* feel that events are caused by fate, powerful others, or other factors out of their control. This orientation has significance in information-seeking behavior, as individuals with an internal locus of control are more likely to seek information about their health problems and choices. Some studies have reported that individuals with an internal locus of control experience more favorable health outcomes than matched subjects with an external locus of control.[6] On the other hand, an external locus of control may work very well for some individuals who prefer to "follow directions of an expert."

Health professionals who are offering educational interventions for their patients or clients need to keep in mind that individuals may not only vary in beliefs regarding the problem and ease of solving the problem (*health belief model*, see above), but they may also vary in the degree to which they believe that their choices and actions will influence the outcomes they experience.

In an interesting study done at the Royal Free Hospital in London, physical therapists sent a letter designed to increase perceived control to 39 first-time patients with a variety of disabilities

May 12, 2005

Royal Free Hospital
222 Hospital Road
Anytown, USA 12345

Dear Sir/Madam:

This is to let you know that you are now being offered physiotherapy at the Royal Free Hospital to help you to overcome your particular health problem. By concentrating on your difficulties, you will be shown how you can control your symptoms and problems as quickly and as effectively as possible.

You may be offered advice and instructions about your symptoms or problems and given a home program. It will be up to you to follow these if you want to recover quickly.

Experience has shown that the more effort you can put in, the more quickly results will be achieved. The therapists are there to help you to resolve your problems.

You may find it helpful to enlist friends and relatives to help you to follow any home program you are given. May we wish you a speedy recovery.

Sincerely,
Royal Free Hospital

Figure 11-1. Written message that increased patient perceived control and satisfaction. (Adapted from Johnston M, Gilbert P, Partridge C, Coolins J. Changing perceived control in patients with physical disabilities: an intervention study with patients receiving rehabilitation. *Br J Clin Psychol.* 1992; 31: 89-94.)

who were scheduled for outpatient physical therapy services. The patients who received the letter reported significantly higher levels of perceived control and were more satisfied with information than the control group who only received a letter about their appointment time.[7] The simple letter in Figure 11-1 illustrates an effective means to influence patient perceptions of locus of control.

Self-Efficacy

Another perspective in understanding health behavior comes from social learning theory.[8] Self-efficacy is an individual's sense that he or she can successfully carry out a particular health behavior needed to result in a desired outcome. Self-efficacy is influenced by one's own past experiences, observations of the experiences of influential others, and valued verbal and emotional support of others.[9] This has tremendous implications for patient education in that we can promote the use of peer counselors who can model the desired behavior in addition to providing emotional support.

Health Promotion Model

Pender[10] built upon some of these ideas and identified modifying factors (demographic, biologic characteristics, interpersonal influences, situational, and behavioral factors) that may influence perceptions of self-efficacy, health status, perceived benefits, and barriers. This model also incorporates internal and external cues to action which further increase the likelihood of our engaging in health promoting behaviors. Educational messages may serve as external cues to influence an individual to continue a behavior. For example, the use of internal cues such as "I feel much better when I exercise," or external cues such as "heart healthy symbols" on a restaurant menu or health information on the evening news increase the likelihood of our continuing these beneficial behaviors.

Trans-Theoretical Model

The trans-theoretical model describes stages that individuals progress through as they change health behaviors.[11] The model includes 5 stages: precontemplation, contemplation, preparation, action, and maintenance, which allow for a nonlinear or even cyclical progression through the 5 stages before sustained behavior change can occur. This model is particularly helpful in understanding change such as starting an exercise routine or stopping smoking. With this orientation to patient education, a practitioner would be aware of the activities that would support the patient in various stages of the change process.[12,13]

Let's look at how this applies.

> Jeanette, a health care professions student feels, that she should begin an exercise program after a class on cardiovascular risk factors. She visits her physician to have her cholesterol checked. She looks through American Heart Association literature, reviews the American College of Sports Medicine Guidelines, and scores over 90% on her class test on the material 2 weeks later. Her friends talk about stopping at the gym almost daily. And she has yet to go with them.

One of the main messages that this model proposes is that if education is introduced when someone is in a precontemplative phase, it won't result in a behavior change. This model is very important when considering the implementation of programs for major changes in life habits, smoking cessation, weight loss, and exercise programs. Practitioners must emphasize readiness and give the patient responsibility and control. Also important to keep in mind when using this orientation is that health behavior may be cyclical and therefore we could expect to see progress and setbacks, and periods of high and low compliance. Tolerance of those ups and downs with a general commitment to "get back on track" seems to be the key to incorporating the health behavior in one's life on a regular basis (Table 11-2).

WHICH APPROACH TO TAKE?

Given the variety of approaches that health behavior theorists have taken to explain why patients choose or don't choose to take recommended action, the practitioner has quite a few things to consider. How can we incorporate this information into good patient education?

PRINCIPLES OF EFFECTIVE PATIENT EDUCATION

Patient education skills are just as critical to our success as the discipline-specific skills and activities that we learn as part of our professional training. They take practice and development. Just as not all patient care skills are applicable to all patients, not all patient education skills are applicable either, but, in general, the following will help to positively influence patient behavior:

1. Build rapport with the patient. This is essential for all other aspects of the process.
2. Communicate clearly and effectively. Focus on the message you want to send.
3. Evaluate the patient's readiness to learn or intention for behavior change.
4. Assess the patient's language skills, beliefs, cultural background, environment, coping skills, and abilities that will help or hinder the change process.
5. Customize your approach to the patient, their readiness and associated needs.
6. Assess barriers (cognitive, emotional, physical, social, or support systems) to carrying out recommendations.

| Table 11-2 |

THE TRANSTHEORETICAL MODEL AND IMPLICATIONS FOR PATIENT EDUCATION

Stage	Patient Readiness for Change	Implications for Patient Education
Precontemplation	Not intending to change	Help client identify personal priorities and lifestyle goals. Establish trust and rapport to eventually provide insight into negative risk behaviors.
Contemplation	Intend to change within 6 months	Provide motivational messages of pros and cons of risk behavior. Tie into goals. Support decision-making and help clients evaluate pros and cons of the behavioral change.
Preparation	Actively planning to change in next 30 days	Seek commitment to risk behavior change and starting date. Support decision to take action with discussion of resources and coping skills.
Action	Has initiated change within the past 6 months	Support behavioral change and adaptive replacement of risk behaviors with new lifestyle practices. Provide information about social and medical resources that facilitate change. Teach self-management strategies to prevent relapse.
Maintenance	Has successfully modified behavior for more than 6 months	Prevent relapse and encourage long-term change. Review skills for managing situations that can trigger relapse to previous behaviors. Reinforce new lifestyle habits and achievement of goals.

Adapted from Basler HD. Patient education with reference to the process of behavioral change. *Patient Education and Counseling.* 1995;26:93-98; and Nolan RP. How can we help patients to initiate change? *Can J Cardiol.* 1995;11(SuppA):16a-19a.

7. Problem solve with patients to generate solutions to apparent problems and concerns.

8. Use appropriate teaching resources (videos, web-based resources, written materials, peer support, other health professionals) to facilitate the learning process.

Notice that the above list does not include giving the patient a poorly-visible photocopy of something you found in the files, or even a computer-generated, custom-made list of exercises. Understanding the *process* of behavior change is the key to effective patient education. Once you have assessed that the patient is ready, willing, and able to make the recommended change, then there is sufficient time to introduce the appropriate instructional materials as reinforcements of the change process. Now, how can you deliver your message in the most effective manner?

INSTRUCTIONAL PLANNING GUIDELINES

Let's look at some ideas used by leading instructional designers. The key elements of any instructional sequence answer the following questions:

1. What is the problem and what are the patient's (learner's) goals?
2. What is the learner's state of readiness for the recommended action?
3. What do you want the learner to know, feel, or do? When? How often? Where? With whom?
4. What is the key content that must be presented to accomplish these outcomes?
5. What learning experiences will help to transmit this content, teach these skills?
6. What key steps, decisions, and activities must the learner do to follow recommendations?
7. What materials can review, supplement, or draw attention to the content or process?
8. How will you know that you've been successful in teaching? How can you evaluate that the learner has learned what you were trying to teach?

Try this exercise as an example. Consider our original problem:

> Our patient has returned seeking treatment for a recurrent skin infection. The patient has already failed to take medication consistently on one occasion. The patient must now undergo a complicated, prolonged course of antibiotic treatment using medications with high potential for toxicity and will not be allowed to work in the hospital due to the possibility of spreading this antibiotic-resistant infection.

Put yourself in the role of the practitioner (physician) in this case:
1. What is the problem and the patient's (learner's) goals?
2. What is the learner's state of readiness for the recommended action?
3. What do you want the learner to know, feel, or do? When? How often? Where? With whom?
4. What is the key content that must be presented to accomplish these outcomes?
5. What learning experiences will help to transmit this content, teach these skills?
6. What key steps, decisions, and activities must the learner do to follow recommendations?
7. What materials can review, supplement, or draw attention to the content or process?
8. How will you know that you've been successful in teaching? How can you evaluate that the learner has learned what you were trying to teach?

PRESENTATION TIPS

Whether you are teaching one-on-one or in a group situation, you may find it useful to incorporate the following ideas in your presentation.

❖ Present the most important content first. (*First, I am going to teach you how to get out of bed.*)

❖ Be brief and emphasize the main point. (*Bend forward as you begin to stand up.*)

❖ Organize the information into topics, clusters, or categories. (*There are three steps to this process.*)

❖ Give specific instructions. (*Test your blood sugar 1 hour prior to meals.*)

❖ Repeat important information in a variety of ways. (*You can see it again here—you have to bend your knees not your back.*)

❖ Present at the comprehension level of the learner. (*We'll review some anatomy terms first before we get into the specifics of the technique.*)

CULTURAL AND LANGUAGE FACTORS IN PATIENT EDUCATION

The Institute of Medicine (IOM), in its 2002 publication, *Unequal Treatment: Confronting Racial and Ethnic Disparities in Health Care*, reported that regardless of a patient's insurance status or income, individuals from racial and ethnic minority groups tend to receive a lower quality of health care than do members of nonminority groups. The study documented that stereotyping, biases, and uncertainty on the part of health care providers all contribute to unequal treatment.[14]

A failure to recognize the influence of language or culture can easily lead to undesirable health outcomes. The IOM report documented numerous examples of poor outcomes related to language barriers and cultural misunderstandings.

For example, findings indicate that patients with limited English proficiency (LEP) are less likely to visit physicians and receive preventive services, regardless of economic status, source of care, literacy, health status, or insurance status.[14] Patients with LEP also report lower rates of satisfaction with their care. Researchers have found that patients who did not speak the same language as their provider were more likely to miss appointments or drop out of treatment. Findings indicate that using interpreters seems to eliminate the likelihood of missed appointments.[14]

The 2001 National Standards for Culturally and Linguistically Appropriate Services in Health Care (CLAS) mandate that health care organizations "ensure that patients/consumers receive from all staff members effective, understandable, and respectful care that is provided in a manner compatible with their cultural health beliefs and practices and preferred language, including access to interpreter services."[15]

Communicating With the Non-English Speaking Patient

Develop sensitivity to verbal and nonverbal language, speech patterns, and communication styles. Incorporate sensitivity to the potential influence of psychological, social, biological, physiological, cultural, political, spiritual, and environmental aspects of the patient or client's experience.

Services for the non-English speaking patient should include informing them that they have the right to receive no-cost interpreter services. Signs and commonly used written patient education materials should be translated for the predominant language groups in a service area.

Try to use the patient/client's preferred language whenever possible. Use interpreters as needed when bilingual clinicians are not available. Interpreters and bilingual staff should have bilingual proficiency and be trained in interpreting. They should have knowledge in both languages of the terms and concepts needed in the clinical encounter. Family members are not considered suitable substitutes for trained interpreters, as they usually lack these skills and knowledge. Avoid using a patient's children or grandchildren as interpreters.

INSTRUCTIONAL TECHNIQUES FOR WORKING WITH GROUPS

Patient education can be done in a group setting as well. There are a variety of instructional techniques that you can use to engage the learner in the learning process.

Lecture

We have all experienced lecture in our formal education. It is most useful when the leader wants to transmit information that the participants do not have.

Lectures are best when they are :
1. SHORT (less than 5 minutes of monologue at a time!)
2. SIMPLE (building on what participants know)
3. VISUALLY INTERESTING (so participants can see concepts and ideas)
4. PARTICIPATIVE (involving participants via questions)

A mini-lecture is helpful to introduce the topic and provide a brief description of the problem and important background material. Participants should be involved as soon as possible to maintain their interest and attention.

Questions

The leader can insert questions in the lecture to stimulate and involve the participants. Asking for agreement/disagreement or for common experiences of participants is an easy way to begin. ("How many of you have experienced this?" or "Does this sound familiar? I see a few of you nodding your heads.")

Demonstration

Lecture can often be enhanced with demonstration of skills or techniques. Demonstration is best followed by practice and a return demonstration. When demonstrating, the leader should be sure that participants can see the demonstration. The leader should take care to illustrate and identify the key points of the demonstrated skill.

Discussion

Discussion provides for participant sharing of knowledge, experience, and skills on the subject. Holding a discussion helps the leader to take advantage of the combined background that the group brings. Discussion is a valuable method to generate many ideas and give participants new approaches to a common problem.

The leader may have several purposes in using a discussion as an instructional method:
1. To gather information. The leader may ask a question ("What are some common causes of back injury?") and get answers from various group members. This way the leader finds out what the group feels and knows and also gets participants involved. If the group does not generate any answers (after a long wait), the leader can contribute, "How about this...? Do you have some additional ideas?"
2. To share experiences. The leader facilitates participants sharing attitudes, experiences, insights. Questions must be focused to keep participants on track. A good opening question starts with an appeal to the individual's experience, "What have you found helpful....?" or "What would you do if...?" Ask open-ended questions.

EXPERIENTIAL TECHNIQUES

This term applies to a variety of techniques that allow learners to experience what you want to teach, rather than just studying or talking about it. Learning occurs via the reactions and emotions participants experience while they participate in the exercise. The leader has a key role in helping participants to analyze their experience and relate it to the objectives of the learning experience.

Role-Play

Role-playing is helpful to provide an opportunity to practice a new process or skill and illustrate different perspectives which one takes on in a "role." It is not "play-acting," as it is intended to simulate reality. Role-playing provides a realistic look at the learner's behavior, emotions, and experience in a "real" situation.

Role-playing is most successful when learners are given a loosely defined situation, a role to play, and attitude or position to take. The role-play should be followed up with a discussion by participants and observer(s). This discussion should help to relate the experience to the skills, concepts, or ideas that it was intended to illustrate and support.

Simulations

Simulations are carefully structured learning activities that assist participants to explore their group working relationships and responses to a variety of situations. The value of using simulations is that if a mistake is made, no one is hurt. Games and simulations must have contingencies built-in for the decisions and actions that participants take. For instance, if a participant makes a decision to proceed with a particular action, there must be feedback that indicates the consequence of that choice. Therefore, the rules and results must be carefully defined.[16]

USE OF TECHNOLOGY IN PATIENT EDUCATION

With the explosion of computer use and web-based information resources, many consumers turn to the Internet for health information. Recent evidence shows that web-based interventions may be effective as a health information delivery system, especially for those with chronic conditions that can be self-managed and for those who lack health care access.[17] Although optimal Web site design goes beyond the scope of this chapter, the principles outlined in this chapter apply to Web-based information. Be aware that health literacy seriously impacts understanding of materials online as well.

EVALUATING WRITTEN MATERIALS

Written materials are important adjuncts to the patient education process. They should be selected or written specifically for the population with whom you are working or the goals of the intervention. Start to collect samples of good patient education materials when you see them.

Your target audience should be able to read and understand the written materials you choose. Be sensitive to technical terms, long sentences, and complex ideas. Watch the use of jargon and translation of medical language to lay terms. Materials should be written at a 6th to 8th grade reading level to reach the most people. Examine the Flesch formula and the Gunning Fog Index for evaluating the reading level of written materials (Tables 11-3 to 11-5).

PUTTING IT ALL TOGETHER

Practitioners who educate patients join in a powerful partnership to achieve goals that each separately could not realize. Through understanding factors that influence attention, readiness for change, motivation, and principles of instructional design and presentation, we are better able to design effective patient education interventions.

REFERENCES

1. Williams MV, Parker RM, Baker DW, Parikh NS, Pitkin K, Coates WC, Nurss JR. Inadequate functional health literacy among patients at two public hospitals. *JAMA*. 1995 Dec 6;274(21):1677-82.
2. Brickman P, Rabinowitz VC, Karuza J, Coates D, Cohn E., Kidder L. Models of helping and coping. *Amer Psychol*. 1982;37:368-384.
3. Kahan M. *Physician Assistants' Models of Helping Behavior and Their Relationship to Perceived Responsibility, Attributions and Patient Education*. University of California Los Angeles, Unpublished manuscript, 1988.
4. Rotter JB. Generalized expectancies for internal versus external control of reinforcement. *Psychology Monographs*. 1966;80:1-28

Table 11-3

THE FLESCH FORMULA

1. For short pieces, test the entire selection. For longer pieces, test at least 3 randomly selected samples of 100 words each. Do not use introductory paragraphs as part of the sample. Start each sample at the beginning of a paragraph.

2. Determine the average sentence length (SL) by counting the number of words in the sample and dividing by the number of sentences. Count as a sentence each independent unit of thought that is grammatically independent, that is, if its end is punctuated by a period, question mark, exclamation point, semicolon, or colon. In dialogue, count speech tags (eg, "he said") as part of the quoted sentence.

3. Determine the word length (WL) by counting all the syllables in the sample as if reading the words aloud. Divide the syllables by the number of words in the sample and multiply by 100.

4. These indices are then applied to the formula to compute the reading ease:
(RE=206.835~1.015 SL-0.846 WL).

   Where RE is the reading ease score, SL is the average sentence length in words, and WL is the average word length measured as syllables per 100 words.

Interpretation of the Flesch Reading Ease Score

Reading ease	Grade	Description of style	No. syllables/ 100 words	Average sentence length
90 to 100	5	Very easy	123	8
80 to 90	6	Easy	131	11
70 to 80	7	Fairly easy	139	14
60 to 70	8-9	Standard	147	17
50 to 60	10-12	Fairly difficult	155	21
30 to 50	College	Difficult	167	25
0 to 30	College graduate	Very difficult	192	29

Adapted from Flesch R. *The Art of Readable Writing*. New York: Harper & Row; 1974:184-186, 247-251.

Table 11-4

THE GUNNING FOG INDEX SCALE

1. Select a sample of writing 100 to 125 words long. If the piece is long, take several samples and average the results.

2. Calculate the average number of words per sentence. Treat independent clauses as separate sentences, "In school we studied: we learned: we improved" counts as three sentences.

3. Count the number of words of 3 syllables or more. In your count, omit capitalized words; combinations of short words like bookkeeper or manpower or verbs made into 3 syllables by adding "-es" or "-ed." Divide the count of long words by the passage length to get the percentage.

4. Add 2 (average sentence length) and 3 (percentage of long words). Multiply the sum by the factor 0.4, and ignore the digits following the decimal point. The result is the years of schooling needed to read the passage with ease. Few readers have over 17 years of schooling, so any passage over 17 gets a Fog Index of "17-plus."

Adapted from Gunning R, Kallan R. *How to Take the Fog Out of Business Writing*. Chicago, Ill: Dartnell Books; 1994.
The Fog Index[sm] Scale is a service mark licensed exclusively to RK Communication Consultants by D. and M. Mueller.

Table 11-5

SAMPLE PATIENT EDUCATION MATERIALS WRITTEN AT DIFFERENT GRADE LEVELS

Written at the Thirteenth Grade Level...

The heart usually receives electrical signals from the sinoatrial node, an area in the top right chamber. In ventricular tachycardia the signals that orchestrate the rhythm originate in the ventricle, located below the atrium. This area of origin results in an erratic beat or rhythm. The erratic beat disables the ventricles from contracting, thus blood is unable to be pumped out adequately. Inadequate blood supply affects all body parts since oxygen and nutrients are located in the blood. When the brain does not receive adequate blood supply, symptoms that include fainting, dizziness, and unconsciousness can occur. Stroke and death are also potential results.

With the knowledge that ventricular tachycardia is an erratic and potentially fatal rhythm that can occur at unpredictable times, physicians usually prescribe medications to control or prevent that rhythm. When medications are unable to keep the erratic beat dormant, the heart may require defibrillation. Defibrillation resets the electrical circuit, allowing the sinoatrial node to once again dominate.

Rewritten at the Sixth Grade Level...

Electrical signals from the heart's pacemaker keep the heart beating in a normal way. The pacemaker is called the S-A node and is found in the top part of the heart. Signals can also come from the bottom part of the heart. If they come from the bottom part, an irregular or rapid beat results. Several rapid and irregular beats are called V Tach. V Tach means the heart is not able to pump blood. When this happens, the body is not able to get the blood it needs. Blood carries oxygen and food to the body. One of the body parts that needs blood most is the brain. When the brain does not get blood, it can make a person feel faint or dizzy. It can also cause a stroke or death.

Doctors order medicines to try to control or stop this irregular or rapid beat. The medicines usually control this type of beat. Sometimes they do not work. The heart may then need to be shocked. The shock is given by a machine called a defibrillator. The shock usually helps the heart to reset its signals. It then beats in a regular way. All parts of the body can then get the supply of blood they need.

Adapted from Evanoski CAM. Sample patient education materials written at different grade levels. *J Cardiovasc Nurs.* 1990;4(2):1-6.

5. Becker MH. *The Health Belief Model and Personal Health Behavior.* Thorofare, NJ: SLACK Incorporated; 1974.

6. Arakelian M. Assessment and nursing applications of the concept of locus of control. *Adv Nurs Sci.* 1980; 3(25):25-42

7. Johnston M, Gilbert P, Partridge C, Coolins J. Changing perceived control in patients with physical disabilities: an intervention study with patients receiving rehabilitation. *Br J Clin Psychol.* 1992;31: 89-94.

8. Bandura A. Self efficacy: toward a unifying theory of behavioral change. *Psychol Rev.* 1977;84:199-215.

9. Bandura A. Human agency in cognitive theory. *Amer Psychol.* 1989;44:1175-1184.

10. Pender NJ. *Health Promotion in Nursing Practice.* East Norwalk, Conn: Appleton and Lange; 1982.

11. Prochaska JO, DiClemente CC. Transtheoretical therapy: toward a more integrative model of change. *Psychother Theory Res Practice.* 1982;19:276-288.

12. Basler HD. Patient education with reference to the process of behavioral change. *Patient Education and Counseling.* 1995; 26:93-98.

13. Nolan RP. How can we help patients to initiate change? *Can J Cardiol.* 1995;11(SuppA):16a-19a.

14. Smedley BD, Stith AY, Nelson AR, eds. *Unequal Treatment: Confronting Racial and Ethnic Disparities in Health Care.* Washington, D.C.: The National Academies Press, 2002.

15. USDHHS. *National Standards for Culturally and Linguistically Appropriate Services in Health Care.* Washington, DC: US Department of Health and Human Services, Office of Minority Health; 2001.

16. Curtis KA. *Instructional Activity Options in Training Programs for Clinical Instructors.* Los Angeles, Calif: Health Directions, 1988.

17 Hirsch SE, Lewis FM. Using the World Wide Web in health-related intervention research. A review of controlled trials. *Comput Inform Nurs.* 2004 Jan-Feb;22(1):8-18.

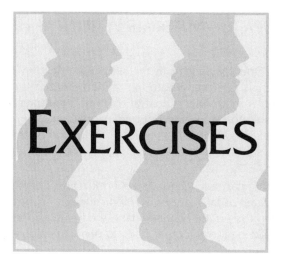

EXERCISES

1. For what types of problems do you hold most patients responsible? List a few of these problems below:

2. Identify a health behavior that YOU put off or don't do (enough sleep, dentist, safe sex, etc). What are your beliefs?

   Enter the answers to these in your journal and be prepared to discuss in class.
   a. Susceptibility to the health threat? (ie, How likely is it that I will have this problem?)
   b. Severity of the health threat? (ie, How serious is this problem?)
   c. Benefits of the recommended behavior? (ie, What will I gain by doing this?)
   d. Barriers or costs of the recommended behavior? (ie, What are the obstacles that stand in my way or the costs to me of taking this action?)
   e. What environmental cues influence you?
   f. What have you seen and learned from others?
   g. In what stage (trans-theoretical model) would you place yourself?
   h. What can you do to influence your own behavior?
   i. What beliefs must you change?
   j. What cues would make it more likely that you'll make the behavior change?
   k. Make an action plan.

3. Identify a health behavior topic relevant to your field (repetitive stress disorders for computer users, preventing low back pain, preventing STDs, low-fat diet, etc).

   Do a mini-survey of 10 people on campus or at your facility about their beliefs on this topic (the cause, the severity of the problem, the effectiveness and ease of prevention or treatment). You can do this as an in-class activity if the instructor assigns it.

   Health behavior:

   Prepare some questions (open-ended) to gather information:

   Summarize your results and discuss in class.

4. Identify a health behavior topic relevant to your field. You can choose the same topic on which you did a needs assessment in #2 above.

   How would you organize a patient education approach?
   a. What is the problem and your goals?
   b. What is the learner's state of readiness for the recommended action?
   c. What do you want the learner to know, feel, or do? When? How often? Where? With whom?
   d. What is the key content that must be presented to accomplish these outcomes?
   e. What learning experiences will help to transmit this content, teach these skills?
   f. What key steps, decisions, activities must the learner do to follow recommendations?
   g. What materials can review, supplement or draw attention to the content or process?
   h. How will you know that you've been successful in teaching? How can you evaluate that the learner has learned what you were trying to teach?

5. Select a patient education pamphlet or brochure with at least 30 sentences and analyze its reading level, using the Flesch Formula and the Fog Index. Be prepared to talk about your pamphlet in a small group.

   What messages specifically influence the reader's perceptions of:
   a The cause of the problem, his or her susceptibility to the problem
   b. The severity of the problem
   c. The effectiveness of his or her actions
   d. Ease of taking those actions
   e. Barriers to those actions

   How would you improve on the brochure?

12

COMMUNICATING WITH PERSONS WHO HAVE DISABILITIES

Kathleen A. Curtis, PT, PhD

OBJECTIVES

1. To emphasize the power of language and the use of words that reflect our innermost values, feelings and thoughts.
2. To explore the negative results of labeling people with disabilities.
3. To distinguish between descriptors often used inappropriately; for example, disability and handicap.
4. To explore models of disability and how our concepts of disability influence our actions.
5. To advocate for people-first language as the humane choice that makes a difference in how we view people with disabilities.
6. To emphasize that individuals with disabilities are human, no more, no less, and to emphasize what an inspiration they are often serves to dehumanize them as paragons of virtue.
7. To emphasize that a person with a disability experiences a problem in context, and the meaning that any problem has to an individual may differ markedly from person to person.
8. To explore how we might identify and counter our ingrained biases from our culture.

Findings from the 2000 Census indicate that 1 in 5 Americans, numbering close to 50 million, report a disability.[1] This may be a chronic disease process such as heart disease, sickle cell anemia, epilepsy, or cancer; a sensory disability, such as a hearing or visual impairment; a physical disability, such as an amputation, paralysis, or problem with pain or movement; a learning disability, such as dyslexia or attention deficit disorder; a cognitive disability, such as confusion or poor memory; or a disability related to a mental health such as schizophrenia or a manic-depressive disorder. Some disabilities are not visible to the casual observer; others are obvious. Some disabilities are stable, some are progressive or intermittent in nature.

How many members of your family have a disability? Rates of disability increase with age, with an estimated 41.9% of older adults, age 65 and older, reporting a disability during the 2000 census.[1] Other estimates report disability rates as high as 50% among older adults.[2]

Disorders of the musculoskeletal system, circulatory, and respiratory systems are the 3 leading causes of disability, accounting for over 40% of all disabilities.[2] Regardless of the type of disability, individuals with disabilities share some common experiences and challenges in their lives. Even in writing a chapter about persons with disabilities, I am making an assumption that all, most, or even some people with disabilities have some common characteristics. That assumption is as wrong as assuming that all people of Italian descent like spaghetti or that people who are tall must be good at basketball. My attempt to provide guidelines is intended to enlighten and stimulate you to examine your attitudes, beliefs, and the subtle and not so subtle limitations that you may inadvertently place on the value of a person, their rights, privileges, and potential contribution to the world, based on the diagnosis or problems they present to you.

LABELS—THE POWER OF WORDS

Health professionals spend many years of education and training studying the characteristics of diagnoses, pathologies, and their typical signs and symptoms. In the seemingly endless task to master the extensive classification of diagnostic categories and subcategories, sometimes we lose sight of the fact that people have these disorders.

Language is a powerful symbol of our understanding of these complex concepts. Our knowledge, attitudes, beliefs, and values determine what we pay attention to and the thoughts we have about what we hear, read, or experience. The language we use reflects, as well as influences, our thoughts, and feelings. Our thoughts and feelings determine, to a large extent, how we act. Moreover, language is not just an issue of political correctness; it influences beliefs, attitudes, expectations, and the course of events.

THE RESULTS OF LABELING

The experience of persons with disabilities throughout time has been largely negative. Summarily, people with disabilities undergo experiences that stigmatize, dehumanize, disempower, and generally discount their needs. Not only do individuals with disabilities face the discrimination of physical barriers in housing, schools, business, and health care, they often face staggering obstacles in both overt and covert discrimination in the job market. In 1995, 16.9 million working-age Americans, or 10.1% of the population aged 16 to 64, reported a work disability due to a chronic condition or impairment. Despite the passage of the Americans with Disabilities Act (ADA) in 1990, two-thirds of those surveyed (67.9%, or 11.4 million people) did not participate in the labor force at that time, meaning that they were neither working nor actively seeking employment.[3] Compared to the current national unemployment rates of less than 6%, this figure is staggering. Although comparable national studies have not been conducted since this time, recent evidence indicates that unemployment has not markedly improved in the past decade for people with disabilities. Let's look at some of the beliefs that may underlie these statistics.

WHAT'S IN A NAME?

Let's consider verbs first. Look at the difference between the active and passive tense. In describing an individual's relationship to an assistive device, one can draw a marked distinction in the meaning of "being confined to a wheelchair" and "using a wheelchair." In other words, active verbs connote control; passive verbs foster victimization and a need to be helped.

There is also an essential distinction between being and having. Can you sense the difference between being a *quadriplegic* and being a *person* who has *quadriplegia*? Bottom line—describing a person as the attributes of their disability connotes an identity solely as the disability. In addition, the emphasis on the disability draws attention to our perception of difference, which most often increases both psychological and social distance. We feel less at one with those we perceive to be most different.

Many terms have been used over the years to refer to people with disabilities. We can also draw a distinction between the terms, *disability* and *handicap*. A disability has been defined as a condition of the person. The term *disability* has been debated, in that by pure definition it connotes a problem with an ability. Some persons with disabilities prefer to define a disability as meaning, "a person may do something a little differently from a person who does not have a disability, but with equal participation and equal results."[4]

Another term, *handicap*, has been used to connote the accrued result of multiple barriers (emotional, physical, social, environmental) imposed by society, which prevent an individual who has a disability from assuming a desired role in society. For example, the characteristic that a person cannot walk quickly from place to place is a feature of a disability. The employer who hires a less qualified applicant who walks more quickly, the landlord who rents to another tenant, the university classroom layout that requires a half-mile walk in the 10-minute break between classes, all help to create the handicap associated with this disability.

Various models have been proposed over the years to define the concepts surrounding disability (Table 12-1). Notice the distinction between problems at the body organ level, the economic level, the functional activity or performance level and the level of the culture or social environment. Health professionals often focus on factors at the body organ and functional level; the person with a disability experiences most life problems because of factors in the economic, cultural, political and social environment. Pay attention as to whether your focus is on the disease or impairment or life experience of the individual with a disability. Be sure to acknowledge individual differences. Few people with similar impairments experience the same degree of disability, activity limitation, or participation restriction. Similarly, the cultural, social, political, and physical environment in which a person with a disability lives may vary widely and strongly influences both the individual's activities and participation in society.

PEOPLE-FIRST LANGUAGE

An established standard of good writing, *people-first language*, requires that the writer identifies the person—the man, woman, child, professor, student, client, physician, receptionist, mother, etc—and then refers to the attribute of having a disability (if it is applicable at all to the discussion) (the man with epilepsy) rather than using the disability as either an adjective (the epileptic driver) or a noun (an epileptic). This distinction, although subtle, makes a profound difference in our focus and perceptions. It empowers and provides information, rather than stigmatizes and labels (Table 12-2).

Language is one conscious choice we can make that does make a big difference. Let's look at some other typical beliefs about people with disabilities.

YOU POOR THING!

Persons who have disabilities are often characterized by the uncontrollable nature of their problem, which leads the potential helper to feel pity for the person. The connotation of the "crippled child" for example, not only breaks some of the above *people-first* language rules, but immediately connotes a poster-child image intended to elicit donations to a well-meaning charitable organization. Social scientists and fund-raisers have known for years that our perception that another person has a problem that is out of his or her control stimulates our desires to help. However, pity turns out to be an emotion that tends to marginalize people with disabilities and interferes with our ability to see them as people who share our aspirations and disappointments, with equal rights and responsibilities to take social and political action.

Table 12-1

MODELS OF DISABILITY

Model	Characteristics of Model	What Health Providers Should Know
Medical	This model denotes a medical etiology that emphasizes the cause of disability as a medical condition or disorder. Disabilities are treated as diagnostic categories. Individuals with disabilities assume a sick role.	Many providers assume that the cause of a disability is a medical condition. Instead, consider how the individual's social or emotional life affects his/her physical health. How do the environment or our social expectations influence the individual's experience of disability? The medical model also minimizes consideration of the social sources of disability, such as stigma, prejudice, and public policy.
Economic	The economic model relates to the individual's inability or limited ability to work. Medical evaluations of disability are used to predict the likelihood of employment. Links functional physical capacity with employment.	Research indicates that employment of persons with disabilities is influenced largely by social and economic trends, not by the nature of their disabilities or their functional capacities.
Functional-Limitation Paradigm	Pathology and impairment refer to an individual's medical condition and the related limitations. In contrast, the term disability refers to social function. It is the interaction of and individual's physical or mental limitations with environmental and social factors that determines disability.	Individuals with physical or mental impairments and functional limitations do not necessarily experience disability in the same ways. Individuals may have a disability in one environment and not in another.
Sociopolitical	At the heart of the disability rights movement is the common understanding that disability is an acceptable form of human variation. In this context, disability is viewed as a policy and civil rights issue, with individuals with disabilities considered an oppressed minority, facing daily prejudice and discrimination. Individuals with disabilities experience architectural, sensory, attitudinal, cognitive, and economic barriers, limiting their full participation in society.	Many health providers see their role as helping individuals with disabilities adapt to the demands of society. Instead, consider the role of policy to alter the barriers of the social, cultural, economic, and political environments in which persons with disabilities live. Facilitate environmental, societal, and political adjustment to accommodate the needs of individuals with disabilities and insure their full participation.

Adapted from: Hubbard S. Disability studies and health care curriculum: the great divide. *J Allied Health.* 2004;33(3):184-188.[5]

Table 12-2

EXAMPLES OF EMPOWERING LANGUAGE

Use This	Instead of This
Persons who have disabilities	Disabled people
Child without a disability	Normal child (in comparing to a child with a disability)
People who have visual impairments	The blind
Uses a wheelchair, crutches, or braces	Confined to a wheelchair; has to use crutches; unable to walk without braces
Individual or person who has (name of the problem	Language such as: Victim of... Suffers from... Afflicted with... Burdened with... Stricken Crippled Diseased Disabled Poor Unfortunate Sick Tragic
Individual who has (describe what the person has accomplished)	Courageous Inspirational Heroic Special
Use people-first language (eg, "a person who has epilepsy") in verbal and written communication, professional journals, laws, and statutes	Referring to the disability as an adjective (the blind man): • A noun (paraplegics, epileptics) • A passive form (help the handicapped)
Ms, Mrs, or Mr	First names or terms of endearment such as "dear" or "honey" when the relationship has the status that you would expect to use a more formal title or address

Adapted from United Cerebral Palsy. *Watch your language fact sheet.* 1991; New York: United Cerebral Palsy Association.

Helping professionals often choose the helping professions out of their desire to help individuals who have experienced misfortune, disabilities, family problems, poverty, and similar challenges in their lives. Although, not all helping professionals agree on the nature of, or the kind of, help that will effect change in the lives of those they help (see Chapter 5 on Effective Helping).

Even helping professionals want to help most those clients whom they see as least capable, least responsible, and least in control of their lives[6,7] (see Chapter 7 on Assertiveness). None of these characteristics are consistent with the image of a healthy, competent, empowered, responsible member of society. As we learned in Chapter 2, helping professionals are often wanting to "fix it" for their clients, an insurmountable and undesirable task given the complexity of our educational, social, and health care systems, and the more lofty goal of empowering clients or patients to fix it for themselves. In contrast, when helping professionals are faced with persistent, unrelenting demands for medication, better care, benefits, equal access to opportunity, or legal rights they often feel powerless or threatened, and may be less likely to help. When health professionals feel angry at their clients it actually may be an indication that they consider their clients to be competent and in control, albeit demanding or intrusive. Unfortunately, it may also cause withdrawal of needed services or less energy spent in moving the client in a positive direction that could further help or empower the client.[6] An interesting dilemma, and one that is up to health care professionals, not patients and clients, to resolve for the good of the patient or client.

Our professional help should be offered in accordance with our perceptions of how likely the client's situation is to benefit from that help. Ask yourself the question, "What type of help would be of greatest benefit and in what ways is this help likely to effect change? Or, How will my action change the individual's ability to participate in society?" Ask the client, "What would be most helpful? What are your goals?" and then listen. Recognize that some of those goals relate to the ways you have been educated to help and some do not. Be clear about what falls within your realm of professional expertise and what must be left for others or the individual to resolve.

YOU ARE SUCH AN INSPIRATION!

At the awards banquet of a national track and field championship for athletes with disabilities, a famous sports figure rises to the podium to give an after-dinner speech. It could be a woman or a man, but let's say it's a man. The speech follows:

> "You people... are such an inspiration. The courage I have seen is remarkable. You have faced the challenges and overcome them. You are all heroes today. You are all winners."

Although well intended, the speaker has distanced the group by immediately emphasizing the distinction of "you people." Further, instead of complimenting the group on their athletic accomplishments, world record performances or victories, the speaker has essentially created different standards for recognition of achievement in this group of athletes with disabilities. In reality, not everyone is a winner. Athletic competition is serious business; it requires long training hours, dedication, commitment, hard work, perseverance, and skill. Of course, there may be a role for courage and inspiration somewhere in the mix, but the point is that athletes who have disabilities share the common experience of commitment, training, successes, and failures with all athletes.

Individuals who have disabilities are human, no more, no less. A person with a disability is not a paragon of virtue, not an exceptional human being, not a person who has overcome adversity, just because he or she happens to have a disability. When we recognize persons who have disabilities for what they have accomplished, for their achievements and victories, using standards that are used for everyone, then we empower them, educate society, and change attitudes about disability.

When we overdo it on praise for minimal achievements, it infers low ability of the achiever. When you are not held to the same standards that everyone else is, it is usually because the evaluator does not feel that you have the capacity to achieve those standards. Not a good message to give, certainly a worse one to receive! Instead, give positive messages that emphasize *what was accomplished* and *what standards* you are using to judge this accomplishment. Indicate where the person stands in progress toward a goal and the end points to be reached if you are using a different standard to evaluate success.

WHAT HAPPENED TO YOU?
TELL ME ABOUT YOUR DISABILITY

In Chapter 6, you learned how to interview patients and clients as part of your professional training. You learn how to ask specific questions which are intended to focus your professional attention on a problem at hand. Your questions assume a clinical orientation, describing signs, symptoms, the onset, and severity of problems. Although helpful for providing information for a specific diagnosis or planning a treatment, these questions might ignore the one essential factor that will determine the importance of all the information you seek. Context!

A person who has a disability experiences a problem in context; in a family, on a wheelchair basketball team, as a student in school, as a colleague, supervisor, or supervisee in a work setting. The client may be with or without social support, financial resources, adequate health care, or housing. Focusing on the clinical aspects of the disability alone in the interview negates the importance of the context, but more importantly may assume that the same common symptoms or problems have the same meaning to all people who have a similar disability.

The *meaning* that any problem has to an individual may differ markedly. One individual may be mortified by unexpected urinary incontinence; another may consider it a minor inconvenience and have strategies in place to deal with the problem quickly and without great emotional cost. Questions like, "How have you handled similar situations in the past?" or "How important is this to you to take care of?" associate competence and ability with the current issues. Never make assumptions about what a problem means to your patient or client. Ask him or her.

Treat the individual as a "culture of one." Avoid reference to disability "groups" to which some individuals belong, such as "Many of my clients who have quadriplegia have skin problems, is this a problem for you?" Instead, ask open-ended, empowering questions like, "What strategies do you use to prevent pressure sores?" Use active listening instead of a relentless list of questions, but most important, talk with the person who has the disability. Listen carefully to his or her story. You've never heard it before, and as you listen, the uniqueness of this particular person and his or her meanings will emerge to assist you in your role as an effective helper.

THE EFFECT OF BIASES AND STIGMATIZATION

Cultural beliefs, the way our lenses are set, including our values, practices, conceptions of illness and acceptable behavior, greatly influence our perceptions of disability. The context in which we live determines the meaning of a disability. For example, Western practitioners tend to conceptualize medicine in a reductionistic and despiritualized fashion, searching for cause and effect relationships that can be explained and controlled.[8] In contrast, Eastern philosophies that may be based in concepts of a life force such as energy or *chi* defy Western scientific explanation, yet may be just as valid to a practitioner of Eastern medicine. Similarly, an individual's illness or disability is understood and given a significance based on the culture in which it occurs.

It is important to understand that we take on social roles to meet the behavioral expectations of influential others. Consider the behavior-shaping influence of the environment on prisoners, institutionalized children, and people who have lived in situations of physical and emotional abuse. Research studies show that people who do not have disabilities often hold attitudes and perceptions that separate them from individuals who have disabilities. For example, a study on over 200 Spanish university students showed that they perceived individuals with hearing and visual impairments to be less communicative, less intelligent, less independent, slower, and less active than individuals with no sensory impairment.[8] In fact, in comparison of the descriptors of individuals with hearing impairments to those with visual impairments, these students perceived that those with hearing impairments were more reserved, less calm, less sociable, less attentive, less prudent, less sure, and less thoughtful than those with visual impairments.[9]

Some researchers in other areas of the world have found that women tend to hold more positive perceptions of individuals with disabilities than men do.[9,10] Interestingly, some studies of the perceptions of individuals who work in medical settings *fail to show* that their attitudes are more positive toward individuals with disabilities than are those of the general public.[11,12] In other words, those who often work with people with disabilities may hold the same prejudices as do lay people.

So, how do we influence attitudes and eliminate negative stereotypes? Some authors argue that even sensitivity training, intentionally provided in professional training programs, may overly emphasize negative perceptions of the difficulties encountered by persons with physical disabilities, rather than providing trainees with a positive perspective of ability.[13] For example, the experiences of students using a wheelchair as a first time simulation experience may provide some awareness of the physical barriers encountered, *but do not seem to reflect the overall generally positive quality of life experienced by persons who use wheelchairs.* This apparent paradox of creating negative attitudes by focusing on the salient differences in the experience of persons with disabilities creates a dilemma for the education of human service professionals such as teachers, health care practitioners, and social workers, people who we want to be sensitive to the needs of and to recognize and foster the abilities of their students, patients, and clients.[5]

How Can We Counter Our Biases?

Recognition of sameness is a key factor. Social psychology tells us that rather than focusing on our differences, it is probably more productive to emphasize our *similarities*. What do we have in common with a person who has a disability? Their age, educational objective, vocational choice, parenthood, daughterhood, sisterhood, status as a student, automobile owner, bus-user, or computer purchaser is often a more unifying characteristic than the apparent (or often unapparent) nature of their disability.

When health care professionals are providing services, they are often forced to focus on the disability or its effects. Don't forget that this *person*, with desires, aspirations, a family, a job, a living situation, is not defined by the nature of his or her disability. Be aware of the many limiting ideas and concepts that prevail in our culture, but also be aware that your cultural beliefs may not be shared by the patient.

Don't Be Afraid to Shift Your Paradigm!

Prior to the late 1970s, wheelchairs were all the same—chrome and exceptionally heavy, with black or blue upholstery. Due to the influence of several young wheelchair users, wheelchair technology totally changed in the late 1970s and innovative lightweight wheelchair designs and colors became optional and available, expressions of one's personality and activity rather than the stigma of inability and confinement. Now the wheelchair market has become competitive; even the wheelchair manufacturers who once produced the heavy, chrome wheelchairs are happy to join in more creative ways of looking at the needs of wheelchair users, in order to stay afloat in this market. Even though the old school eventually shifted, they lost a significant portion of the lightweight wheelchair market. Moral of the story: Listen, believe, don't allow yourself to be limited by stereotypes and expectations.

Legislative and Economic Aspects of Disability

In the past 30 years, we have seen many legislative acts that affect the quality of life of individuals with disabilities. Below are a few examples of the major pieces of legislation that provide the basis for the rights of persons with disabilities in the United States. Unfortunately, although there is legal protection in many situations, we still have a long way to go in changing public beliefs

Table 12-3

KEY LEGISLATIVE ACTIVITY AND DISABILITY ISSUES

Legislation Affecting Persons With Disabilities

Rehabilitation Act of 1973: Mandated no discrimination by federally funded agencies against workers with disabilities and affirmative action requirements for federally funded employers.

Americans with Disabilities Act of 1990: Mandated reasonable accommodations to ensure the integration of people with disabilities in the private sector, including employment, telecommunications, transportation, and public services and accommodations.

Telecommunications Act of 1996: Required manufacturers of telecommunications equipment and providers of telecommunications services to ensure that such equipment and services are accessible to and usable by persons with disabilities, if readily achievable.

Legislation Affecting Children With Disabilities

PL 94-142: Education for All Handicapped Children Act of 1975: mandated a free and appropriate education and the least restrictive environment (ie, mainstreaming). Annual IEP's (Individual Educational Plans) are developed for all children with disabilities.

PL 101-476: Revised provisions of PL 94-142 to include children with autism and brain injury and included training and technology provisions for education of children with disabilities.

IDEA Improvement Act of 1997: Gave parents and school districts more autonomy in determining children's needs for special education services through a mediation process, further defines services available to infants and toddlers, and provides disciplinary sanctions for students who engage in criminal misconduct, unrelated to disability.

that it serves *all* people to make entrances to buildings barrier-free, it serves all people to actively foster opportunities for employment for individuals with disabilities and to provide diagnostic and treatment services to the millions of children and adults with disabilities who live in poverty (Table 12-3).

Fostering economic opportunity is not only the right thing to do, it is also good business! On a personal note, for example, I was struck by the experience I had at the 1996 Atlanta Paralympic Games, which followed the Olympic Games by several weeks. At the beginning of the Paralympic Games, there were many leftover Olympic souvenirs on sale and many street vendors who were profiting from the influx of thousands of competitors with disabilities, their coaches and sport organizers, their friends, families, and spectators from over 100 countries. Paradoxically, the Olympic pavilion, which housed many large companies and exhibitions, decided to close and tear down their exhibits and stores while the Paralympic Games opened, creating an eyesore and a racket! They not only lost out on the opportunity to sell millions of dollars of merchandise, they also missed the chance to influence the international market and reap the benefits of the economic power of thousands of individuals with disabilities from all over the world.

STILL A LONG WAY TO GO

Although legislation has protected the rights of individuals with disabilities, we still live largely in a world that does not yet meet their needs nor recognize their potential power as a group. Adequate income, education, health insurance, housing, and employment still largely remain challenges for members of our community who have disabilities (Table 12-4).

Table 12-4

COMMON NEEDS AND ISSUES FOR INDIVIDUALS WITH DISABILITIES

Major Problems Identified by Americans With Disabilities*	The Details
Affordability and availability of assistive devices	Wheelchairs, prosthetic and orthotic devices, walking aids, home equipment are all very expensive to purchase and/or repair and largely unavailable to rent. Since these devices mean independence to many persons with disabilities, lack of access to technology limits functional potential.
Accessibility of commercial services, facilities, restrooms, parking	Private businesses, restrooms, and parking are largely inaccessible in many areas. This may include the lack of curb cuts, snow removal, gravel, sand, and rough terrain.
Legal rights to public housing, transportation, social support agencies, programs and systems	Despite legal rights to these services, lack of information, prejudices, institutional barriers, and shortages prevent many individuals with disabilities from accessing these services.
Employment accommodations, discrimination	Although the ADA has improved employer understanding of their responsibilities to provide reasonable accommodations, it still does not keep the employer from discriminating against potential employees with disabilities in the hiring process.
Health care insurance and services inadequate for needs	Many health care providers refuse to treat Medicaid or Medicare patients. Respite care and attendant care is largely unfunded. Many individuals cannot buy health care insurance because of their disability or pre-existing conditions.
Auto, life and liability insurance costs	Insurance companies often discriminate based on disability, offering more expensive premiums.
Stigmatization, asexualization, grouping	The media portray individuals with disabilities in a negative, asexual and unrealistic way. People with disabilities are often not portrayed as individuals who exist beyond the definition of their disability.
Fixed incomes; poverty	Many individuals with disabilities exist on supplemental security income (SSI) and live below the poverty level.

*Summarized from the results of a survey of 13,000 individuals with disabilities in 10 states. Described in: Nagler M. *Perspectives on Disability*. Palo Alto, Calif: Health Markets Research; 1993.

Adapted from Suarez DeBalcazar Y, Bradford B, Fawcett S. Common concerns of disabled Americans: Issues and options. In: Nagler M. *Perspectives on Disability*. Palo Alto, Calif: Health Markets Research; 1993.[14]

AGING WITH A DISABILITY

The life expectancy for persons with disabilities has increased markedly, resulting in many people with severe disabilities reaching middle age and older age groups. Age-related changes, when combined with pre-existing impairments, often create secondary disabilities, which if left unrecognized or untreated, many impair quality of life and independence.[15]

Health care professionals must be aware of screening for recent loss of function in individuals with long-term disabilities. Routinely asking questions such as the following may identify a secondary problem before it becomes a serious health threat.

Have you noticed...
- ❖ Any increased fatigue or pain during daily activities?
- ❖ A change in your posture?
- ❖ Difficulty sleeping?
- ❖ Any change in your weight?
- ❖ Any change in your sensation?

WOMEN WITH DISABILITIES

Over 20 million women with disabilities experience some unique challenges. Statistics show that they differ from both men with disabilities and from women without disabilities in that they have increased social isolation and less access to higher education. They also have higher unemployment rates and even those employed earn lower incomes.[16]

A women's perspective on disability can be appreciated in the words of author Nancy Mairs, who writes about the image of the perfect body and perceptions of disability:[17]

> *"The 'her' I never was and am not now and never will become. In order to function as the body I am, I must forswear her, seductive though she may be, or make myself mad with self-loathing. In this project, I get virtually no cultural encouragement. Illness and deformity, instead of being thought of as human variants, the consequence of cosmic bad luck, have invariably been portrayed as deviations from the fully human condition, brought on by personal failing or by divine judgment."*

Women with disabilities have been documented to have limited access to medical services, education, and vocational opportunities. These issues influence their health, as they often lack information, financial resources, and health services to meet their unique needs.

Despite the needs, there are many barriers that reduce the quality and accessibility of services for women with disabilities. Physical and communication barriers often limit access to health care settings, despite the requirements of the Americans with Disabilities Act (ADA). In many cases, women also lack adequate transportation and support services to get to health care appointments.

Women with disabilities often have less access to breast health services than any other group of women. Women with disabilities are at a higher risk for delayed diagnosis of breast and cervical cancer, primarily for reasons of environmental, attitudinal, and information barriers. They report difficulties in receiving women's health services such as mammograms and Pap smears, reproductive health/birth control, STDs, and services to address specific issues of aging. In addition to reproductive health needs, women with disabilities frequently experience a lack of privacy and autonomy while receiving health care, high rates of violence, and abuse and unmet mental health needs.[18]

Strategies that eliminate barriers to care include providing education to women and their health care providers and identifying solutions such as appropriate communication techniques, accessible equipment and available services. Health care practitioners can make a difference treating women with disabilities as women first, with health needs, perspectives, and issues that they share with all women.

WHAT CAN YOU DO TO MAKE A DIFFERENCE?

The following exercises are designed to help you raise your awareness to recognize the perceptions and biases you hold about individuals with disabilities. You are morally obliged to make an active effort to recognize the abilities of all people. Be aware of the influence of your language. Set a personal goal to empower individuals with whom you have contact and support access to health care, educational opportunities, employment, housing, and transportation. Don't be satisfied with being an 8-hour-a-day advocate for people with disabilities!

REFERENCES

1. *2000 US Census Summary Tables.* (QT-P21. Disability Status by Sex: 2000). Available at http://factfinder.census.gov. Accessed April 2, 2005.
2. Kraus L, Stoddard S, Gilmartin D. *Chartbook on Disability in the United States, 1996. An InfoUse report.* Washington, DC: U.S. National Institute on Disability and Rehabilitation Research. Available at: http://www.infouse.com/disabilitydata/disability/index.php. Accessed April 2, 2005.
3. LaPlante MP, Kennedy J, Kaye S, Wenger B. *Disability and Employment—Disability Abstract #11.* San Francisco, Calif: Disability Statistics Rehabilitation Research and Training Center, University of California, San Francisco; 1997.
4. Kailes J. Watch your language, please. *J Rehabil.* 1985;51(1):68-69
5. Hubbard S. Disability studies and health care curriculum: the great divide. *J Allied Health.* 2004; 33(3):184-8.
6. Curtis KA. Role Satisfaction of the physical therapist in the treatment of the spinal cord injured person. *Phys Ther.* 1985;5:197-200.
7. Kahan M. *Physician Assistants' Models of Helping Behavior and Their Relationship to Perceived Responsibility, Attributions and Patient Education.* University of California Los Angeles, Unpublished manuscript; 1988.
8. Banja JD. Ethics, values and world culture: the impact on rehabilitation. *Disability and Rehabilitation.* 1996;18(6):279-284.
9. Cambra C. A comparative study of personality descriptors attributed to the deaf, the blind and individuals with no sensory disability. *Am Ann Deaf.* 1996;141(1):24-28.
10. Gannon PM, MacLean D. Attitudes toward disability and beliefs regarding support for a university student with quadriplegia. *Int J Rehabil Res.* 1996;19:163-169.
11. Lys K, Pernice R. Perceptions of positive attitudes toward people with spinal cord injury. *Int J Rehabil Res.* 1995;18:35-43
12. Eberhardt K, Mayberry W. Factors influencing entry-level occupational therapists' attitudes toward persons with disabilities. *Am J Occup Ther.* 1995;49(7):629-636.
13. Grayson E, Marini I. Simulated disability exercises and their impact on attitudes toward persons with disabilities. *Int J Rehabil Res.* 1996;19:123-131.
14. Suarez DeBalcazar Y, Bradford B, Fawcett S. Common concerns of disabled Americans: issues and options. In: Nagler M. *Perspectives on Disability.* Palo Alto, Calif: Health Markets Research; 1993.
15. Klingbeil H, Baer HR, Wilson PE. Aging with a disability. *Arch Phys Med Rehabil.* 2004 Jul;85(7 Suppl 3):S68-73; quiz S74-5. Review.
16. Jans L, Stoddard S. *Chartbook on Women and Disability in the United States.* Available at: http://www.infouse.com/disabilitydata/womendisability. Accessed April 9, 2005
17. Mairs N. *Waist High in the World: A Life Among the Non-Disabled.* Beacon Press; 1996
18. Nosek MA, Howland CA, Rintala DH, Young ME, Chanpong GF. *National Study of Women With Physical Disabilities: Final Report.* Houston, Tex: Center for Research on Women with Disabilities; 1997.

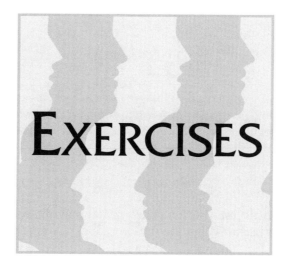

EXERCISES

1. Identifying your attitudes and beliefs:

   What beliefs do you have about the following conditions? What beliefs do you think most people have?

	Your Beliefs	Others
Epilepsy		
Cerebral palsy		
Quadriplegia		
Cataracts		
Cancer		
Brain injury		
HIV-positive		
Congenital heart disease		

2. Replace each of the following statements with "people-first" language:

   He is a quadriplegic.

   It is a fund-raiser for the mentally retarded.

   The blind man came in last.

   The developmentally disabled children.

Congenitally-dislocated hips (speaking of babies).

Confined to a wheelchair.

Stroke victim.

Stricken with Lou Gehrig's disease (amyotrophic lateral sclerosis).

Cystic fibrosis kids.

3. Find an article or advertisement in a magazine that portrays an individual with a disability. Comment on that portrayal. What stereotypes does it reinforce? What positive messages come out of it?

4. Watch one of the following films/videos. Analyze the experience and portrayal of individuals with disabilities in the film. Discuss in class.
   a. *Waterdance* (1992, Columbia/Tristar)
   b. *Born on the 4th of July* (1989, Universal)
   c. *Coming Home* (1978, MGM)
   d. *The Wedding Gift* (1994, Miramax)
   e. *Whose Life is It Anyway?* (1981, Warner Bros.)
   f. *The Terry Fox Story* (1983, HBO)
   g. *My Left Foot* (1989, Miramax)
   h. *Passion Fish* (1992, Miramax)
   i. *Regarding Henry* (1991, Paramount)
   j. *Do You Remember Love* (1985, CBS)
   k. *The Other Side of the Mountain (Parts 1 and 2)* (1975 & 1978, Universal)
   l. *The Other Sister* (1999, Touchstone)
   m. *I Am Sam* (2001, New Line)

13

SEXUALITY AND DISABILITY: EFFECTIVE COMMUNICATION

Sherrill H. Hayes, PT, PhD

OBJECTIVES

1. To define sex, sex acts, and sexuality.

2. To emphasize the importance of understanding one's own sexuality, values, and beliefs in order to communicate effectively in the clinical setting.

3. To review the process of becoming a patient and the negative effects of institutionalization on sexuality.

4. To understand myths and misconceptions regarding both sexuality and disability, and how these may affect both the patient's as well as the practitioner's viewpoints and comfort levels.

5. To introduce experiences of the patient that may compromise his or her image of self as a sexual being and precipitate feelings of shame.

6. To discuss the importance of self-esteem, self-image, and self-actualization with respect to rehabilitation.

7. To review normal sexual arousal cycles for the male and female, and the impact of certain disabilities on sexual functioning.

8. To discuss the role of the rehabilitation professional with respect to sexuality and the disabled.

9. To understand and utilize the principles of the PLISSET model as a structure for identifying one's knowledge base, comfort, and skills in sexuality and disability.

10. To stress the importance of effective communication and therapeutic presence through case studies designed to prevent shaming experiences, maintain privacy, and promote sexual integrity of the patient.

As a way of introducing you to this content, take a moment now and turn to Exercise 1 at the end of this chapter, and complete the true-false Pre-Test. Then read the chapter *before you check your answers*. Then complete the test once more as a Post-Test. Check your answers as a last step in your learning process.

INTRODUCTION

Myths and misunderstandings often arise around groups of people who display 3 charac-teristics: 1) they are a minority; 2) members are clearly identifiable; and 3) society harbors fears or aversion toward them. Many physically disabled people meet all 3 criteria and thus become objects of social bias.[1]

Over the last 50 years, there has been a virtual revolution in Western society pertaining to sexu-ality and roles of males and females. The "typical" family core of the male working outside and the female staying home with the children has changed to the more common rule of both parents working outside the home. Additionally, we have seen a large increase in single-parent families, same sex relationships, and same sex parents raising children. Sexual behaviors have also changed, from relatively little premarital sex, to the "free love" of the 1960s and 1970s, to the current trend of more of a series of longer lasting relationships or "serial monogamy," largely owing to the AIDS epidemic beginning in the 1980s. Lastly, these relationships may be heterosexual, homosexual, or bisexual in nature.

Concomitantly, there has also been an increase in the number of people with disabilities, owing to improved medical interventions, providing increased survival for injured persons, or persons with chronic disabling conditions.

Finally, there have been major inroads in the field of sexual dysfunction and infertility, which have dramatically improved the lives of both able-bodied persons and persons with disability or chronic illnesses. For example, treatments for erectile dysfunction are widely known and even advertised in the media; in vitro fertilization is common; and electro-vibration and electro-ejacula-tion techniques have dramatically improved fertility in some males with spinal cord injury.

Let's begin with 3 important definitions:

1. Sex: Maleness/femaleness; one of the 4 primary drives (along with hunger, thirst, and avoidance of pain) that originates in the subcortex and are modified by learned responses in the cortex.

2. Sex acts: Any behaviors involving the secondary erogenous zones and genitalia, such as kissing, hugging, caressing, and fondling, with sexual intercourse being only *one* kind of sex act.

3. Sexuality: The combination of sex drive, sex acts, and all those aspects of personality con-cerned with learned communications and relationship patterns. There are many levels to sexuality: conversation, shared activities and interests, various expressions of affection and intimacy, and sexual intercourse. Some persons equate sexuality with intimacy. *Everyone* is capable of intimacy—young or old, male or female, able-bodied or disabled.

Any discussion regarding sexuality should consider the broad picture, and definitions of *sexual-ity* vary. Common thoughts regarding sexuality often focus on what happens in bed—or the sex acts—as the essence of sexuality. Some see sexuality as being "the major way people define and present themselves to others as people, and as men and women."[2] Another definition of sexuality involves "the way one dresses, the way one carries oneself, the way one looks at others and oneself, the way one speaks to other people, the way one touches other people and oneself."[3] Yet another definition includes "the many facets of an individual's personality, including affection, companion-ship, intimacy, and love."[4]

What all of these definitions display is the universality of the emotional importance of sexuality, able-bodied, or disabled. Some also feel that because of the relationship of sexuality to self-esteem and body image, that it is an important part of rehabilitation.[5] Since self-esteem is so important to a person's psychological well-being, and since disability affects the way a person feels about themselves, it is logical to see that a damaged self-esteem will also affect their sexuality. Self-image and self-efficacy are also important considerations, and are affected by disability. Additionally, dis-ability and illness affect both the injured person and his or her partner.

In previous chapters, the importance of developing listening skills and effective communication in the practitioner-patient relationship were presented. Identification of who owns the problem and communicating about emotion-laden topics is certainly evident with issues of sexuality and self-image in the rehabilitation process. According to Sipski & Alexander,[6] communication within the health care system should have 6 goals, all of which are essential when addressing the topic of sexuality and disability:

1. To establish rapport.
2. To determine a basic medical and interpersonal history.
3. To assess the role and nature of relationships in the patient's life.
4. To identify what changes have occurred since the onset of the disability or illness.
5. To determine how those changes have been explained to the patient and how the changes have affected quality of life.
6. To communicate in such a way so that questions are encouraged.

Sexuality continues to be a sensitive topic that most clinicians are uncomfortable addressing with their patients. There are at least 2 major reasons for this discomfort: 1) lack of training in the area of sexuality; and 2) the subject of sexuality is an area where the professional's own personal values and biases are based on their own upbringing, values, and life experiences. For many professionals, it is difficult to separate their own values and attitudes on sexuality from those of their patients in order to be objective. It therefore is not surprising that the subject is rarely addressed, addressed inappropriately, or simply dismissed.

Attitudes of health professionals toward sexuality have been studied, though most of these studies have been with nurses, and few with physical or occupational therapists. In studies of nursing students, it has been found that they are less knowledgeable and more conservative than other students.[7] In rehabilitation nurses, increased religiosity was correlated with decreased knowledge of sexuality and more conservative sexual values.[8] Nursing faculty have been found to be unprepared to teach this content, thus it was ignored or limited in content (usually reproduction only).[9] While studies of other health professionals are limited, one could assume that many of these professionals have similar origins and values. Indeed, in one of the few studies of rehabilitation professionals, it was found that the majority (79%) thought sexuality was as important as other aspects of rehabilitation, but few (7%) were comfortable addressing sexuality with their patients.[10] The reasons for this discomfort were a lack of knowledge, or an assumption that "someone else does it."

Since sexual identity, self-concept, and self-worth are so strongly linked, if one is impaired, all are affected. Additionally, impaired sexual function has a direct adverse effect on medical, psychological, and vocational rehabilitation of an individual, and addressing this issue can have a positive effect on overall rehabilitation of a patient with a disability or chronic illness. Certainly, knowledge building in the areas of anatomy and physiology, human sexual response, disability-specific effects, cultural variables, religion and values, and dispelling of myths and stereotypes should be presented. Skills training should address effective and active listening (see Chapter 6), interviews and assessment skills (see Chapter 10), and values clarification (see Chapter 3); discussion and modeling of compassion, patience, perceptiveness, and integrity are also valuable. Because of the close bonds patients develop with rehabilitation professionals, especially therapists, due to the intensity of contacts and type of care, these therapists are in a unique position to respond to their patients, often more so than the physician.

THE PLISSIT MODEL

The PLISSIT model (an acronym for Permission, Limited Information, Specific Suggestion, and Intensive Therapy) by Annon[11] is a model that ideally is utilized by all members of the health care team in conversing with people with disabilities who are questioning about sex and sexuality. In this model, all members of the team are educated to feel comfortable enough with their own sexuality and have enough knowledge to function at the first two levels of the model (ie, permitting discussion of the topic of sex and sexuality and having enough knowledge about sexuality and about various specific disabilities to provide limited information). Additionally, they should know enough about their limits, or "know what they do not know," in order to properly refer the patient to another more knowledgeable professional. The reader is referred to the reference for specific information, but each element will be briefly described here.

Permission

Permission is a valuable tool to help patients deal with basic issues of self-esteem, personal worth, and body image. At this level, the practitioner gives both overt and covert messages to the patient who inquires about sex, provides permission through his or her responses to the patient's questions, offers more information when the patient is ready, or introduces the topic in a nonthreatening manner (eg, using bridging statements [see pp. 227]). Here, the health care practitioner is being open and accepting of the topic of sex and gives the patient permission to inquire without embarrassment.

Limited Information

At this second level in the model, the practitioner provides general and basic education such as anatomy and physiology, dispelling of myths, and describing general ways in which others in similar situations resolved their own problems. At this level, it is important that the practitioners know their own limitations (in knowledge, skill, and comfort), and refer the patient to others when the patient's needs exceed their own limits.

Specific Suggestions

In this third level, the practitioner assists the patient with more specific needs or concerns, by suggesting or providing specific ways to resolve a problem (eg, specific positions for sexual intercourse, erectile dysfunction, management of bowel or bladder problems), or specific effects of medications or surgeries. For functioning at this level, the practitioner should have additional education, expertise, or experience in sexuality and disability beyond others on the team, as well as being astutely aware of his or her own limitations in knowledge, comfort, or skills.

Intensive Therapy

This level is usually beyond the rehabilitation setting, and requires psychotherapy, relationship counseling, or surgical or invasive procedures (penile implants or injection therapy). Referral to these professionals is usually coordinated outside the inpatient setting.

As can be seen, the PLISSIT model provides a structure for an effective team approach, and for individuals to identify their own level of appropriate practice, as well as a process that assists one to identify areas for future professional growth. Case presentations are particularly helpful in identifying options for management and problem solving, as well as mentoring opportunities for practitioners (see Case Study exercises on page 239).

SEXUALITY AND THE HEALTH CARE PROFESSIONAL

Although not widely recognized or spoken of, a relative sexism in the "hospital family" continues to exist, where the physician is subconsciously related to as a "father," the nurse, physical therapist, occupational therapist, or other health professional who is female as a "mother," and the patient treated as a "child." It is also important to acknowledge that health professionals are sexual beings as well. We cannot "turn off" our sexuality (our maleness, femaleness) when we enter a clinical setting. It is also important to recognize that health care professionals between the ages of 25 and 35 are in the developmental stage of desire for a sexual partner; just about every encounter among staff, and sometimes among patients and staff, tends to be seen through the lenses of sex and sexuality. It is not uncommon for the middle-aged male patient to be sexually attracted to the younger female physical therapist or nurse, or for the female patient to be similarly attracted to the male physician or physical therapist. Phrases such as "the dirty old man," or the "oversexed female" are often heard in clinical settings, when patients overtly exhibit this normal attraction to the opposite sex, who may happen to be a health care professional. Acknowledging this natural part of our own humanness is a first important step toward self-awareness. Acknowledging the patient's natural expressions of his or her innermost concerns (eg, "Am I still attractive?") is also central to a holistic approach to treating the patient as a whole person.

SEXUALITY AND DISABILITY

Hospitalization—The Process of Becoming a Patient

Becoming a patient in today's medical care arena involves many processes that threaten one's independence and dignity, and one's very sense of self-identity. The transformation of a *person* into a *patient* begins with several predictable events:[12]

1. Answering the same seemingly innocuous questions from several people about personal information (name, address, social security number, insurance, age, weight, reason for admission).
2. Undressing and donning the "neuter" hospital gown (affording little in the way of propriety).
3. The surrendering of all personal effects.
4. The application of the familiar wristband for identification.
5. The transportation via wheelchair to a room with a bed and a chair, even when one is capable of walking unaided.

Whether the hospitalization is for a minor procedure or a life-threatening illness, this process remains the same. The point I want to emphasize here is the ubiquitous custom of forced dependence of individuals who have previously been in control of their lives outside the hospital, but who are forced to lose their identity and sense of self when they become a patient. Suddenly they are no longer Mary Smith, CEO, or John Jones, Esq, but Mrs. Smith or Mr. Jones, or even worse, Mary and John. The ultimate insult occurs when they become "room 22, bed 2," and this process occurs in just about every inpatient setting in the entire country.

Following the initial round of the admission process and settling into the hospital routine is the process of myriad evaluations by different health care practitioners assigned to the patient's care—nurses, physicians (including residents, interns, and medical students), and rehabilitation professionals and their assistants and students. All are asking similar questions about the patient's personal and medical history, doing physical examinations, and ordering both invasive and noninvasive procedures in the process of establishing a diagnosis or treatment regimen.

All of these assessments are believed to be necessary and important in the process of diagnosis and treatment of the patient's problem. However, what is often overlooked in this process is the privacy of the individual, and often there is a consistent lack of concern about personal modesty and humility, as the patient is questioned, examined, prodded and probed in often intimate places. Significantly, the patient's problem may involve areas of the body that reflect one's sexuality, such as the breast, uterus, or prostate. When the areas of the body are the cause of the hospitalization, there is an inevitable increased sense of invasion accompanying the process of assessment. If surgery is imminent, whether a mastectomy, hysterectomy, or prostatectomy, there is a significant, unspoken fear about the patient's sense of self after the surgery.

Table 13-1

EFFECTS OF DISABILITIES ON SEXUALITY AND SOME EXAMPLES

Effects on Sexuality	Examples
Interference with sexual function due to physiological changes or tissue damage	Spinal cord injury (SCI); diabetes; prostate cancer
Treatment may result in a change in body image, which may seem incompatible with maintaining a sexual relationship	Mastectomy; orchiectomy; ostomy; amputation
Pharmacological agents may interfere with sexual function	Antihypertensive medications; chemotherapy; insulin.
Physical symptoms (fatigue) may interfere with or hamper sexual performance	Cancer patients on chemotherapy or radiation therapy; rheumatoid arthritis; multiple sclerosis (MS)
Anxiety related to illness may interfere with sexual response	Post-myocardial infarction (MI); cancer patients; genital herpes; HIV+
Depression or grief may be associated with impaired libido or sex drive	Post-MI; hysterectomy; mastectomy; cancer; MS
Illness may necessitate physical separation from a partner	SCI; Post-CVA; HIV+; AIDS

Body Image

Any patient who experiences trauma, surgical removal of a body part, or treatment which results in disfigurement or loss of a body part experiences a disturbance of his or her body image. Body image disturbances may occur when there is a discrepancy between the way in which one had mentally pictured the body, and the way the body is currently perceived. This conflict often arouses anxiety and fear of rejection. The response of loved ones is thought to exert a significant influence on the patient's ability to reintegrate his or her new body image. Body image distortion may elicit feelings of unacceptability, thus negatively influencing the person's perception of self as a sexual being, and in turn influencing sexual function.

Effects of Illness on Sexuality

Illness may influence one's sexuality in many different and diverse ways, as shown in Table 13-1. It is important for health care practitioners to be aware of how various disease processes or drugs may affect their patients' physiological functioning, as well as their own sense of self. There are several excellent and comprehensive resource textbooks for health care practitioners (see Suggested Readings on page 236).

Acting Out Sexually

When patients consciously or unconsciously test the response of others to themselves as sexual beings, they may act out as a means of gaining control of a situation in which they feel dependent. For example, flirtatious behavior is often exhibited as a way to attract attention. What the patient may be expressing is the effect of sexual deprivation or separation from a sexual partner or significant other. Also, they may simply be seeking out validation of themselves as attractive or desirable. Chapter 8 on Neurolinguistic Psychology offers communication alternatives to help professionals set strong boundaries and break rapport if this acting out becomes sexual harassment.

Cultural Variables

As was described in Chapter 9 on Cultural Sensitivity, it is important for health care professionals to be aware of different cultural customs and beliefs in the patients they are treating. Often, without thinking of it consciously, different customs are considered odd, strange, or silly, when in fact they should be merely considered different. Greater emphasis on cultural diversity is evident in most professional curricula nowadays, which is certainly needed in the multicultural environment encountered by practicing clinicians today.

In many cultures, there are certain proscriptions that may modify an individual's response to hospitalization and treatment. For example, in certain Latin cultures, illness is believed to be a manifestation of weakness. Loss of blood is thought to impair sexual vigor. Protection of the wife's modesty is seen as a duty of a good husband during physical examinations. Any or all of these cultural dictates may be misinterpreted by uninformed health care professionals as stubbornness or stupidity unless cultural differences are understood.

Likewise, if a practitioner is not accustomed to being in the presence of same-sex couples, they may find themselves acting in ways that are judgmental or unkind, and not conducive to therapeutic presence. Same sex couples have very similar needs and concerns as heterosexual couples, and efforts should be made to make them feel comfortable and understood.

Basic Rules for Effective Communication About Sexuality and Rehabilitation

As a clinician, the following 3 basic rules will assist you in communicating with therapeutic sensitivity.

1. *Prevent shaming experiences.* Shame implies admitting to oneself that part or all of the self is unacceptable. Shaming experiences can be prevented by providing both physical and psychological privacy, carefully reading body language, and listening to words to avoid "touchy" areas, and explaining that the given situation is not intended to embarrass, but is necessary for effective care.

2. *Maintaining privacy.* During hospitalization, personal autonomy and the limitation and protection of information is usually jeopardized. In order to emphasize confidentiality, it is often wise to acknowledge to patients that you realize that some things are difficult to discuss, then provide some dimension of privacy, and always show respect as a means to address this problem. Make use of curtains and close doors whenever possible

3. *Do not make judgments.* Chapters 2, 3, and 4 emphasize that we all have our own values, and there are some individuals whose values may be in conflict with our own. Accept that people are different, and maintain a professional decorum without inflicting your own values on others, verbally or nonverbally. Be aware if you are a person who readily displays facial expressions that reveal dissatisfaction with different values than your own.

Improving Communication—Bridge and Barnum Statements

It is obvious to all health care professionals that not all questions are easy to be asked, some questions need to be asked more than once, and not all answers will be the same to different health care professionals. This is especially true with the topic of sexuality. Bridge statements (including questions) facilitate the transition from easy, comfortable topics to those that are difficult or awkward. They move from the general to the specific, emphasize the professional relationship between the patient and the therapist, and focus on permission giving and permission seeking. Some examples are:

❖ "Has anyone talked to you about how your illness can affect your ability to have sex?"

❖ "How has your (MS, arthritis, CVA) changed the kinds of things you and your partner do together?"[6]

❖ "Many people with amputations have concerns about their sexual attractiveness. Is this a concern of yours?"[6]

Although Bridge statements are a means to solicit information and improve communication, Barnum statements can hinder information and create anxiety. Barnum statements are overly general, and empty of content, though fashioned to be encouraging or optimistic. Some examples are:

❖ "You are in the best hospital for your condition." (To an anxious patient)

❖ "Come on smile—it's a wonderful day."[6]

❖ "How is your love life?"[6]

Barnum statements minimize and depersonalize the patient's problem, and do not help the professional understand the problem from the patient's perspective. Though often heard in rehabilitation settings, they should be avoided.

Understanding Normal Human Sexuality

We are all sexual beings, able-bodied or not. The onset of disability does not eliminate sexual feelings any more than it eliminates hunger and thirst. Both sexuality and disability remain taboo areas that are *not* discussed without anxiety or discomfort. Health professionals, in assisting people with disability to rehabilitate, must remain aware of this anxiety and become involved in the sexual adaptations required of their patients. We cannot treat the whole patient without effective support and counseling in this important area.

Myths

As reflected in the quote from Cole[1] at the beginning of this chapter, people with disabilities fit the 3 criteria that would characterize them as being "different" from those in the general population. People with disabilities are a minority, readily identifiable, and others often feel uncomfortable as a result of their presence. Most people in ethnic or racial minorities have experienced all of these criteria at some point in their lives, and the similarities are striking.

It was only recently, with the various revolutions that transpired following the turbulent 1960s, that significant research was done to investigate the effect of disability on sexuality. During the 1970s and early 1980s there was a rash of medical, psychological, and behavioral investigations that added greatly to our body of knowledge about sexuality and disability. Prior to this period, there were many myths perpetuated by the media, as well as educational publications, which did little to explore the true realities and capabilities of sexual functioning in persons with disabilities. Furthermore, there was little in the medical literature regarding sexuality and disability, further perpetuating the myth of asexuality in these individuals.

It is also important to recognize that prejudice against disabled people is longstanding in our culture and in others, and is not merely a phenomenon of the 20th century. One need only consider some of the most well-known literary works to realize that many of the loathsome characters in literature had some kind of disability. *Lady Chatterley's Lover*, for instance, depicts the paraplegic as "sexually incapable and hopeless," while familiar children's fairy tales depict various "monsters:" Captain Ahab of *Moby Dick* was an amputee, Captain Hook of *Peter Pan* had a prosthesis, and Quasimodo from *The Hunchback of Notre Dame* had a deformity we now recognize as severe kyphoscoliosis. All of these characters were referred to as "grotesquely deformed and evil." Is it any wonder that many of us grow to harbor feelings of revulsion or pity for anyone with a disability?

The stigmatization of people with disabilities has been sustained for many years in our own subconscious. It is also pertinent to recognize that for many individuals who sustain a traumatic disability, such as an amputation or spinal cord injury (SCI), that they themselves may have harbored feelings of revulsion toward the disabled prior to their injury. These attitudes or feelings may have been built on fear, ignorance, or prejudice. In effect, these preconceived beliefs may result in considerable self-prejudice, hampering their own self-acceptance. This further complicates the acceptance of their "new" body image for their own self-esteem. In a society such as ours, with so much emphasis placed on beauty, health, and physical fitness, it is easy to see how physically disabled people may feel ostracized in today's sexual arena and low on a scale of sexual desirability. Finally, it is important for health professionals to recognize that people are not "handicapped" intrinsically. As pointed out in Chapter 12, a person with a disability becomes handicapped when he or she is restrained from usual social interaction by barriers, social and architectural, that prohibit participation in normal daily activities.

Self-Esteem

According to Abraham Maslow,[13] sex is one of the basic physiological needs that must be met, in addition to air, water, food, shelter, and sleep. All are needed in order for an individual to move toward self-esteem and self-actualization.

Taking Maslow's theory to practical application, Anderson and Cole[14] did groundbreaking research with respect to examining the interrelationship of sexual success, work success (meaningful employment), and the self-esteem of an individual with a disability. They found that if there was perceived success in sexual activity, the person with a disability reported a higher self-esteem and fewer feelings of castration. If there was success in work life, there was less tolerance for dependency and thus a higher self-esteem. And if there was success in both areas, the individual had a high self-esteem, fewer medical complaints, and less need for medical and social support.

Another meaningful point with respect to success in sexual relations relates to the importance and significance of the sexual partner or significant other. The significant other plays a pivotal role in the acceptance of a changed body image for a person with a disability. As Rosenbaum so eloquently stated:

> *What becomes apparent when the direct genital urge toward physical release is lost are the many other needs that can be met or expressed through sexual activity—the need for touching, for reassuring body contact, to be held and to hold, to express love and caring through caressing and kissing. These become especially important when the body has been damaged and the individual is attempting to integrate and accept a new and altered body image. We all need the acceptance of another to make the image of ourselves whole and more loveable.[15]*

So, the acceptance of the partner is important in allowing and assisting the re-integration of the disabled person in a "new" body image. Additionally, and of no less importance, is the attitude of the health care professional toward his or her patients. Self-esteem and self-confidence depend on feedback from the environment and those around the patient. If professionals project a sensitive, honest, and truthful attitude, the patient can be encouraged to discover a new sense of self, without anxiety. If, on the other hand, the patient and his or her questions are not addressed openly and honestly, or are brushed off in a shaming experience, the patient's adjustment and acceptance will be dealt a significant blow, and their recovery will be compromised.

NORMAL HUMAN SEXUAL RESPONSE—NEUROPHYSIOLOGY

In a culture and era when sexuality seems to scream from billboards, magazines, and movie theaters, it is amazing how little education those in the health care professions actually receive with respect to normal human sexuality. Understanding sexuality and disability, especially as it relates to the person with SCI, requires an understanding of the normal sexual response and its components. These components, and the male and female response cycles, are found in Table 13-2.

Table 13-2

THE NORMAL SEXUAL AROUSAL CYCLE—MALE AND FEMALE COMPONENTS

1. Excitation

Excitation develops from any source of bodily or psychic stimuli, and with adequate stimulation, leads to further excitation. This first phase may be interrupted, prolonged, or ended by distracting stimuli.

Male	Female
Rapid engorgement and erection of the penis	Clitoral glans enlarged
Tensing and thickening of the scrotal skin	Vaginal lubrication
Elevation of scrotal sac	Nipples become erect, breast size may enlarge
Occasional nipple erection	"Sexual flush" may be seen (rash on chest to breast)
Elevation of heart rate (HR) and blood pressure (BP)	HR and BP increase

2. Plateau

Often called the "consolidation period." A period of intensified sexual tension; also affected by distracting stimuli.

Male	Female
Increased penile circumference	Lower 1/3 of vagina constricts, upper 2/3 balloons (creates a "squeezing" action)
Increase in testes size	Clitoral glans retract
Continued increase in muscle tension, HR, RR, and BP	Uterus elevates
"Sexual flush"—rash over face, neck, and chest	"Sexual flush" may spread to entire body
	Increase in muscle tension, HR, RR, and BP

3. Orgasm

An involuntary climax of sexual tension increment. It is really only a few seconds of the sexual response cycle, during which vasocongestion and myotonia are released. There is a greater variety of intensity and duration in the female.

Male	Female
HR, RR, and BP increase further	Further increase in generalized muscle tone, HR, RR, and BP
Expulsive contraction of the penile urethra	Involuntary rhythmic muscle contraction in perineal muscles
Ejaculation (internal bladder sphincter closes, preventing retrograde ejaculation)	Involuntary contraction, spasm of muscle groups
Involuntary muscle contraction of perineal muscles	May be multiple orgasms (unlike males)

4. Resolution

The period when involuntary changes occur that restore the individual to the pre-excitatory state.

Male	Female
Gradual reversal of anatomical and physiological changes	Gradual reversal of anatomical and physiological changes
Males require a refractory period before another cycle occurs.	Females usually do not have a refractory period, and may begin another cycle immediately.

In men, it is important to note the following facts regarding erection and ejaculation, based on neurophysiology.

There are 2 centers for erection within the spinal cord:

1. Psychogenic (T11-L2)—mental arousal, psychic stimuli (or, "whatever turns you on")
2. Reflexogenic (S2-4)—local arousal, reflex sensory-motor feedback loop

Ejaculation is mediated by both the sympathetic nervous system (T11-L2) and the parasympathetic nervous system (S2-4), as well as the somatic nervous system. The 2 kinds of erection are not separate in the normal male response cycle, but become important in understanding sexual function in the man with SCI.

SEXUALITY AND SPINAL CORD INJURY

Sexuality is affected more with spinal cord injury (SCI) than with any other disease or pathological condition. The patient's first question usually is "Will I live?" The second question (often unexpressed) is, "How will this injury affect me sexually?"

There are far too many exceptions within each spinal cord level to state, with any certainty, what any one patient's sexual disability will be. What should be emphasized is that sexual activity may or may not involve genital sensation, and ultimately, sexual satisfaction per se is a cerebral event, and therefore can be achieved by everyone.

Spinal Cord Injury—Sexual Function in Men

SCI is a devastating injury to anyone, but there are significant effects with respect to sexuality that affect men more than women, and these are summarized in Table 13-3. As one can see from the table, for levels above the cauda equina, the ability to achieve and sustain an erection is generally maintained, as long as there is local stimulation to activate the feedback loop for reflexogenic erection. Ejaculation is more rare, and fertility is a problem, although there have been recent major breakthroughs (electro-vibration and electro-ejaculation) in this area.

What is also important with respect to males with SCI, is the entire socialization of males and masculinity in our culture. It is known that males are socialized very early into expected gender roles and behaviors. "Performing" is of primary importance, and strength, self-reliance, success, sexual interest and prowess, independence, aggressiveness, and dominance are all important male attributes. Indeed, their manhood is often tied to their penis, and having erections is directly related to masculinity. Sexual education and sexual comparisons go on all the time. With these messages, it is no surprise that if one's ability to achieve an erection is impaired, as it certainly is in a male with SCI, that this is a devastating blow to his manhood and his self-identity. It is yet another disability to contend with, in addition to the SCI, and one which must be addressed in the rehabilitation arena.

Spinal Cord Injury—Sexual Function in Women

There has been a distinct sexual bias in the literature regarding female sexuality, although it is true that the majority of persons with traumatic SCI are young men. Women with SCI are often dismissed, since their fertility is unaffected for the most part, and thus many people mistakenly believe that they do not suffer the overt sexual disability that is seen with men. Often, they are told that their sexuality is "unaffected." In fact, women experience the same differences and inabilities, neurophysiologically, as do men. The female sexual cycle is similar to that of the male, thus the lubrication, engorgement, and contraction components of the sexual response cycle are affected. Recent research has shown that women with complete SCI's with UMN lesions will have reflexogenic lubrication but not psychogenic lubrication, similar to their male counterparts with the same type of injuries.[16] Yet, because these problems are not as "overt and obvious" as when a man is unable or has difficulty in achieving erection, women are mistakenly viewed as unaffected.

Table 13-3

SPINAL CORD INJURY—EFFECTS OF SEXUAL FUNCTION IN MEN*

Quadriplegic	*Paraplegic#*	*Cauda Equina Lesions*
Reflexogenic—intact	Reflexogenic—intact	Reflexogenic—arc may be disturbed (below L2)
Psychogenic—not intact	Psychogenic—not intact	Psychogenic—intact (T11-L2)
Ejaculation—rare	Ejaculation—rare	Ejaculation—moderate chance
Fertility**—almost nil	Fertility—almost nil	Fertility—may be present, but with sperm problems (retrograde ejaculation, temperature problems)

*There is a distinct difference between complete and incomplete lesions of the spinal cord, with effects from incomplete lesions being far less predictable than from complete lesions.

#Essentially, there is no difference between a quadriplegic or paraplegic male with respect to sexual capability and fertility. The major difference is in the greater area of intact skin sensation and motor ability (trunk, arms, abdomen).

**Since ejaculation is rare, fertility is severely affected; however, fertility can be greatly assisted today with technological advances such as electro-vibration, electro-ejaculation, and artificial insemination.

Immediately after a traumatic SCI, a woman's menses may be halted, but her menstrual cycles will usually return within 6 months, and fertility is therefore unaffected, unlike men. Labor and delivery present complications, however, due to the inability of a woman with SCI to sense labor contractions or to push during the expulsion phase of labor. Cesarean birth is usually not necessary since the uterus is an involuntary muscle capable of contracting despite loss of innervation. However, due to the inability of the woman to push and potential problems of emboli or autonomic dysreflexia, vaginal births are rare, though not impossible.

Obviously, sexuality is much more than childbearing, but information usually given in a rehabilitation setting is often overly clinical, focusing on bowel and bladder routines and focusing more on the physical act of intercourse, removed from the context of the entire relationship. While it is true that the greatest concerns of women focus on the physical (bowel or bladder accidents) and the psychological (satisfying the partner, being attractive), the latter usually diminishes over the time, but the former persists, partially due to the emphasis placed by professionals, who tell them "to expect bowel and bladder accidents and other negative possibilities." If women with SCI are told repeatedly of the negative consequences during rehabilitation, a time when their self-esteem and self-confidence is already challenged, it is no wonder that many are not encouraged, or even scared to face a relationship. Warnings about possible problems should be realistic, but not overwhelming. Discussion of these issues should be done in a nonjudgmental way, in order to promote self-confidence and self-acceptance.

In the literature relating to the human sexual response, Masters & Johnson have contributed greatly to our understanding of this basic human need. One of the things they noted is that the "human sexual response is a *total body response*, rather than merely a *pelvic phenomenon*. There are changes in cardiovascular and respiratory function, as well as reactions of the skin, muscles, breasts, and rectal spincter. This is also an important distinction, since it is commonly reported that many individuals with SCI actually experience orgasm, although usually of a different type than they experienced prior to their injury. As mentioned previously, it is believed that orgasm is more strongly a cerebral event, and not totally dominated by pelvic activity. Individuals with SCI are often taught to use various methods of "assignment," "fantasy employment," "memory," and "recall," and report that they experience a sensation that, while different, is nonetheless satisfying.

SEXUALITY AND MYOCARDIAL INFARCTION

With respect to sexuality and myocardial infarction (MI), there is still much discrepancy in the literature. Either little information is given (and what is given is often "too conservative") or conflicting information is given, making it difficult for patients to decide whether it is safe or not to resume sexual activity after a heart attack.

Much of the discrepancy in the literature about sexuality and the post-MI patient is related to discrepancies in the maximal heart rate during sexual activity. In their studies of human sexual response, Masters & Johnson recorded couples' heart rates, respiratory rates, and other physiological responses during sexual intercourse and found that heart rates escalated to 180 beats per minute during intercourse. They therefore concluded that sexual activity is "heavy cardiac work." Following the results of this study, many cardiologists and other physicians, when asked by their patients, related these findings and cautioned against any excessive cardiac work for their post-MI patients.

What was missing in this information for cardiac patients was the fact that the Masters & Johnson studies were conducted on healthy, young college students in their early 20s. The average post-MI patient in the mid-1980s was a man in his 50s, married for 20 or more years to the same spouse. Hellerstein and Freidman[17] saw this discrepancy and pursued their own study, similar to that of Masters & Johnson, except using post-MI couples in their 50s. Their results were dramatically different, as they found the maximal heart rates to be 120 beats per minute, roughly the equivalent of climbing 2 flights of stairs, and actually lower than heart rates during a football game or during a heated argument in the office. They concluded that, for the "typical post-MI patient," with their spouse of 20 or more years, and a frequency of sexual intercourse of 1 to 2 times per week, sexual activity was not the wild, amorous fit of passion seen often in the movies, and did not constitute "heavy cardiac work." They stressed, however, that there were likely distinct differences for a man who has recovered from a heart attack and is conducting an extramarital affair. The heightened anxiety, coupled with guilt, could likely result in increased heart rates into a dangerous range, often culminating in what has come to be referred to as DIS, or "death in the saddle," though this has been attributed to less than 1% of death due to coronary artery disease (CAD).

Recent studies have shown promising results of a gradual return to sexual activity, though all have shown a reduction in frequency of sexual activity when compared to the pre-MI state, for both males and females.[6]

The focus on SCI and post-MI patients in this chapter is largely due to the amount of literature in these areas, but almost any kind of disease process or treatment can have an effect on a person's sexuality, as shown in Table 13-4.

Drugs Which May Interfere With Sexual Function

Many pharmacological agents can affect sexual performance either directly or indirectly, a factor which has been increasingly noted in the media today. Normal sexual function depends on multiple physiological mechanisms, including vascular, hormonal, neurologic, and psychological processes, all of which can be altered by medications. Again, there is a gender bias in much of the literature, with few studies evaluating adverse effects on female sexual response. The most common adverse side effect is erectile dysfunction (and presumably the female counterpart of inadequate lubrication during sexual intercourse). Some of the more common drug families and their effects are listed in Table 13-5.

CONCLUSION

Self-image and self-esteem are major considerations in the sexual rehabilitation of a person with a disability. When one's sense of self is seriously disrupted by the trauma of a spinal cord injury or

Table 13-4	

OTHER CONDITIONS THAT MAY CAUSE PROBLEMS OR DIFFICULTY WITH SEXUAL INTERCOURSE

Condition	Problem
Genital lesions	May cause difficulty with penetration or painful intercourse (dyspareunia)
Respiratory disease	May impair the ability to breathe adequately or limit positions used to engage in sexual intercourse
Cardiac disease	May involve poor circulation to the genital area, angina with exertion, or decreased libido due to medications; denial, anxiety and depression
Neurological diseases (stroke, MS, Parkinson's)	May involve components of the nervous system, altering sensation or motor ability (erection, lubrication); may also have spasticity, impairing range of motion; decreased libido; language deficits
Amputations	May limit some positions due to inability to assume them; may be a "physical turn-off" or "fetish" for the partner
Arthritis	Limitations due to joint mobility and/or painful joints limiting activity
Ostomies	May limit some positions due to pressure on ostomy site; may be a "physical turn-off" to the partner
Severe burns	May be limited in joint range of motion (ROM), difficulty in assuming some positions due to limited mobility; may be a "physical turn-off" to the partner
Scleroderma	May be limited in joint ROM, difficulty in assuming some positions due to limited mobility; loss of elasticity of skin may hamper intercourse or cause painful intercourse; may be a "physical turn-off" to the partner
Cancer	Physical and emotional disturbances; primary sexual organs may be affected (disfigurement, body image); treatment options (chemotherapy, radiation therapy or surgery) may cause impairment; fatigue, nausea, vomiting; anxiety and depression

any other disability, it is more important than ever to help the patient re-establish a positive self-concept. Responding to an individual's sexual concerns can go a long way toward re-establishing a feeling of self-worth, which is essential to rehabilitation in general. Rehabilitation has traditionally emphasized the comprehensive management of the *total patient*. The basic premise is to help each patient to use all of his or her strengths and assets to the maximum in forming a new self-image based on positive factors, and to help the patient to focus on areas of worth instead of deficiency.

It is unfortunate that the patient's sexuality, with its potential as a positive integrating force in building a new image of self and body, has been neglected for so long. Many professionals do not volunteer information to the patient because the patient has not asked. Since the subject of sex is viewed with discomfort by both the patient and the professional, they are caught in the dilemma of who will initiate the communication. It is easy to ask questions regarding the patient's home, family, number of stairs to climb, etc; it is not easy to ask questions about the patient's customary sex life. Hence, patients are afraid of asking, and professionals are not comfortable with asking, or answering when asked. Yet it has been shown that increased knowledge about a subject enhances

> **Table 13-5**
>
> # DRUG FAMILIES
>
> *Drug Category*
>
> | | |
> |---|---|
> | Cardiovascular drugs | Psychotropic drugs |
> | Antihypertensive agents | Antidepressants |
> | Sympatholytic | Tricyclic antidepressants |
> | Reserpine, beta-blockers | MAO inhibitors |
> | Diuretics | SSRIs |
> | Thiazides | Lithium carbonate |
> | Anticholesterolemic agents | Antianxiety agents |
> | Digoxin | Neuroleptics |
> | Antiarrhythmic drugs | Phenothiazines |
> | Stimulants/anorectics (weight control, ADD) | Butyrophenones |
> | Anticonvulsants | Anticancer drugs |
> | Antiulcer drugs | |

feelings of comfort about the subject matter. Perhaps by providing health care professionals with at least the minimal information, and suggesting where to look for more information, comfort levels in providing this necessary care will improve.

Physical therapists and occupational therapists are in excellent positions to coordinate discussions about sexuality, for they are members of the disciplines around which total rehabilitation evolves, especially for the individual with SCI. Therapists must be comfortable with their own sexuality, however, through adequate knowledge and an accepting, nonjudgemental attitude. Attitudes around sexual expression may communicate a message that encourages adjustment and growth, or may accomplish the opposite and actually inhibit patients from taking positive avenues of action, and thus discourage a desirable outcome. Harmful attitudes can, in effect, add a new disability to the pre-existing one for the patient. If a therapist is uncomfortable with a patient's questions, at the very least he or she should refer the patient to another person who could answer the patient's questions and render the assistance and advice that the patient is seeking. To ignore the subject, or downplay it, only further handicaps the patient, exposes him or her to a shaming behavior, and closes down any further communication regarding this important component in his or her self-esteem. All rehabilitation professionals should be comfortable communicating within the first 2 components of the PLISSIT model, and should be knowledgeable about referring to other professionals if more specific information is requested that is beyond their knowledge or comfort levels.

In conclusion, Cole & Cole perhaps said it best, as they listed guidelines for professional practitioners and patients in learning about the sexuality of physical disability:[18]

> *Absence of sensation does not mean absence of feelings... the presence of deformities does not mean absence of the desire...the inability to perform does not mean the inability to enjoy... Sexual health cannot be separated from total health.*

The following exercises will assist you in understanding your knowledge and attitudes that will facilitate your therapeutic presence in helping patients reconcile unwelcome changes in their ability to be sexual following injury or illness.

REFERENCES

1. Cole TM. In: Rosenzweig N, & Pearsall FP. *Sex Education for the Health Professional—A Curriculum Guide.* New York, NY: Grune & Stratton; 1978:88. (

2. Chipouras S. Cornelius D, Daniels SM, Makas E. *Who cares? A handbook on sex education and counselling services for disabled people.* Austin Tex: PRO-ED; 1979.

3. Trieschmann RB. *Spinal Cord Injuries: Psychological, Social and Vocational Rehabilitation.* 2nd ed. New York, NY: Demos, 1988.

4. Rotberg A. An introduction to women, aging, and sexuality. *Phys Occup Ther Geriatr,* 1987;5(3):3-12.

5. Ducharme SH, Gill KM. *Sexuality After Spinal Cord Injury. Answers to Your Questions.* Baltimore, Md: Paul H. Brooks Publishing; 1997.

6. Sipski ML, Alexander CJ. *Sexual function in people with disability and chronic illness: a health professional's guide.* Gaithersburg, Md: Aspen Publications; 1997.

7. Medlar T, Medlar J. Nursing management of Sexuality Issues. *J Head Trauma Rehab.* 1990;5(2):46-51.

8. Wilson PS, Dibble SL. Rehabilitation nurses' knowledge and attitudes toward sexuality. *Rehab Nurs Res.* 1993;2(2):69-74.

9. Gender AR. An overview of the nurse's role in dealing with sexuality. *Sexuality & Disability.* 1992;10(2):81-89.

10. Ducharme S, Gill KM. Sexual vales, training, and professional roles. *J Head Trauma Rehab.* 1990; 5(2):38-45.

11. Annon J. The PLISSIT model: a proposed conceptual scheme for the behavioral treatment for sexual problems. *J Sex Educ Counsel.* 1976;2:1-15.

12. Woods NF. *Human Sexuality in Health and Illness.* 2nd ed. St. Louis, MO: CV Mosby Co; 1979.

13. Maslow A. *The Further Reaches of the Mind.* New York, NY: Viking Press; 1971.

14. Anderson TP, Cole TM. Sexual counselling of the physically disabled. *Postgrad Med.* 1975;58:117-123.

15. Rosenbaum M. Sexuality and the physically disabled: the role of the professional. *Bull NY Acad Med.* 1978;54:501-559.

16. Sipski ML, Alexander CJ, Rosen RC. Physiological parameters associated with psychogenic arousal in women with complete spinal cord injuries. *Arch Phys Med Rehab.* 1995;76: 811-818.

17. Hellerstein H, Friedman EH. *Medical Aspects of Human Sexuality.* 1969;March.

18. Cole TM, Cole SS. The handicapped and sexual health. In: Comfort A, ed. *Sexual Consequences of Disability.* Philadelphia: George F. Stickley Co; 1978.

SUGGESTED READING

Ducharme SH, Gill KM. *Sexuality After Spinal Cord Injury. Answers to your questions.* Baltimore, Md: Paul H. Brooks Publishing; 1997.

Hazeltine FP, Cole SS, Gray DB. *Reproductive Issues for Persons With Physical Disabilities.* Baltimore, Md: Paul H. Brooks Publishing; 1993.

Masters WH, Johnson V. *Human Sexuality.* Boston, Mass: Little Brown & Co; 1966.

Krotoski DM, Nosek MA, Turk MA. *Women With Physical Disabilities—Achieving and Maintaining Health and Well Being.* Baltimore, Md: Paul H. Brooks Publishing; 1996.

Rosenzweig N, Pearsall FP. *Sex Education for the Health Professional—A Curriculum Guide.* New York, NY: Grune & Stratton; 1978.

Sipski ML, Alexander CJ. *Sexual Function in People With Disability and Chronic Illness: A Health Professional's Guide.* Gaithersburg, Md: Aspen; 1997.

RECOMMENDED MOVIES

Commercial

Waterdance (1992, Columbia Tristar)
Coming Home (1978, MGM)
Born on the Fourth of July (1989, Universal)

Educational/Training

Sexuality and Spinal Cord Injury (Kessler Rehabilitation Institute, NJ)

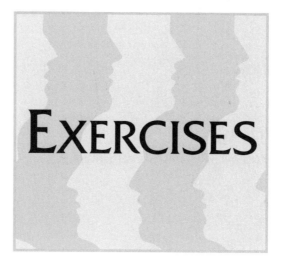

EXERCISE 1: PRE-TEST—SEXUALITY AND DISABILITY

1. Respond to the following questions. Answer each question True or False.

   a. Sexual activity is as important as walking to some of those with paraplegia.

   b. The menstrual period of a woman with a spinal cord injury (SCI) will cease after the trauma and never resume.

   c. Orgasm can be reached in men and women with SCI by stimulating parts of the body other than the genitals.

   d. Erection in most men with SCI can be maintained as long as stimulation is present.

   e. Men with SCI must remove in-dwelling catheters before engaging in penile-vaginal intercourse.

   f. If the man with SCI can ejaculate, he is likely to be fertile.

g. Cesarean sections are necessary in women with SCI because their uterine muscles will no longer contract.

h. Fertility in the man with SCI is low, but fertility is unaffected for the woman with SCI.

i. In SCI, erection occurs more often in persons with complete lower motor neuron lesion than in those with complete upper motor neuron lesions.

j. Sperm from a man with SCI can be obtained via electro-ejaculation and stored until there is enough for artificial insemination.

k. Muscle spasms in the extremities during sexual activity can result in either loss or facilitation of an erection.

l. A persistent abnormal erection without sexual desire (priapism) is most common with cervical cord injuries.

m. The alteration in the bodies' heat regulatory mechanism could affect fertility of the man with SCI.

Answers: T: a, c, d, h, j, k, l, m   F: b, e, f, g, i

EXERCISE 2: PATIENT-PRACTITIONER INTERACTIONS

A series of case studies follows. Each involves an actual patient-practitioner scenario that may be encountered in the clinical setting. Divide into groups and discuss how you would handle the following interactions. Discuss the case study as it is written among yourselves, but *first* write down how you would handle the patient's or other professional's requests before your discussion. Employ your understanding of the PLISSET model in framing your response. Use your active listening skills and effective communication skills when presented with difficult and emotion-laden questions. Avoid using less than helpful responses, such as those mentioned in Chapter 6 (reassurance, judgmental responses, defensiveness), and remember that indifference is the most unhelpful response.

1. A 37-year-old divorced woman with a complete C6-7 lesion requests assistance from the sex counselor. She wishes to have sex with a male friend but is afraid that "I won't be able to move my hips and clasp my legs around him." The sex counselor approaches you, the physical or occupational therapist, for specific information on the woman's hip movement capabilities, and asks for possible assistance with pillow supports under her pelvis and legs, and for some method of helping her hold her ankles together to clasp the male. What are your feelings as the sex counselor asks for this information?

2. A 49-year-old man with complete paraplegia and his 37-year-old wife expressed great concern about involuntary urinary and bowel discharge during sex play. The patient is on intermittent catheterization, and uses a condom catheter during the daytime. The patient's wife approaches you for suggestions about alternate positions to avoid undue pressure or irritation for both partners. You verified the patient's sexual functioning status with the sex counselor before discussing these questions with the couple. How does this request make you feel? (Remember, feelings are one word). What information must you have in order to respond to their request?

3. An 18-year-old female patient with spina bifida is engaged in a lighthearted conversation with a male physical therapy aide about the latest fashions and clothing styles while doing her exercises in the gym. Discussion focuses on the difference between "sexy" and "sensuous" clothing, and the patient turns to you for your opinion. What are you feeling? What would your response be? Does your Code of Ethics inform you on appropriate boundaries in this situation? If so, what are they?

4. A 28-year-old single man with complete C6 quadriplegia with limited hand motion and grip, asks you, a male, for advice about a way to masturbate to see if he still had the ability to ejaculate. How do you feel about this question? How would you respond? If you are a woman, how would you tell your male colleagues to respond?

5. A 21-year-old single man with quadriplegia turns to you, a woman, to express his embarrassment over his constant erections (priapism), which are particularly noticeable while doing mat exercises. How would you feel? What would be an appropriate way to respond to him? Role play this interaction in your group.

6. An 18-year-old woman with complete T4 paraplegia is planning on going to her high school prom and then wants to spend the night afterward in a hotel with her boyfriend. She asks you, a female, for suggestions for different positions that she could use for sexual intercourse with her boyfriend. Before the accident they were sexually active, and she is unsure what she is able to do now. Also, due to problems with thrombophlebitis, she is no longer able to take birth control pills and asks what other birth control method is possible. How would you feel? What would you respond? If you are a man, how would you tell your female colleagues to respond?

7. The wife of your 54-year-old patient with a previous MI asks to speak with you outside the PT gym. Her husband is about to be discharged home, and she is uncertain about resumption of sexual activities due to his heart condition. Before his MI, they engaged in sexual intercourse 2-3 times per week for most of their 26-year marriage. She is afraid that he might have another heart attack if they resume sex. How would you feel? What advice would you give her?

8. A 57-year-old female patient with severe rheumatoid arthritis asks you about sexual activity, now that her disease has progressed to severe joint immobility and pain. Previously, she and her husband had always favored the missionary position, but that has become impossible due to her lack of hip range of motion. How would you feel? Where would you direct her to go for the information she needs?

9. A 29-year-old female patient with severe low back pain approaches you with questions about positions for sexual intercourse which would not aggravate her back pain. You know that she has limited flexibility in her low back, either in flexion or extension. How would you feel? What would you do first to respond to her?

Chapter **14**

COMMUNICATING WITH THE DYING AND THEIR FAMILIES

Carol M. Davis, PT, EdD, MS, FAPTA

OBJECTIVES

1. To clarify the importance of this topic to the maturation of the health professional.
2. To emphasize the importance of the therapeutic communication skills of touch and active listening.
3. To assist the reader to clarify current values around dying and death and to identify current values around dying and death and to identify current comfort with the topic.
4. To delineate the knowledge and skill needed to facilitate a life of quality for the dying patient.
5. To describe the developmental stages health professionals go through as they learn to cope with the anxiety of caring for dying patents.
6. To emphasize the importance of a written living will as illustrated by the Terri Schiavo case.

No one likes to contemplate death, except perhaps those for whom living has become entirely too painful. But to deny death totally throughout one's life, to refuse to reflect on the certainty that one day life will end for each one of us is to avoid a wonderful opportunity for enriching the quality of one's life. You've heard the phrase; "The unexamined life is not worth living." Elisabeth Kübler-Ross has written:[1]

> It is the denial of death that is partially responsible for people living empty, purposeless lives; for when you live as if you'll live forever, it becomes too easy to postpone the things you know that you must do. You live your life in preparation for tomorrow or in remembrance of yesterday, and mean while, each today is lost. In contrast, when you fully understand that each day you awaken could be the last you have, you take the time that day to grow, to become more of who you really are to reach out to other human beings.

Camus said, "There is only one liberty... to come to terms with death. After which, everything is possible."[2] Ernest Becker, in his Pulitzer prize winning book, *The Denial of Death*,[2] writes, "Of all the things that move men [and women], one of the principal ones is his [her] death... All historical religions address themselves to this same problem of how to bear the end of life."

This may seem like an unlikely chapter for a book aimed at facilitating professional socialization, but I believe it deals with a topic that is most critical to the maturation of health professionals. To grow into one's profession requires personal growth along with professional growth. To deal with death greatly enhances this life task.

Some of you who have already lost a loved one will know what I mean when I say that this experience is unique in its ability to "grow one up" rapidly. James Agee, in *A Death in the Family*[3] recounts a tale of fresh grief as experienced by several members of one family following the sudden death of the husband and father in a car accident. Mary, the victim's wife, stands in front of a mirror ready to place the mourning veil over her face as she dresses for the funeral. She thinks to herself:

> *I am carrying a heavier weight than I could have dreamed it possible for a human being to carry, yet I am living through it... She thought: this is simply what living is; I never realized before what it is... now I am more nearly a grown member of the human race; bearing children, which has seemed so much, was just so much apprenticeship. She thought that she has never before had a chance to realize the strength that human beings have to endure.*

THE EXISTENTIAL FEAR OF DEATH

Children are not born with a fear of death. At about age 3, children begin to deal with object loss and experience both fear at the disappearance of the mother and joy at playing peek-a-boo. It isn't until age 10 or so that we begin to realize what it means for "life to disappear forver."[2] In fact, if fear of death were held constantly conscious, we would be unable to function normally, so we repress it, and by adulthood the common thought is, "I know I'll die one day, but I'm having too much fun living to worry about it."[2]

We can ignore our fears of death, or we can carefully absorb them and repress them in what Becker describes as our "life expanding process."[2] With each victory in life comes a feeling of indestructibility, of proven power. Each time we notice the strength of our bodies, recover from the flu, avoid an automobile accident, or narrowly escape an injury or, more phenomenal yet, escape death, we further prove that we are indestructible. In addition, as we grow into secure and loving relationships with partners, parents, and children, we feel secure support and appreciation for our existence and a warmly enhanced sense of self acts to further repress the fear of our inevitable death. A healthy self-esteem doesn't have time to ponder death, we believe.

Only when death confronts us in remarkable ways do we even consider our own mortality. Besides near-death experiences, perhaps the deepest assault to our repression of the fear of death as health professionals is to care for a patient or a cherished family member who is close to the moment of death.

WHY CONCERN OURSELVES WITH DEATH AND DYING IN HEALTH CARE?

To come to terms with imminent death is one of the most difficult tasks human beings ever have to face, and we face it absolutely alone. No one can take our death away from us, nor give us the courage to die. However, the role others play at our side during this intense time can be either tremendously helpful or cruelly fragmenting and hurtful.

The quality of the help we render to those who are dying and their families has everything to do with our own ideas, values, and fears about death, and until we clarify those ideas and values and confront our fears, we will be apt to increase the burden that is already almost too great to bear.

When death is imminent, we will be governed by what is deep inside of us, and our patients or loved ones will either benefit or suffer. If our fears of death predominate, we will deny the inevitable or defend fiercely against it. Out of our inner anxiety will emanate denial statements such as "Oh hogwash! You're healthier than I am! You're going to live forever!" or "Don't talk like that, Silly. It makes me depressed."

If our fears get stirred up too much, and our denial starts to break, we can expect anger and aggressive and passive aggressive assaults against those who are suffering. Just before we took my father home from the hospital to die (he was given 6 to 8 weeks more to live after fighting cancer of the larynx with brain metastasis for the greater part of 2 years), the young nurse came to my father's hospital room and harshly asked, "Are you the daughter?" When I replied, "Yes, I'm John's daughter," he cautioned me as he flipped a vial of pills in front of my face, my father's medication for pain: "Now, don't give this to him when he asks for it, give it like the label says. I can't help it if he's in pain; he has to learn to endure it. If you give him medication every time he asks for it, and he comes back here to my unit, I'll have to be in his room ever hour or so, and I have 30 other people who need me just as much as he does."

I felt frightened and assaulted in that moment by a person who had supposedly studied to be a healing professional. The more our behavior is governed by our denial and fear of death, the greater the chance that we will add to the already overwhelming burdens of the patient and the family as they struggle with one of life's deepest pains.

Author and dancer Isadora Duncan lost both her young children in a tragic accident in which a taxicab carrying them both fell in the water and they were drowned. After the accident, she fled to her friend, the Italian actress Eleanora Duse, at her villa in Italy. Her friend knew how to help her grieve and did not offer platitudes, or sit with her in embarrassed silence, offering her ideas and activities to "take her mind off her worries." She allowed Duncan to feel what had happened to her, to experience her loss. Duncan writes in *My Life*:[4]

> *The next morning I drove out to see Duse… She took me in her arms and her wonderful eyes beamed upon me such love and tenderness that I felt just as Dante must have felt when, in "Paradisio," he encounters the Divine Beatrice.*
>
> *From then on I lived at Biareggio, finding courage form the radiance of Eleanora's eyes. She used to rock me in her arms, consoling my pain, but not only consoling me, for she seemed to take my sorrow to her own breast, and I realized that if I had not been able to bear the society of other people, it was because they all played the comedy of trying to cheer me with forgetfulness. Whereas Eleanora said: "Tell me about Deidre and Patrick," and made me repeat to her all their little sayings and ways, and show her their photos, which she kissed and cried over. She never said, "Cease to grieve," but she grieved with me, for the first time since their death, I felt I was not alone.*

As a health professional, you will not be called upon to provide this level of support and caring. However, once people have matured and confronted their innate fears of death, we find that their ability to comfort and support the dying in whatever way is needed in the moment develops into quite profound skill and sensitivity. When we get beyond our defenses about death, we can then learn how to be therapeutically present for the dying. Life affirmation replaces death denial, and our actions are characterized by an intrinsic belief that life, moment to moment, is good and that we have the power to do something about the quality of a person's life, moment to moment. We realize that, even in the face of inevitable death, the support and comfort of family and mature healing professionals can actually help the patient transform his or her last days into some of the most rich and meaningful of his or her entire life. Confronting our fears of death is not easy, and we reflexively avoid it. But when we face this task with courage, we experience a quality of growth that is unparalleled in our development, personally and professionally.

Quality of Life Is More Important Than Quantity

Each one of us will die. We're only here for a short time on earth that we know of. The average life expectancy of about 75 to 81 years may seem like forever to us when we are young, but as we approach that age, we will wonder where the years went. Dying is a holistic experience. All of a person is involved—the physical part of us "gives up the ghost;" the intellectual often struggles with meaning, the emotional with the deep feelings of the inevitability of this moment, and the spirit is released to continue on in a journey that we can only speculate about.

The lucky ones among us will have time to prepare for death. I believe this preparation time is a cherished gift, not just because it feels good to be able to tie up loose ends, to tell our dear friends how much life with them has meant to us, to make final arrangements, etc. In most cases, when you know your time is very limited, and you accept the inevitability of your death, the quality of that time increases exponentially. You become as liberated as a 4-year-old in your intentions and in your communication. You ask for what you want, and you say what you really feel without the concern for whether someone will think ill of you, or not like you. This is a tremendously freeing experience. Commonly felt anxieties are replaced with living each moment just as you wish, for these are your last moments here on earth, and they are very precious, for few of us feel that we really know what lies beyond death. Genuine, heartfelt feelings are expressed. There is no time for superficialities or small talk, unless one chooses. Every conversation reflects deeply held thoughts and values. Great wisdom is passed along without fear of being accused of egocentrism. In fact, the predominant feeling becomes, "What is to be feared now?" The ultimate fear has been confronted. The goal becomes how to live well the remaining time, rather than how to avoid death. This acceptance does not happen all at once, but takes place in stages over time, as I'll discuss in just a moment.

When we, as health professionals, take the opportunity to work with the dying, the quality of our lives can also improve. However, we find it far easier to be present to the dying who have accepted the inevitability of their imminent death, than to work with patients and families who refuse to face inevitable death, and live each day working furiously to maintain denial or controlling the anxiety of the inevitable. There are few worse situations in life than to try to be present in a therapeutic way to a patient or family who is denying imminent death. This situation most often develops out of a mistaken fear that the patient (or family) will lose hope, and the patient will give up the will to live. Studies reveal the opposite.[5] Depression and the loss of hope may appear as part of the coping of dealing with dying, but these feelings usually do not last long, and are replaced by hope for more realistic things. For example, patients will maintain their hope for a miracle all the while accepting the inevitability of death. Then, more pragmatically, they will shift their emphasis to, for example, the hope to live long enough to see a child be married, or return home to see loved ones or pets.[5]

Stages of Loss

Elisabeth Kübler-Ross, in her well-known book, *On Death and Dying*,[5] describes what we can expect to experience as we go through the loss of a loved one, or experience our own dying. People initially experience a denial at the news of impending or actual death of a love one. The most extreme forms of denial include total repression of the news or actually losing consciousness.

Denial is often followed by anger. Once we allow the news to begin to penetrate, intense feelings of anger can be expected to emerge. Health care workers must take care not to personalize this anger, but to allow patients to fully experience it and express it. This is made more difficult in society that does not tolerate emotional outbursts of any kind.

Following anger, the patient often experiences a brief bargaining phase in which a kind of a deal is cut with life, or with fate, or God. For example, one will hear such thoughts as, "Okay, I know I'm going to die soon, but please let me live long enough to see my children get married." Or "If I can live, I'll never smoke another cigarette again."

Often the next stage that emerges is depression. Patients become quiet and more lethargic, reacting to the undeniability of this news as they live with it day after day. They keep to themselves, often refusing to see visitors or speak to certain family members. Reactive depression then leads into a preparatory depression in which patients quietly reflect on the sadness of their fate, and prepare for inevitable death.

Finally, patients move into acceptance of their fate, and begin to live life as a precious gift. Not everyone reaches this stage before dying, and very often these stages do not occur in a linear sequence. It is quite common to hear a patient who seems to have worked through the stages into acceptance say, for example, "Next year I'm going to plant a different garden. I'm tired of the same old flowers. I'm going to rethink the whole layout and do it the way I always wanted to."

Thus, the dynamics of coping with inevitable death take on a certain predictable rhythm and character, *but each person copes in his or her unique way*. It would be wrong to suggest that each and every person follows the same identical linear pattern of coping stages. Likewise, family members go through their own unique stage processes, and it can become quite complex just trying to keep track of where each person is in the process of accepting one person's imminent death. The patient may be in acceptance, but her husband may still be angry. Children may need to deny until the end. It takes great sensitivity and acceptance to be willing to be therapeutically present to each of these people and requires that we choose to believe that each one is doing the very best he or she can, at the moment, to cope. It is not our role to force "reality" onto them.

Most important, be careful not to use this knowledge of the various stages as a way of diminishing the importance of certain statements and removing them from the context of their meaning. For example to say, "Oh, he's just in the anger stage. He'll get over that" as a way to avoid meaningful interaction is not a wise use of this knowledge.

PREDICTABLE RESPONSES FROM CAREGIVERS

Working with the dying can become a great challenge, depending on the extent to which we have confronted our own fears, and the extent to which the patient and family have accepted the inevitability of the imminent death. What data exist to help us understand our natural responses to this caregiving challenge? How can we be guided to offer a healing response no matter what the atmosphere surrounding the patient?

Beatrice Harper has studied the development of health professionals' ability to cope with the anxiety surrounding the death of their patients.[6] Figure 14-1 and Table 14-1 illustrate the five stages of coping that she observed in social workers as they dealt with their anxiety about dying patients. She observed that the nature and intensity of anxiety of caregivers shifted in a developmentally predictable way from Stage I: Intellectualization, characterized by the need to deny and intellectualize death, to the inevitable Stage V: Deep Compassion, characterized by the development of the ability to give of oneself and a feeling of comfort in relation to oneself, the patient, the family, and the tasks of caregiving.

This figure can help you anticipate and analyze your responses when you first confront a patient who is dying. I offer it to assure you that your therapeutic skill in caring for the dying will develop and improve, and to remind you that caregiving for the ill involves a personal as well as professional growth process. You should not expect yourself to be an expert in this area from the very start.

Figure 14-1. Coping with professional anxiety in terminal illness. Reprinted with permission from Harper B. *Death: The Coping Mechanism of the Health Professional.* Greenville, SC: Southwestern University Press; 1977.

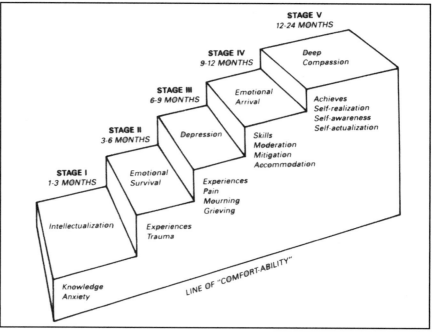

THERAPEUTIC PRESENCE IN THE ATMOSPHERE OF DENIAL OF IMMINENT DEATH

The atmosphere of death denial is very uncomfortable. As was mentioned above, there seems to be an aura of fear surrounding the patient and family member; a false cheerfulness pervades that is edged with an iciness of the need to control every situation, every conversation. Instead of feelings of liberation, genuineness, and authenticity, we feel surrounded by paranoia, fear, defensiveness, and nervous chatter. Silence is often avoided, as is warm eye contact.

When we contribute to the conspiracy of silence, we condemn a patient to the pain of facing death alone.[6] Our task is not to judge those who need to deny death, or to contribute to that conspiracy. Rather, we can help more by accepting their fear, and by realizing that their need to deny is very likely well intentioned.

Active listening skills are imperative, as well as use of touch.[7] Health professionals would do well to find out what the patient has been told, and what the patient's response to what he or she has been told has been. Knowing what the patient has been told allows health professionals to support and interpret the health care team's plan of treatment. How the patient feels dictates the main thrust of the treatment approach.

Whether the patient has accepted the imminence of death or not, our approach to caring remains essentially the same. Debra Flomenhoft, a physical therapist who died of cancer, wrote the following important suggestions after having undergone treatment for over a year, in "Understanding and Helping People Who Have Cancer" published in *Physical Therapy*.[7]

1. Don't be afraid to say the wrong thing, and don't keep silent out of that fear. This is interpreted as avoidance and rejection. Instead of worrying about the content of your response, reach out to the patient and show your support by actively listening and allowing the patient to talk.

2. Learn to recognize your feelings and the effect these feelings may have on the communication process. Direct your predictable anger at something other than the patient.

Table 14-1

STAGE CHARACTERISTICS AND DIFFERENCES OF THE SCHEMATIC GROWTH AND DEVELOPMENT SCALE

STAGE I	STAGE II	STAGE III	STAGE IV	STAGE V
Professional knowledge	Increasing professional knowledge	Deepening of professional knowledge	Acceptance of professional knowledge	Refining of professional knowledge
Intellectualization	Less intellectualization	Decreasing intellectualization	Normal intellectualization	Refining intellectual base
Anxiety	Emotional survival	Depression	Emotional arrival	Deep compassion
Some discomfort	Increasing discomfort	Decreasing discomfort	Increasing comfortableness	Increased comfortableness
Agreeableness	Guilt	Pain	Moderation	Self-realization
Withdrawal	Frustration	Mourning	Mitigation	Self-awareness
Superficial acceptance	Sadness	Grieving	Accommodation	Self-actualization
Providing tangible services	Initial emotional involvement	More emotional involvement	Ego mastery	Professional satisfaction
Utilization of emotional energy on understanding the setting	Increasing emotional involvement	Overidentification with the patient	Coping with loss of relationship	Acceptance of death and loss
Familiarizing self with policies and procedures	Initial understanding of the magnitude of the area of practice	Exploration of own feelings about death	Freedom from concern about own death	Rewarding professional growth and development
Working with families rather than patients	Overidentification with the patient's situation	Facing own death	Developing strong ties with dying patients and families	Development of ability to give of one's self
		Coming to grips with feelings about death	Development of ability to work with, on behalf of, and for the dying patient	Human and professional assessment
			Development of professional competence	Constructive and appropriate activities
			Productivity and accomplishments	Development of feelings of dignity and self-respect
			Healthy interaction	Ability to give dignity and self-respect to dying patient
				Feeling of comfortableness in relation to self, patient, family and the job

Reprinted with permission from Harper B. *Death: The Coping Mechanism of the Health Professional.* Greenville, SC: Southeastern University Press; 1977.

3. When patients ask the hard questions, like, "Why me?" don't respond by trying to "fix it." Patients aren't looking for answers as much as they are expressing grief and anger. Allow that expression. Supportive listening is the best response.

4. Recognize the importance of touch, even as simple as a handshake or a touch on the shoulder. Communicate with touch and eye contact that you care, and that you are there to listen and to do whatever you can to maintain or improve the quality of the patient's life.

5. Don't assume that patients want to talk about their illness. Ask the patient if he or she wants to talk about his or her illness before initiating a discussion.

6. Never assume that you know what the patient is feeling. Ask instead, "Am I right that you are feeling...?"

7. Communicate confidence in your therapeutic skills both verbally and nonverbally. This is essential for patient trust. Answer the patient with authority and no hesitation, and if you don't know the answer, simply say, "I can't answer that, but I will find out who can."

8. Don't try to anticipate which stage of coping patients are in, or that they will progress through the stages in exact linear sequence. Accept patients where they are, each day, with caring and understanding. Try to view the impending death from the patient's perspective, not from the theory of dealing with loss.

9. Take care not to contribute to isolation of the patient as death nears. Once a relationship has been established, work to maintain it, even if the required therapy is minimal, or the patient has been discharged from your service. Stopping in to say hello, no matter how busy you are, will mean a great deal.

10. Help patients maintain hope at all costs. Maintaining hope is not in direct conflict with being realistic. The value of hope far exceeds the need to face the truth of the inevitable. One can feel hope in spite of imminent death, and it is important to nurture and sustain it, being both realistic and hopeful at the same time. Learn to communicate honestly and frankly, always with hope.

11. Take care of your own emotional needs to prevent professional burnout so that you can continue to communicate care, sympathy, and support to the patient and family. If you need help in dealing with your feelings, get it. Your patient can't wait for you to grow at your own pace.[7]

What do dying patients want and deserve to have with regard to care? Table 14-2 illustrates "The Dying Person's Bill of Rights," which was developed by the Southwestern Michigan Inservice Education Council.[8] Read each item carefully. They represent the minimal goals for care by which we all should be guided.

HOSPICE CARE

One effective way of helping to assure therapeutic effectiveness in caring for the dying is the Hospice movement. Hospice is not a building, but a philosophy of care that promises that the patient will die with pain controlled to the greatest possible extent, and that the quality of life will become the primary focus of all treatment. Interdisciplinary team members each contribute to the care of the patient by direct services, often in the home, and by teaching family members and volunteers how to ensure that the quality of life for the patient remains as high as possible. Pain is controlled while maintaining alertness. Death is accepted as inevitable, and family members are encouraged to talk openly with patients in preparation for the time of death.

In addition to effective control of pain, it is important for the physical and occupational therapist to teach the patient and family how to keep the "lived world" of the patient as large as possible for as long as possible. By "lived world," I mean the world that is accessible to the patient to live in. Traditionally our lived world shrinks from almost limitless possibilities (given funds and opportu-

Table 14-2	

THE DYING PERSON'S BILL OF RIGHTS

I have the right to be treated as a living human being until I die.

I have the right to maintain a sense of hopefulness, however changing its focus may be.

I have the right to be cared for by those who can maintain a sense of hopefulness, however changing this might be.

I have the right to express my feelings and emotions about my approaching death, in my own way.

I have the right to participate in decisions concerning my case.

I have the right to expect continuing medical and nursing attention even though "cure" goals must be changed to "comfort" goals.

I have the right not to die alone.

I have the right to be free from pain.

I have the right to have my questions answered honestly.

I have the right not to be deceived.

I have the right to have help from and for my family in accepting my death.

I have the right to die in peace and dignity.

I have the right to retain my individuality and not be judged for my decisions, which may be contrary to the beliefs of others.

I have the right to expect that the sanctity of the human body will be respected after death.

I have the right to be cared for by caring, sensitive, knowledgeable people who will attempt to understand my needs and will be able to gain some satisfaction.

Adapted from Barbus A. The dying person's bill of rights. Presented at: *The Terminally Ill Patient and the Helping Person*, South Western Michigan Inservice Education Council; Lansing, Mich; 1975.

nity to travel) to confinement to a chair or bed in one room as we age and become unable to move about. Range of motion, ambulation with support, bed mobility, getting up for meals, even placing the bed in the living room in front of a window all help to prevent the lived world of the patient from shrinking to a circle on the ceiling above the bed, as some patients have reported. The quality of life has every bit to do with how much of the world is available for us to experience.

Family members are encouraged to be around the patient as the patient requests. Pets are allowed to be close by. The atmosphere becomes one of living life fully.

Pain control is made possible through finely titrated narcotics, massage and exercise to the patient's tolerance, and the use of transcutaneous electrical stimulation to the nervous system (TENS). Data show that patients respond very favorably to this modality, especially in the presence of severe, intractable pain often accompanying imminent death.[9]

Importance of a Living Will—The Schiavo Case

Throughout the latter part of 2004 and early 2005, the media in the United States detailed the struggle of Terri Schiavo, a young woman in Florida who had been in an irreversible coma for over 10 years and was being cared for in a hospice. Her husband wanted to honor her verbal wishes to not have her life extended by extraordinary means under these circumstances, but since Ms. Schiavo never wrote down her wishes in a living will or end-of-life document, her parents contested her husband's decision to remove her feeding tube and allow her to die and took their case to the Florida Supreme Court. The Court ruled that her husband had the final authority, not her parents, and ruled in favor of the husband. The parents appealed, but lost in court, and Terri Schiavo died peacefully a week after the removal of the feeding tube, with her husband at her side.

There were many lessons learned from this case. Primary is the importance of writing down and sharing with close family members your wishes for end of life care as specifically as you can. This is an ethical dilemma between beneficence and autonomy. It seemed as though everyone wanted to do for Terri Schiavo what they felt she wanted, but no written instructions were made to help them. The court ruled that her husband had more recent and intimate knowledge of her wishes than her parents, but her parents had been caring for her for the better part of the last decade of her life, and found great meaning in that process. They held out hope that one day she would wake up and heal from this crisis.

Unfortunately, the main fact that the media failed to mention, time after time, in many of the debates was that those who believed Terri Schiavo would wake up one day and be back to her old self didn't know or chose to ignore for personal reasons that this was impossible, given the MRI images of her brain. Her ventricles had expanded to the point that the greater percentage of her cranium was filled with fluid; insufficient gray matter existed to support meaningful cognition.

Terri Schiavo went into cardiac arrest as a result of a metabolic electrolyte imbalance in her early 20s, most likely due to a life long struggle with anorexia. When young people are doing their best to be approved of and loved by others, the last thing on their mind would be to create a living will. The fear of death, or the superstition that thinking about one's death will bring it on, must be faced to confront this issue in a mature way. Perhaps Terri Schiavo's gift to others will be to point out the extreme dangers of anorexia and to emphasize the critical importance of creating a living will and communicating to your loved ones your wishes if you should lapse into irreversible coma or brain death.

OTHER ISSUES

This chapter does not have the space to deal with several important issues that accompany a consideration of death. The moral issues of "mercy killing" or euthanasia (both active and passive), suicide, the unique needs of persons with AIDS, and the current fascination with past lives as described by Dr. Brian L. Weiss[10] are just 4 issues that would require greater attention than this chapter can give them. After the fear of death is confronted, it becomes easier to read and study such topics independently. All are critically important to one's development as a healing professional.

Finally, there exists some controversy around the topic of near-death experiences as researched by Moody[11] and colleagues and around the person of Elisabeth Kübler-Ross.[12] Any consideration of death must, by necessity, incorporate the spiritual, for to ask, "Why have I lived?" is a spiritual question. It is within this category of awareness that much criticism was leveled at Kübler-Ross. I would encourage you to read about this controversy and form your own opinions. Once you have experienced the death of one who resides in your innermost circles of self, these readings, indeed, this entire chapter, will likely assume new meaning. For now, deal with this material seriously and as best you can.

Victor Frankl,[13] a survivor of 2 Nazi death camps, has said, "Everything can be taken from a man [or woman} but one thing: the last of the human freedoms—to choose one's attitude in any given set of circumstances, to choose one's own way."[13] To accept death as a necessary part of life is not resignation; it is surrender to an opportunity to grow into one's own complete humanness.

I conclude with the following thoughts from Elisabeth Kübler-Ross:[1]

> *We are living in a time of uncertainty, anxiety, fear, and despair. It is essential that you become aware of the light, power, and strength within each of you, and that you learn to use those inner resources in service of your own and others' growth. The world is in desperate need of human beings whose own level of growth is sufficient to enable them to learn to live and work with others cooperatively and lovingly, to care for others—not for what those others can do for you or for what they think of you, but rather in terms of what you can do for*

them. If you send forth love to others, you will receive in return the reflection of that love; because of your loving behavior, you will grow, and you will shine a light that will brighten the darkness of the time we live in—whether it is in a sickroom of a dying patient, on the corner of a ghetto street in Harlem, or in your own home. Humankind will survive only through the commitment and involvement of individuals in their own and others' growth and development as human beings. [Through this commitment will come]… the evolution of the whole species to become all that humankind can and is meant to be. Death is the key to that evolution. For only when we understand the real meaning of death to human existence will we have the courage to become what we are destined to be.

CONCLUSION

This text is devoted to helping you as health professionals grow to be mature and healing in your very nature, so that your actions with those needing your help will be healing and therapeutically whole. Elisabeth Kübler-Ross has said, "For only when we understand the real meaning of death to human existence will we have the courage to become what we are destined to be."[1]

The goals for this chapter, therefore, are for you to confront your own fears about death at whatever level you can at this time in order for you to become more aware of whom you are to be. By way of reflection on this content and completing the exercises, you will conduct a current values clarification about death, recognizing your experiences of death-denying rather than life-affirming ways.

What should our goals be with persons who are facing imminent death? In sum, what we want to achieve with dying patients includes the following:

- ❖ Assist the patient to remain in control of most decisions concerning daily life for as long as possible.
- ❖ Keep the patient's "lived world" (the world available for the patient to move about) as large as possible for as long as possible by helping the family learn to transfer or assist with ambulation or wheelchair management, assist with transfers out of bed, move the bed to an appropriate place to avoid isolation.
- ❖ Control pain with medication, activity, imagery, and TENS, yet allow maximum alertness.
- ❖ Along with other health care team members, perform professional skills with self-confidence and patience, being sure to include the patient and family in the therapeutic process.
- ❖ Provide support for loved ones and family, realizing each is in different stages of coping with the impending loss of a loved one.
- ❖ Utilize active listening skills and touch as our primary forms of communication, allowing the dying person to have control over the topics and length of conversations.
- ❖ Avoid the desire to want to "fix" anything.
- ❖ Be willing to stand by, to touch, to reach out, and to risk in the face of our own fears.
- ❖ Clarify in writing, following these exercises, your wishes at the end of your life.

No easy task. Stanley Kellerman, in *Living Your Dying*,[14] says, "There's big dying and there's little dying…" As health professionals we confront loss of health and mobility as a "little death" rather regularly. In your day-to-day patient care, always remember that people cope with little deaths similarly to big deaths.

So now move on to the exercises, and don't forget to journal about what you're feeling, and about what you've learned.

REFERENCES

1. Kübler-Ross E. *Death—The Final Stage of Growth.* Englewood Cliffs, NJ: Prentice Hall; 1975.
2. Becker E. *The Denial of Death.* New York: The Free Press; 1973.
3. Agee J. *A Death in the Family.* New York, NY: Grosset and Dunlap; 1957.
4. Duncan I. *My Life.* New York, NY: Liveright Publishing Corp; 1955.
5. Kübler-Ross E. *On Death and Dying.* New York, NY: Macmillan; 1969.
6. Harper B. *Death: The Coping Mechanisms of the Health Professional.* Greenville, SC: Southeastern University Press; 1977.
7. Flomenhoft DA. Understanding and helping people who have cancer. *Phys Ther.* 1984;4:1232-1234.
8. Barbus A. The dying person's bill of rights. Presented at: *The Terminally Ill Patient and the Helping Person.* South Western Michigan Inservice Education Council; Lansing, Mich; 1975.
9. Reuss R. Hospice: one PT's personal account. *Clin Manag.* 1985:4(6):28-37.
10. Weiss BL. *Many Lives, Many Master.* New York, NY: Simon and Schuster; 1990.
11. Moody R. The light beyond. *New Age Journal.* 1988;May-June:55-67.
12. Nietzke A. The miracle of Kübler-Ross. *Human Behavior Magazine.* 1977:206-211,254.
13. Frankl V. *Man's Search for Meaning.* New York, NY: Washington Square Press; 1963.
14. Kellerman S. *Living Your Dying.* New York, NY: Random House; 1974.
15. Worden JW, Proctor W. *Personal Death Awareness.* Englewood Cliffs, NJ, Prentice Hall; 1976.

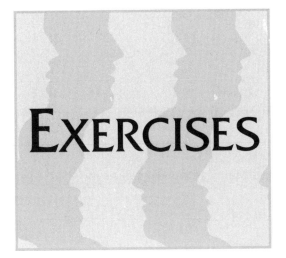

EXERCISES

EXERCISE 1: PERSONAL DEATH HISTORY

Answer the following history questions below.

1. The first death I ever experienced was the death of:

2. I was ___ years old.

3. At that time I felt:

4. I was most curious about:

5. The things that frightened me most were:

6. The feelings I have now as I think of that death are:

7. The first funeral I ever attended was for:

8. The most intriguing thing about the funeral was:

9. I was most scared or upset at the funeral by:

10. The first personal acquaintance of my own age who died was:

11. I remember thinking:

12. I lost my first parent when I was:

13. The death of this parent was especially significant because:

14. The most recent death I experienced was when _____ died _____ years ago.

15. The most traumatic death I ever experienced was:

16. At age _____ I personally came closest to death when:

17. The most significant loss I have ever had to endure was:

    Because:

What insights come to you as you review your answers, or as you discuss your answers with a classmate? What do these answers have to do with your current ideas about death? The next exercise will help you clarify your current ideas.

Adapted from Worden JW, Proctor W. *Personal Death Awareness.* Englewood Cliffs, NJ, Prentice Hall; 1976.

EXERCISE 2: VALUES AROUND DEATH AND DYING

In order to better clarify your current feelings, attitudes, and beliefs concerning death and dying, please reflect on and respond to the following questions:

1. When I die, I believe that (what will happen?):

2. I would rather die (suddenly and without warning…or after being given a period of time in which to say goodbye to loved ones? What beliefs make me say this?):

3. When I die, I'd like the following to be done. (Be as specific as possible. Make a list.):

4. The person I want to be in charge of this process is:

   Because:

5. The worst possible thing that could happen to me around my dying and death is:

6. As a health professional, the best thing I can do for my dying patients and their families is:

   Because:

EXERCISE 3: LIFE LINE

Draw a line that best represents your total life span. At the end of the line, mark the year, and your age, at the point of your death. Indicate the ups and downs of your life by labeling them with words and dates.

1. Reflections:

   a. How does it feel to consider the total span of your life? Remember, feelings are one word, like anxious or exciting, not "I feel like my life..."

   b. How would you characterize your life so far? More "up" than "down," or the reverse, or neutral? What are the major forces that have contributed to this assessment?

   c. Did you have difficulty actually marking the date of your death? Some people think this a difficult, if not impossible, task. If you did, why? Why not?

   d. Do you have certain life goals that you can identify? If so, identify them, and then comment on how well you feel you are progressing toward them. Indicate what goals you expect to have achieved at certain points along your lifeline.

2. Journal about this experience.

STRESS MANAGEMENT

Carol M. Davis, PT, EdD, MS, FAPTA

OBJECTIVES

1. To define burnout and explore personal sources of stress.
2. To explore the effects of stress on the body and on our perceptions of situations.
3. To discuss the negative effects of health care reorganization on quality of care and provider stress.
4. To discuss the stress development model.
5. To describe external and internal factors which contribute to the build-up of stress in professional helpers.
6. To emphasize the importance of one's thoughts on the quality of life.
7. To explore mechanisms that interfere with the build-up of stress, and thus help us to control the negative effects of stress.

One of the most powerful rewards of the healing professions is the tremendous job satisfaction it brings. Most people enter the helping professions in order to work with people who need help in overcoming illness or disability, or to help well people stay well and fit. The expectation is that it is a career in which one assumes that each day will be interesting and rewarding and expects to feel a great deal of personal satisfaction and meaning in helping others. Few people ever anticipate or prepare for the tremendous amount of stress that is inherent in the helping professions. Despite the deepest feelings of caring and altruism, caring for people who need help can bring with it great emotional and physical exhaustion to those who do not prepare for it.

STRESS

Let's take a closer look at stress in general. Stress is a value neutral word, that is, it need not indicate something negative. In fact, stress is simply a response to being alive, and the human organism requires certain stress in order to have something to respond to, to live.

What we perceive as negative stress results from our inability to solve a problem or to reach a goal that is believed (or feared) to be unattainable. We feel out of control, and tension arises from attempts to figure out how to get back in control and reach our goal.[1] It's like standing at the bottom of a huge mountain and not knowing how in the world we'll ever manage to get to the top.

This kind of stress has effects on our perspective of the situation, and it has effects on our bodies. When we feel the anxiety of negative stress, we tend to misread the situation at hand, we tend to blow things out of proportion, take on unrealistic guilt or internalize and personalize thoughts that have little to do with us. For example, let's say you feel under the stress of seeing 5 more patients in the next 15 minutes (an unattainable goal), and a colleague comes into your office and is noticeably upset about something. There's a high likelihood that one of your immediate responses to your colleague would be, "Oh great! What did I do now?"

The fact is that often you are not the cause of another person's anger or frustration, and you increase your stress by making that erroneous assumption. Under stress you've simply distorted a situation and, depending on the energy of your paranoia, blew it all out of proportion. Stress distorts our ability to see the world as it truly is, and this distortion then increases our stress, causing a positive progression or escalation of our anxiety. The greater the existing stress, the more likely the addition of more stress. In other words, a positive feedback loop is established.

Stressors Commonly Experienced by Health Care Professionals

The health care profession underwent massive change in the last 2 decades of the last century and currently continues to reflect those changes. The impact of managed care on the quality of care of patients has a mixed review, but for the most part, patients now report more depersonalized care, are disappointed with the quality of the care they are receiving, particularly the lack of individual time spent with their providers, and resent the increasing cost of health insurance.[2,3] A study examining the impact of the changing health care environment on fieldwork education in occupational therapy revealed that stress was increased by increased productivity expectations, number of hours worked, and time spent in documentation, with a decrease in job security, time for continuing education and quality of patient care.[4] In a study of primary care physician practices, patients reported a lower rating on the quality of care from physicians in managed care practices.[5] In a literature review in 2003, the most common sources of workplace stress for nurses included more intense workload, conflicts with leadership/management style, professional conflicts in general, and the emotional cost of caring.[5] In sum, it is a sign of the times that the environment of health care has changed significantly to become more stressful for health care professionals and their patients, and it will take a quantum shift for health care to once again be characterized by healing and less by business practices. When patients become a means to an end for profit, the stress on health care professionals who want to serve those in need becomes enormous when they are forced by organizations to pay more attention to the "bottom line."

Stressors Commonly Experienced by Students

Purtilo discusses ongoing anxieties commonly related to student life.[1] Remember that negative stress is experienced in the presence of a fear that a goal that we've set is unattainable. She reports that students respond most dramatically to 3 anxiety-provoking questions throughout their education:

1. *Am I good enough*? Not only troublesome just before exams, but also an ongoing fear related to questions of moral and intellectual competence—in other words, this is an issue of self-esteem and can be fueled by constant comparison of oneself to "more talented" classmates and professionals.

2. *Do I have what it takes?* Similar to question 1, this relates to perceptions of and fears about one's physical and emotional limits. This anxiety rears its ugly head the first time a student feels faint while in a hospital, or experiences the exhaustion of long hours of work without breaks.

3. *Can I pay?* The cost of tuition is steadily rising without a concurrent increase in financial aid. The anxiety of having to take out another loan, take on another job, or quit altogether weighs on students and often affects their performance in classes and clinics.

Life issues go on while students are in school, and as the age of students entering the professions increases, life issues become more complex, with families and partners to be concerned about. For example, illnesses, pregnancies, having to move, and marital and/or parent problems don't automatically disappear while the student finishes his or her education. These anxieties feed into the base level of life stress and can markedly affect students' abilities to learn.

Physical Effects of Stress

Stress takes its toll physically, as well. Now that medicine has made great strides in eradicating infectious disease, most illnesses are of chronic nature, and most chronic diseases have been found to be greatly influenced by stress. When we perceive stress, the endocrine system goes into action. This was quite useful when we depended upon the sympathetic nervous system for our survival in the jungle. "Fight or flight" was at one time our only alternative in stressful situations, most of which were, indeed, life threatening. However, it seems as if our nervous system has not kept up with our progress as a civilized society. Few wild animals threaten our survival, but in some situations we respond as if that were exactly the case.[6] This outpouring of adrenaline and other neuro-peptides acts as a stressor on our bodies.[7] Peoples' physical responses differ. Some suffer from headaches, others from diarrhea, nausea, cardiac palpitations, etc. Over time, organ systems break down under this constant stress, and the result might be diabetes, high blood pressure, ulcers, colitis or arthritis, or chronic fatigue.

Stress Development Model

The key to understanding stress and preventing its negative effects lies in understanding the following model:

Life situation → Perception → Emotion → Physiological Response → Disease

The life situation is *not* the key component in this model; it is the perception that I have that this life situation is a tiger that is going to eat me unless I get out of here fast, or fight like crazy for my survival. Some people live all day every day as if there were a tiger just around the corner. They have learned a worldview that life is a hostile place and one must always be on guard.[6] (Remember that Chapter 2 gives us insights into how people learn this worldview.) Others simply periodically find themselves in situations where they realize that their stress is too high, that the worldview has been distorted, and that it is time to get a grip on things and time to do what we must to get back in control of their lives.

How Misperceptions Develop

When there is, indeed, a misperception of the current situation, it is most often a result of the influence of past experience. We become programmed in a sense, based on unfortunate things that have happened to us in the past and thus we misperceive what is happening right now and we fear the unknown of the future. As a result, we allow history or old data to distort the present and our anxiety mounts.

Thought is at the heart of all stress. Actually, our thoughts create our reality in the largest sense. When you think of it (pun intended), there are 4 kinds of thoughts. Only one kind of thought is truly beneficial to the quality of our lives—positive thoughts. Thoughts that are focused on optimism, possibility, connection with others and the world, gratitude, appreciation, and love are thoughts that will develop a feeling of oneness, confidence, and hopefulness. However, too often we are consumed by negative thoughts, wasted thoughts (if only I had...) and neutral thoughts (thoughts needed to get through the day). Thoughts lead to feelings that lead to attitudes, which lead to actions and behavior, which lead to habits, which lead to destiny.

The key, then, to changing the negative effects of stress is to examine carefully the nature of our thoughts and our misperceptions. Negative thoughts leave us feeling exhausted, worried, frustrated, drained, combative, and angry. Positive thoughts leave us feeling hopeful, appreciative, optimistic, caring. We have an internal mechanism that can help us recognize immediately if our thoughts are helpful or stressful. If we can interrupt the stress build-up by changing what we think and what we believe about what is happening, then the emotion will be more realistic, and the sympathetic nervous system need not be overstimulated. By reaching for the positive thought, and making the best of a situation, we can literally transform our day from stressful to uplifting, but this takes practice.

Learning to "stay in the present" is a place to start. As soon as we begin to feel anxious, we should take a deep breath and simply say to ourselves, "Stay in the now. Do not be influenced by the past that is gone forever, or the future that has yet to happen. Listen carefully to what is going on now. Do not personalize or react. Listen."[6] This is not an easy thing to do, for our reactions are firmly set in place by years of habitual ways of thinking. To interrupt these ingrained habits takes conscious practice and commitment to change. The skill of staying in the "now" is best learned by purposefully quieting your mind. This can be done by learning meditation techniques such as Transcendental Meditation,[7] or by practicing tracking your breath for 10 to 30 minutes every day. Sit quietly and practice focusing 100% of your concentration on the breath as it flows in and out of your nostrils. Quiet the "monkey-chatter" in your brain, let all thoughts float away in imaginary bubbles, and simply breathe. Soon your body will relax, and your parasympathetic nervous system will help you to slow down and feel more centered and peaceful.

BURNOUT

Burnout is a term that has been popularized to indicate a state of emotional and physical exhaustion that results from intense and long-standing professional stress. Christina Maslach first described burnout in 1976.[8] Interestingly, the subjects in her investigation were human service personnel, or people helpers. The fact is, that when we agree to help people, there are always professional demands that seem impossible to meet and this creates stress and tension that builds over time. This professional stress and tension has been termed "burnout," and it is a dynamic process that is fed by a negative self-concept and negative job attitudes, which result in a loss of concern for people, a withdrawal from interaction, and alienation from the work environment.[9]

Signs and Symptoms of Burnout

Health professionals enter the professions with enthusiasm and optimism and often soon realize that the demands of the work far exceed their expectations. The common response is to double the effort, with little change in productivity.[5] Soon fatigue and discouragement set in.

The stress of the intense emotional demands of health care interaction builds, and a common coping mechanism is to distance oneself, or become emotionally detached from work.[9] Detachment is often unconscious and can take the form of actual physical withdrawal, spending shorter time with people, or emotional withdrawal, objectifying people, for example, by labeling them. A patient with back pain becomes "the low back in 343."

Other signs of burnout are the drawing of crisp boundaries between work and home; compartmentalizing one's life sharply; and demonstrating less creativity in treatment, offering more rigid, "by the book" responses to problems, lowering the risk of making a mistake. Feelings of personal inadequacy from not achieving (often unrealistic) goals can result in self-dissatisfaction, which results in projected anger and frustration. People tend to stay away from you because of your "short fuse."

At-home burnout can contribute to marital tension. There is a tendency to engage in compulsive behavior (addictions) to numb oneself from stress, so use of food, drugs, sex, and alcohol may increase. Physical signs such as headaches, stomach ailments, or problems with elimination begin to appear. Sleep may be disturbed. By this time one is well on the way to increased absenteeism and begins to job hunt or seriously considers applying to graduate school, often believing that finding the right "place" to work, or be, will solve all of these problems.

Table 15-1 illustrates that the symptoms of burnout permeate several areas of our lives and build over time, and, as they escalate, they can be seen to fall into 4 stages. Stage One, Enthusiasm, characterizes the symptoms of early burnout mentioned before. Without appropriate intervention, a person inevitably progresses to Stage Four, which carries many of the symptoms of a full-scale depression.[10] Stage Four burnout is a serious condition, and very often professional help is needed to free oneself from this situation.

Causes of Burnout

Factors that lead to burnout can be grouped into internal and external causes. External causes include conditions in the workplace that make it virtually impossible to experience consistent success such as:

1. Work overload
    a. Understaffed conditions
    b. Overload of too many of one type of patient or one type of activity; not enough variety.
    c. Inability to use professional skills and creativity due to lack of time.
2. Role ambiguity
    a. Less than clear guidelines of boundaries of responsibility.
    b. Nebulous expectations not communicated clearly.
3. Role conflict
    a. Several professionals perceive they are responsible for achieving the same goal. Especially apparent in multidisciplinary team situations in which there is inadequate communication.
    b. Physicians make all decisions with no regard for input from other professionals.[10]

Internal causes of burnout are more difficult to identify and often are more challenging to influence. They include:

1. Professional's self-esteem. How individuals view themselves personally and professionally has impact on their work. Low self-esteem facilitates imagined feelings of failure.
2. Inability to set clear boundaries between personal and professional needs. Unclear ideas about the motives for wanting to help people (ie, the desire to "fix it" for people rather than encouraging autonomy) results in inadvertently contributing to patients' neediness and dependence on health care workers, which results in a feeling of becoming too close, or trapped in a relationship with a patient.
3. The establishment of unrealistically optimistic goals for patients and the failure to meet them, which lowers self-image, a common event from overachieving new graduates. Intervention and guidance is required from mentors or supervisors.[10]

	Table 15-1

MANIFESTATIONS OF BURNOUT IN OCCUPATIONAL THERAPISTS

Components	Stage 1: Enthusiasm	Stage 2: Stagnation	Stage 3: Frustration	Stage 4: Apathy
Personal characteristics	Do I invest my whole self in my work?	Am I beginning to question whether I like my job and whether it meets my personal needs?	Am I not only questioning the value of my job but also the value of the entire profession?	Am I feeling totally disinterested in my job?
	Do I set extremely high goals for myself?	Am I beginning to see that there are limitations in my work environment?	Do I blame myself when a patient does not improve or return to treatment?	Do I avoid work by using all of my sick time? Am I disinterested in patient progress?
Modality use	Do I work toward increasing my repertoire of activities and/or attempt to create new program ideas?	Do I find myself using the same activities over and over again?	Is my stress so great that I no longer feel creative?	Do I always let the patients choose their activity, even when another modality may be more therapeutic?
	Do I verbally discuss with my patients the purpose of an activity and the progress that I have observed?	Do I focus with the patient on only one or two aspects of their performance?	Do I look at product versus process?	Am I disinterested in my patient's response to the modality selected?
Use of theoretical	Am I interested in learning about new theories and applying them to my practice?	Do I prefer to use the theory base with which I am most comfortable? Do I attempt to use new concepts after discussion with peers and supervisors?	Do I find new theories to be a waste of time and more professional jargon?	Do I find myself using no theoretical base at all?
Interdisciplinary relationships	Do I attempt to engage other disciplines in the activity process?	Do I get annoyed when people from other disciplines ask to observe my groups?	Do I feel competitive with other team members and avoid talking to them outside required meetings?	Do I feel there is no need to deal with my team about unresolved issues because nothing helps?

continued

Table 15-1 (cont)

Components	Stage 1: Enthusiasm	Stage 2: Stagnation	Stage 3: Frustration	Stage 4: Apathy
	Do I work to increase communication among team members and to effectively resolve conflicts?	Do I feel that my domain is being stepped on by other team members?	Do I find myself expressing my anger about the team to the other therapists in my department?	
Education	Do I enjoy the opportunity to educate others about what I do as an occupational therapist?	Do I get tired of always having to explain my practice?	Am I beginning to resent the need to always educate others, especially team members?	Do I avoid having to explain what to do?
Budget	Do I find it easy to adapt to a low budget by finding creative ways to use limited supplies?	Am I becoming tired of the constant need to adapt my programs to supply and budget constraints?	Do I find myself frequently complaining to my coworkers and supervisor about our limited budget and supplies?	Have I given in to our low budget by limiting my program to only those supplies that are readily available?
Response to supervision and increased responsibilities	Do I look forward to supervision and the opportunity to improve my job performance?	Do I become anxious when my supervisor suggests a change or that I take on additional responsibilities?	Do I resent changes implemented within the department and frequently discuss my resentment with my peers?	Do I avoid work because of what will happen next?
Professional development	Do I actively pursue workshops, seminars, and courses to improve my skills?	Do I find that outside of work I always choose to pursue activities other than continuing education?	Do I find suggestions to pursue continuing education to be an imposition? Will I pursue these activities only on work time?	Am I disinterested in professional activities and continuing education?
	Do I put a lot of energy into my professional organizations?	Am I questioning the value of the profession and its organization?		

Reprinted with permission from Apter LC, Kolodner EL. Professional burnout—are you a candidate? *Phys Ther Forum*. 1987; 6:10.

INTERVENTION

Previously we've discussed the importance of perception in handling stress. Cultivating an ability to "stay present" or "stay in the now," resisting the habit of interpreting present, ongoing events from past history or fear of the future will greatly assist one in remaining clear and realistic from moment to moment. Asking clarification questions and employing active listening skills will reduce the tendency to personalize and take undue responsibility for others' problems. Learning to inventory one's thoughts by checking on how you feel is critical to replacing negative thoughts with more energetic and hopeful thoughts that feel better.

However, the next step in reducing the problem of burnout is recognition that it is occurring, that it is happening right now to you, and choosing to believe that you have the power to stop its escalation. Since burnout has both internal and external antecedents, intervention must take place in both areas.[9]

Externally or organizationally, lowering staff-patient ratios is critical, as is allowing for time away from contact with patients. Time doing less stressful work, such as record keeping, reading journal articles, planning patient research, student education, or quality assurance activity are effective ways to lower the stress exacerbated by intense interaction with people.[8]

Required use of vacation time also helps those who tend to overwork and deny the presence of burnout.[10] Mixing of patient loads and scheduling of regular staff rotations also help reduce the stress of seeing too many of one type of patient.[10]

Organizationally sanctioned support groups are also an effective way to help reduce stress.[11] In these sessions, discussion of feelings is more important than discussion of patient problems.[12] Many health professionals keep fears and feelings of personal failure to themselves, but most will welcome the opportunity to discuss frustrations concerning patients, especially if the organization encourages this opportunity for all its members.[12]

In rehabilitation we must maintain a constant awareness that strict adherence to the medical model of diagnose, treat, discharge "cured" very often does not apply to our patients. Most patients we see have multiple chronic illnesses, and we must learn how to expect an appropriate amount of effort from them, maintaining a somewhat more realistic goal than a hope for a cure.[10] Patients' values and hopes must be clearly delineated and integrated into any plan of care.[13]

Studying burnout and its prevention while still in school gives you an added advantage before you get caught up in the confusing situations that your first position offers. Internally, or personally, health care professionals must develop a realistic view of helping and learn effective ways to handle repeated, intense, emotional interactions with people.[10] Regular exercise is critical in reducing stress. A lunch break that is taken away from the patient care milieu and that includes a brisk walk, bike ride, or swim has immediate and long-term positive benefits. Sufficient sleep and a nutritional diet also serve to keep one's internal stress low.

The logical, systematic left brain is the seat of the anxiety that leads to burnout. It is the left brain that can't seem to figure out how to get the goal met. The right brain, however, is the source of relief from this pressure. The right brain functions by way of pictures, symbols, colors, and dreams. Meditation and activities that balance left and right brain activity and engage the right brain in activities such as daydreaming or imagery for relaxation during breaks in the work day also help.[13] Tracking your breath, as described earlier, is one such activity.

Above and beyond all, however, is the importance of each health professional carefully examining his or her own needs in becoming a health care worker in order to identify and curtail the tendency to overwork that is so common among us.[10] Workaholism is just as addictive as alcohol, food, and drugs. We engage in compulsive behavior in order to keep from dealing with our problems or from feeling the pain of normal growth and development. When work is used to keep us from growing, everyone suffers. Unfortunately, unlike drugs and alcohol that do not carry public sanction, workaholics are often praised for their dedication and allow themselves to be taken advantage of by others.

Eventually workaholics come to the realization that they are receiving from their efforts far less than they are contributing, and often this awareness leads to a temporary decrease in activity, but unless the original pain and need for personal growth are examined and confronted at this time, a new addictive behavior will move in rapidly to fill the void. Remember that Chapter 2 focuses on the need to not only confront compulsive behavior, but to locate and communicate with the abandoned child within all of us to begin the healing process before real change can be experienced.

PREVENTION

Since stress occurs from the perception of the inability to successfully achieve goals, one way to prevent this from occurring is to set goals that are predictably attainable. Stewart [11] writes, "Unless the goals of therapy are agreed upon in the beginning, the therapist and the patient can be forced to work together over a long period of time attempting to achieve goals which are not shared by both." When working with patients, Stewart suggests the following steps to help lower stress:

1. Establish a clear contract with the patient. This should contain an explicit description of the goals and responsibilities of both parties, should take into account the patients' values and priorities.

2. Do not promise more than you are prepared to deliver to the patient, the family, or referring practitioner.

3. Be aware of the patients' feelings of dependency, loneliness, and fears of abandonment. Deal with feelings with active listening, encouraging open discussion. Give plenty of advance notice before taking time off or separating from patients in any way.

Another skill that is useful in helping to keep control over the work environment is assertiveness training, for those who lack the skills needed to communicate ideas for change. Learning how to speak up from a position of personal confidence can help revitalize an entire work setting.[13] Chapter 7 will assist you in developing these skills.

CONCLUSION

Health professionals are responsible for clearly understanding the patients' problem, and, perhaps most important and most stressful, we are responsible for teaching the patient how to avoid future problems; we are responsible for helping people take responsibility for themselves and their health. This can be the most demanding of our obligations to those we serve. We must learn to handle situations that fail to respond to our interventions. We must learn to set realistic limits as to what we're willing and able to do to facilitate change. We must learn to face the inevitability of terminal illness and death. Each of these realities in health care, if perceived as failure, will cause stress, as the ideal, hoped for goal of cure and wellness is unattainable. We set ourselves up to experience burnout if curing is our only goal in health care.

When one enters the health professions, there must be an early commitment to taking care of oneself in order to prevent the negative effects of inevitable stress. In a previous chapter we discussed that people can be seen to be composed of 4 quadrants: the physical, the intellectual, the emotional, and the spiritual. To avoid stress, one must keep a healthy balance of activity and growth in all four quadrants. This would include a commitment to eat well, get enough rest and sleep, get regular exercise, time away from people, emotional confirmation and support, and dedication to play and fun. Many of us who become health professionals who grew up in troubled homes have had to be serious from the very start, and we lack the ability for spontaneous play. If that is true, we must find others to help us. Our healthy survival depends on it.

The exercises are designed to help you identify the amount of stress you are currently experiencing and how that stress affects you physically.

REFERENCES

1. Purtilo RB, Haddad A. *Health Professional/Patient Interaction*. 6th ed. Philadelphia, Pa: WB Saunders; 2002.
2. Barr DA. The effects of organizational structure on primary care outcomes under managed care. *Ann Intern Med*. 1995;1:122(5):353-359.
3. Tu HT. More Americans willing to limit physician-hospital choice for lower medical costs. *Issue Brief Cent Stud Health Syst Change*. 2005; Mar (94):1-5.
4. Casares GS, Bradley KP, Jaffe LE, Lee GP. Impact of the changing environment on fieldwork education: perceptions of occupational therapy educators. *J Allied Health*. 2003;32(4):246-51.
5. Grembowski DE, Patrick DL, Williams B, et al. Managed care and patient related quality of care from primary physicians. *Med Care Res Rev*. 2005;62(1):31-55.
6. Keyes K. *Handbook to higher consciousness*. Coos Bay, Ore: Living Love Publications; 1975.
7. Chopra D. *Ageless Body, Timeless Mind: The Quantum Alternative to Growing Old*. New York, NY: Harmony Books; 1993.
8. Maslach C. Burned-out. *Human Behavior*. 1976;5:16-22.
9. Wolfe GA. Burnout of therapists inevitable or preventable? *Phys Ther*. 1981;61:1046-1050.
10. Apter LC, Kolodner EL. Professional burnout—are you a candidate? *Physical Therapy Forum*. 1987; 6:6-10.
11. Stewart TD. Psychotherapy and physical therapy common grounds. *Phys Ther*. 1977;57:279-283.
12. Pines A, Maslach C. Characteristics of staff burnout in mental health settings. *Hosp Community Psychiatry*. 1978;29:233-237.
13. Davis CM. The "difficult" elderly patient: stressful effects on the therapist. *Topics in Geriatric Rehabilitation*. 1988;3:74-84.

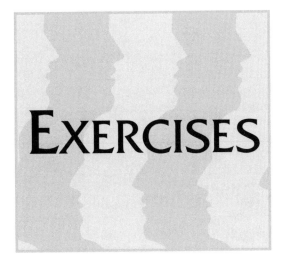

EXERCISES

EXERCISE 1: RECOGNIZING

1. I realize I am stressed when:

   which makes me feel:

   and I react by:

   Afterwards, thinking about it calmly and quietly, I realize and tell myself next time I may choose to:

2. Signs and symptoms of burnout for me:
   a.

   b.

   c.

   d.

   e.

3. Coping mechanisms that I use now within my environment:
   a.

   b.

   c.

   d.

   e.

4. Three things I did last week to take care of myself:
   a.

   b.

   c.

EXERCISE 2: MAJOR SOURCES OF STRESS IN STUDENTS

Purtilo mentions that there are 3 major sources of anxiety for students:[1]
1. Am I good enough? (basically)
2. Do I have what it takes? (physically, emotionally)
3. Can I pay?

First of all, do you agree that these are stressors for you? What would you add to that list? Are there life issues that cause you stress, for example, developing identity and finding a life partner? Is the task of breaking away from your home and parents a major stress for you? Are you concerned that you may have chosen the wrong profession? Do you have a habit of procrastination that gets you into trouble rather consistently? Make a personal list of stressors and prioritize them. Assign relative stress points to each item. Now, journal about how those stressors affect you each day physically, emotionally, mentally, and spiritually. For each stressor, list any actions you might be able and willing to take right now to minimize their negative universe, and learn to put away anxiety about things you have no control over. Carrying a list of constant worries around in your mind or on your back makes it difficult to be present to the world and to people. Develop the habit of taking regular inventory of what you're worried about, what you can do about it right now, and what you must "offer up" and get off your mind. Make it a goal regularly to flush your mind and your heart of anxieties that are not appropriate or welcome. You'll feel lighter if you do.

Table 15-2

MEASURE YOUR STRESS QUOTIENT

This stress-rating chart, designed by Dr. Thomas H. Holmes, provides a measurement of the stress in your life. Check the events that have happened to you in the past year and then add up the total.

Event	Value	Event	Value
Death of Spouse	100	Death of Close Friend	37
Divorce	73	Change to Different Line of Work	36
Marital Separation	65	Trouble with In-Laws	29
Jail Term	63	Outstanding Personal Achievement	28
Death of Close Family Member	63	Spouse Begins or Stops Work	26
Personal Injury or Illness	53	Starting or Finishing School	26
Marriage	50	Change in Living Conditions	25
Fired from Work	47	Revision of Personal Habits	24
Marital Reconciliation	45	Trouble with Boss	23
Retirement	45	Change in Work Hours, Conditions	20
Change in Family Member's Health	44	Change in Residence	20
Pregnancy	40	Change in Schools	20
Sex Difficulties	39	Change in Church Activities	19
Addition to Family	39	Change in Social Activities	18
Business Readjustment	39	Mortgage or Loan Under $10,000	17
Change in Number of Marital Arguments	35	Change in Sleeping Habits	16
Mortgage or Loan Over $10,000	31	Change in Number of Family Gatherings	15
Foreclosure of Mortgage or Loan	30	Change in Eating Habits	15
Change in Work Responsibilities	29	Vacation	13
Son or Daughter Leaving Home	29	Christmas Season	12
Change in Financial Status	38	Minor Violation of the Law	12
		Total	___

Score:

0 to 149	Mild stress	30% chance of illness
150 to 299	Moderate Stress	30 to 80% chance of illness
300+	Severe Stress	80% chance of illness

Adapted from Imes T, Rahe R. The social readjustment rating scale. *J Psychosom Res.* 1967;11:231.

EXERCISE 3: HOLMES STRESS QUOTIENT INVENTORY

The emphasis in this chapter has been on revealing the effects of negative stress on the body and on the emotions. Hans Selye has identified that both positive and negative stressors affect people. Thomas Holmes has published research that correlates the effects of both positive and negative stress. Certain stressors are given a relative value or quotient with regard to their potential effects. Complete the Holmes Stress Quotient Inventory in Table 15-2. How vulnerable are you to the effects of stress at this point in time? What stressors would you add to update this inventory, and what points would you give them? Which ones would you delete?

Table 15-3

PHYSICAL STRESS SYMPTOM SCALE

In the space provided, indicate how often each of the following effects happens to you either when you are experiencing stress, or following exposures to a significant stressor. Respond to each item with a number between 0 and 5, using the following scale: 0=Never, 1=Once or twice a year, 2=Every few months, 3=Every few weeks, 4=Once or more each week, 5=Daily.

Cardiovascular Symptoms
____   Heart pounding
____   Heart racing or beating erratically
____   Cold, sweaty hands
____   Headache (throbbing pain)
____   Subtotal

Respiratory Symptoms
____   Rapid, erratic or shallow breathing
____   Shortness of breath
____   Asthma attack
____   Difficulty in speaking because of poor breathing control
____   Subtotal

Gastrointestinal Symptoms
____   Upset stomach, nausea, or vomiting
____   Constipation
____   Diarrhea
____   Sharp abdominal pains
____   Subtotal

Muscular Symptoms
____   Headaches (steady pain)
____   Back or shoulder pain
____   Muscle tremors or hand shaking
____   Arthritis
____   Subtotal

Skin Symptoms
____   Acne
____   Dandruff
____   Perspiration
____   Excessive dryness of skin or hair
____   Subtotal

Immunity Symptoms
____   Allergy flare-up
____   Catching colds
____   Catching the flu
____   Skin rash
____   Subtotal

Metabolic Symptoms
____   Increased appetite
____   Increased craving for tobacco or sweets
____   Thoughts racing or difficulty sleeping
____   Feelings of crawling anxiety or nervousness
____   Subtotal

____   OVERALL SYMPTOMS TOTAL
(Add all seven subtotals)

Scale:
0 to 5: No predisposition in that symptom
6 to 13: Slightly higher risk of disease in that symptom
14+: Likely to experience psychosomatic disease in that symptom

Adapted from Allen R. *Progressive Neuromuscular Relaxation.* College Park, Md: Autumn Wind Press; 1979.

EXERCISE 4: PHYSICAL STRESS SYMPTOM SCALE

In most families, people react to stress in similar ways. The data is inconclusive as whether this is primarily due to genetic weakness or learned behavior, but it is common to see several people in a family respond to stress with similar symptoms. The Physical Stress Symptom Scale in Table 15-3 will help you identify which organs or systems are most vulnerable to stress. You may want to compare your results with other members of your family.

EXERCISE 5: HOW TO THINK IN A HEALTHIER WAY

Recognizing unhelpful negative thoughts is the first step to stopping them. The best way to change your thinking is to write negative thoughts down and come up with alternatives. The key is to recognize, through negative feelings, that you are thinking negative thoughts, then change those thoughts, and reach for the better thought to pull you up on the emotional scale toward positivity.

Track your thoughts:

Situation: Late for class. Lost track of time. Traffic was unforgiving. No place to park.

Feelings/Body Responses:	**Negative Thought:**	**Alternative Thought:**
Sick to my stomach, down on myself, anxious that I will be embarrassed in front of the group.	I'm not good enough. I'll never be successful. I can't be trusted.	I'm under a lot of stress. I'm making too much of this one incident.

Now it's your turn.

Situation:

Feelings/Body Responses:	**Negative Thought:**	**Alternative Thought:**

AFTERWORD

MY FINAL CONCLUSION, WITH BEST WISHES

One of the goals of this text, and the growth that is expected to accompany working through this text, is to help you grow in self-awareness in order to be less susceptible to professional burnout. Only you can evaluate your current worldview, your current level of self-esteem, you current ability to alter harmful perceptions that contribute to negative stress—and only you can change your self-esteem, only you can alter the perceptions about yourself, about the world, and about other people to the end that you experience a deep sense of personal confidence and satisfaction in your self and in your work. That is my wish for you. You, your patients, and, indeed, the world will benefit from the positive energy that you will convey.

You've got a start toward self-awareness and personal growth. Don't stop. Find ways to continue to take regular personal inventory of your self-esteem and your stress levels. Use your journal to stay on top of feelings that would become buried in the overwhelming amount of work you've agreed to do. Make a personal commitment to ongoing growth in all 4 of your quadrants, and keep a check on the imbalances.

The Signs of Maturation

How will you know when you're succeeding at the maturation process? Someone very wise once offered this description. Life will become more enjoyable, and you will become less worried about making mistakes or not being liked. Relationships will become more important to you than things. You will accept criticism gratefully and graciously, glad for the opportunity to improve. You will not indulge in self-pity, but will begin to see the marvelous opportunities for growth that misfortune and pain often bring. You will not expect special consideration from anyone. You will be aware of your emotions, and you will rarely feel the need to react impulsively in a tense situation. You will meet emergencies with poise; your feelings will not be hurt easily. You will accept responsibility for your own actions without needing to make excuses, readily acknowledging that you are still growing and learning.

You will have grown beyond dualistic, "all or none," "black or white" thinking about the world, and you will be able to tolerate ambiguity. You will recognize that people are doing the best they can, that no one is all bad or all good. You will come to know that true humility is not feeling less important than others are, but believing that everyone else is every bit as important as you are.

You will be less impatient with reasonable delay. You will be willing to adjust yourself to others and their needs. You will be gracious losers and will endure defeat without whining or complaining. You will not worry about things you have no control over, and you will learn how to take control of appropriate things with confidence and sensitivity.

You will not need to boast or call attention to yourself. You will feel sincere joy at the success of others, outgrowing both jealousy and envy. And you will be open-minded enough to thoughtfully listen to the thoughts of others.

Above all, you will not tolerate the mistreatment of human beings by those who are careless in their interactions, especially with those who are ill. You will take personal responsibility to help people realize the negative effects of their fragmenting interactions on you and on others, and you will kindly ask them to change their behavior for the good of all concerned. Best of luck to you as you set out to make the world, and yourself, each better than they were when you started.

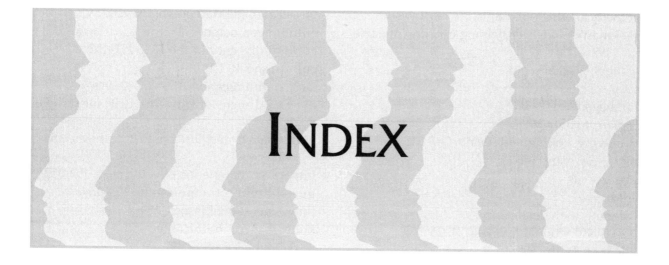

INDEX

acceptance, stage of loss, 247
accountability, 36
active listening, 99, 119, 211
addictive behavior, 25–26
adolescents, interviewing, 169
Adult Children of Alcoholics (ACOA), 24, 26
African American population, 153–154
aggressive behavior, 113
Al-Anon, 26
Alcoholics Anonymous (AA), 26
altruism, 36, 63
ambiguity, 7
Americans with Disabilities Act of 1973, 206, 213, 214
anger
    assertively dealing with, 118
    stage of loss, 246
Anglo-European culture, 154
Asian culture, 155
assertiveness skills
    action, 120–121
    advantages, 119–120
    aggressive behavior, 112–113
    assertive behavior, 113
    assertive responses
        examples, 113
        types of, 114

attribution theory, 114–116
communication challenges, 110
dealing with anger, 118–119
DESC format, 117–118
gender differences, 110–111
learning, 116–117
myths about, 120
nonassertive behavior, 112
personal power
    challenges, 111
    improving, 109
    stressful situations, 111–112
personal rights, 112
training, 109–110
attitudes, 153
attribution theory, 114–116
auditory (A) systems, 138
autonomy, 60, 66

baby boomers, 159
Bandler, Richard, 134
bargaining phase, stage of loss, 247
Bateson, Gregory, 134
Becker, Ernest, 243
behavior, 153
"being" half of life, 3
belief systems, 153

beneficence, 60, 63, 66
Benjamin, Alfred, 172–173
biases, 211–212
biomedical ethics, 57–58
Brickman's models of helping and coping, 190–192
burnout, 264–267

Camus, Albert, 243
Caplan, Arthur, 57
caregiving, coping with death, 247–248
caring. *See* compassion
case law, 66
children
    coping with death, 247
    in dysfunctional families, 24–25
    fear of death, 244
    nervous systems, 18
clarification, 99
clinical decisions, 55–56
closed (dysfunctional) families, 23
code of ethics, 38–39
codependence, 25–26
codes of ethics, 60–61
collectivistic cultures, 154
Combs, A.W., 86
communication skills. *See also* interviewing; therapeutic communication
    definition, 132
    with disabled patients, 205–206
    quantum perspective, 133–134
compassion. *See also* empathy
    definition, 36
    for oneness with all of life, 7
    therapeutic use of self, 38–39
compensatory model of patient education, 191
compulsive behavior, 26
confidentiality, 60
confrontive response, 116
congruence, 100
controllability, 114
coping mechanisms, confronting mortality, 246–248
core values, 38–39
courage, 6
creativity, 34
cross-cultural interactions, 154
"crossing over" phenomenon, 6

cultural factors in patient education, 197
cultural sensitivity
    belief systems, 153
    biases and stigmatization, 211–212
    cultural competence, 152
    cultural diversity in the U.S., 151–152
    culture shock, 149–151
    face communication, 156–157
    hidden dimensions or implicit meanings, 157–158
    high context and low context cultures, 154–156
    impact on therapeutic effectiveness, 152–153
    intercultural communication, 153–154
    intergenerational issues, 159
    nonverbal communication, 158
    in patient education, 197
    personalismo, 158
    related to health care, 154
    somatization, 159
    time and space issues, 157
    universal aspects of health care, 159–160

death. *See also* self
    atmosphere of denial of imminent death, 248–250
    caregivers' responses, 247–248
    confronting our mortality, 245
    "crossing over" phenomenon, 6
    dying person's bill of rights, 251
    existential fear of, 244
    health care concerns, 244–245
    hospice care, 250–251
    imminent, 245–246, 248–250, 253
    importance of a Living Will, 251–252
    preparing for, 246
    quality of life and, 243–244, 246
    stage characteristics, 249
    stages of loss, 246–247
    therapeutic presence, 248–250
defensiveness, 97
    demonstration techniques in patient education, 198
denial, stage of loss, 246
deontological systems, 59–60
deontology, 62, 67
depression, confronting mortality, 246
depression, stage of loss, 247

DESC format, 117–118
developmental psychology, 40
dilemmas, 56
disability. *See also* sexuality and disability
   aging issues, 214–214
   biases and stigmatization, 210
   communication strategies
      active listening, 211
      considerations, 205–206
      empowering language, 209
      labels and word choices, 206
      people-first language, 206
      vocabulary, 206–207
   helping disabled patients, 215–216
   legislative and economic issues, 212–214
   models of, 208
   women with, 215
discernment, 64
discursive ethical reasoning, 58
discussion techniques in patient education, 198
diversity, 7
"doing" half of life, 3
doubt, 7
drug families, 235
dualistic thinking, 7
Duncan, Isadora, 245
dying person's bill of rights, 251

economic issues, 212–214
effective communication, 217–218
ego, 5–6, 8
ego-based emotions, 156
emotions
   acknowledging, 8
   emotion-laden interchanges, 97
   recognizing, 7–8
   therapeutic communication, 96
empathy
   definition, 8
   in interactive processes, 85
   in the interpersonal interaction processes, 83–84
empowering language, 209
enlightenment model of patient education, 191
entrepreneurial spirit, 34
environmental issues, 58
Erickson, Milton, 134

Erikson, Erik, psychosocial theory of development, 18, 19–22
ethics. *See also* moral values
   biomedical ethics versus everyday ethics, 57–58
   challenges, 37–38
   components of ethical action, 58
   definition, 55
   ethic of care, 64–65
   ethical consciousness, 39–40
   ethical distress, 65
   ethical principles, 70
   ethical situations, 56, 69
   ethical system, 58–60
   laws and statutes, 65
   nondiscursive approach to ethical dilemma resolution, 62–63
   RIPS professional analysis model, 66–68
   rules of veracity, 67
   solving ethical problems, 67–68
   virtue ethics, 63–64
ethnic groups, 153–154
ethnocentrism, 160
everyday ethics, 57–58
excellence, 36
exercises
   assertiveness skills, 122–129
   communicating with the dying and their families, 255–258
   cultural sensitivity, 163–165
   effective communication, 102–107
   effective helping, 90–93
   family history, 28–31
   helping disabled patients, 217–218
   interviewing, 175–186
   moral values, 73–77
   NLP (neurolinguistic psychology), 143–146
   self-awareness, 10–14
   sexuality and disability, 238–241
   stress management, 271–275
   values as determinants of behavior, 45–53
   external locus of control, 192–193

face communication, 156–157
family history
   characteristics, 19
   codependence, 25–26
   dysfunctional, 23

healthy, 23
    role in self-esteem, 18–22
    styles of relating, 17
fear-based axioms, 63
fellow feeling, 85
fidelity, 60
Flesch formula, 199–200
Flomenhoft, Debra, 248–250
Frankl, Victor, 252
Freud, Sigmund, 5

Generation X, 159
gestalt therapy, 134
Gilligan, Carol, 40, 41–42, 61–62, 156
Glaser, Jack, 67
"good boy-nice-girl" orientation, 42
goodness of our humanness, 6–7
greeting cards, 25–26
Grinder, John, 134
growth, 7, 8. See also self-awareness
Gunning Fog Index, 199–200

handicap, definition, 206
Harper, Beatrice, 247
healing attitude, 168–169
health behavior
    definition, 190
    health promotion model, 193
    patient's noncompliance, 189–190
    theories
        health belief model, 192
        locus of control, 192–193
        self-efficacy, 193
    trans-theoretical model, 194
health care professionals. See also assertiveness
        skills; stress management
    active listening, 99
    beliefs of effective helpers, 87–88
    common stressors, 262–263
    communicating with disabled patients, 206–
        210
    communication skills, 96–97
    confronting fear of death, 244–245
    discussing sexuality and disability, 223
    emotion-laden interchanges, 97
    generic abilities, 132
    goals, 81–82
    interpersonal interaction processes, 83–84

less than helpful responses, 97–98
    role of self-esteem, 23–25
    self-awareness, 26
    self knowledge, 26
    setting appropriate boundaries with patients/
        clients, 85–86
    sexuality and, 224–225
    therapeutic communication, 83, 86, 95–96
    therapeutic use of self, 4, 38–39, 82
    values underlying therapeutic responses, 98
health care system, economically driven, 34–35
health literacy, 190
hidden dimensions, 157–158
high context cultures, 154–156
higher self, 6
hostility curve, 118–119
human sexual response, 229–231
hypertension, 153–154

"I" statements, 100, 117, 118
identification, 84
implicit meanings, 157–158
individual process, 69
individualism, 34
information gathering, 171–172
instructional planning guidelines, 195–196
instrumental relativist orientation, 42
integrity, 8, 36, 62. See also ethics; moral values
intensive therapy level, PLISSIT model, 224
interactive processes, 85
intercultural communication, 153–154
intergenerational issues, 159
internal locus of control, 192–193
interpersonal concordance, 42
interpersonal interaction processes, 83–84
interpersonal values, 36–37
interviewing
    adolescents, 169
    example of nonhelpful interview, 173
    healing attitude, 168–169
    helpful attitude and skillful questioning, 168
    information gathered, 171
    nonverbal communication, 171–172, 171–172
    older patients, 170
    phrasing, 170
    skills required, 167–168, 172–173
    stages of, 170–171
    timing, 170

intimacy, 85–86
introjected values, 33–35

judgmental responses, 97
Jung, Carl, 5, 6
justice, 60, 67

kickbacks for referrals, 68–69
kinesthetic (K) systems, 138
Kohlberg, Lawrence, 40–42
Kübler-Ross, Elisabeth, 243, 246–247, 252–253

language factors in patient education, 197
"law and order" orientation, 42
leading, 137–138
lecture techniques, 197–198
legalism, 39
legislative issues, 212–214
life affirmation, 245
limited information level, PLISSIT model, 224
litigation, 135
Living Will, 251–252
locus of control, 192–193
low context cultures, 154–156

malpractice suits, 135
Maslow, Abraham, 229
maturation, 277–278
MCOs (managed care organizations), 65–66
Mead, Margaret, definition of culture, 152
meaning of life, questions, 3
medical model of patient education, 191
Medicare, 67
metabeliefs, 58
Middle Eastern cultures, 157
Millenials, 159
Miller, Alice, 23, 25
moral character, 58
moral developmentalists, 62–63
moral judgment, 58, 70
moral model of patient education, 191
moral motivation, 58
moral sensitivity, 58
moral temptations, 56
moral values. *See also* ethics
    components of moral action, 59
    consistent moral behavior, 63–64

discernment as a virtue, 64
identifying and resolving dilemmas
    alternatives, 57
    clinical decisions, 55–56
    nondiscursive approach, 62–63
    problem ownership, 98, 100
    problem-solving process, 69–70
    professional codes of ethics, 60–61
    suggested process for solving ethical prob-
        lems, 67–68
    types of decision-making opportunities, 56
    utilization of principles, 61–62
ingredients of moral decisions, 58
moral awareness versus moral consciousness,
    43
moral decision-making, 40–42
morality of justice, 156
vs nonmoral values, 35–36
problem-solving process, 68–69
underlying therapeutic responses, 98
mortality, 244. *See also* death
myocardial infarction, 233

Narcotics Anonymous (NA), 26
Nash, Robert, 62
National Standards for Culturally and Ling-
    uistically Appropriate Services in Health
    Care (CLAS), 197
near-death experiences, 244, 252
needs vs values, 35
negativity, 7–8
nervous systems, of children, 18
neurophysiology, 229–231
NLP (neurolinguistic psychology). *See also* com-
    munication skills; rapport; therapeutic
    communication
    historical perspectives, 134–135
    map vs territory it describes, 141
    meaning of communication, 135
    positive descriptive statements, 140
nondiscursive ethicists, 62–63
nonmaleficence, 60
nonmoral values, 35–36
nonverbal communication, 155, 158, 171–172
North American societies, 154
nutrition, 150–151

objectivist approach, 39
occupational therapists. *See* health care professionals
older patients, 170
oneness with life, 7
open (healthy) families, 23
Overeaters Anonymous, 26

pacing, 137–138
parental dysfunction, 24
passive responses, 113
patience, 8
patient education
    cultural and language factors, 197
    experiental techniques, 198–199
    health literacy, 190
    instructional planning guidelines, 195–196
    instructional techniques for working with groups, 197–198
    presentation tips, 196
    principles, 194–195
    responsibility for, 190–192
    sample materials for different grade levels, 201
    technology in, 199
Pellegrino, Edmund, 43, 61–62
pelvic phenomenon, 232
people-first language, 206
Perls, Fritz, 134
permission level, PLISSIT model, 224
persona, definition, 5
personal gain, 63
personal integrity, 62
personalismo, 158
Piaget, Jean, 18, 40
pity, 83–84
PLISSIT model, 223–224
Powell, J., 85
PPOs (prepaid health organizations), 65–66
practice acts, 65
preparatory depression, 247
presentation tips, 196
principle-oriented ethical systems, 59–60
principled ethical reasoning, 58, 61–62
privacy, 60
problem ownership, 98, 100
problem-solving process, 68–70
problems, 56

professionalism
    codes of ethics, 60–61
    ethics, 37–38
    professional duty, 36
    proficiency, 4
    values, 36
PRS (preferred representational systems)
    predicates, 138–139
    watching eye movements to ascertain, 139–140
pseudotolerance, 160
psychology of the self, 4–7
psychosocial theory of development, 19
punishment and obedience orientation, 42
Purtilo, Ruth, 67

quality of life, 243–244, 246
questioning techniques in patient education, 198

rapport ("bedside manner")
    definition, 131
    establishing, 135
    matching, 136–137
    pacing and leading, 137–138
Rath's seven requirements for a value, 40
reactive depression, 247
Realm-Individual Process-Situation Model, 67
realm principle, 69
reassurances, 97
reflection, 7, 99
Rehabilitation Act of 1973, 213
reincarnationists, 6
relational holism, 133–134
relativism, 39
representational systems, 138
Rest, James, 67
restatement, 99
results-oriented ethical systems, 59–60
RIPS professional analysis model, 66–68
Rogers, Carl
    on beliefs of effective helpers, 86–88
    list of introjected values, 34
    on self-awareness, 7, 9
    on self-transposal, 84
role-playing techniques, 198–199
rules of the house, 7
rules of veracity, 67

Satir, Virginia, 134
Schiavo, Terri, 251–252
self, 6, 8. *See also* death
self-awareness
    desire for, 4
    of health professionals, 26
    lack of, 7–8
    personal choices, 3
    psychology of the self, 4–7
    signs of growth in, 9
    through action, 26
self-centered behavior, 7
self-efficacy, 193
self-esteem
    acting assertively, 114–116
    definition, 24
    face communication, 156
    of health professionals, 23–25
    influence of family history, 18–22
self-examination, 86–87
self-interest, moral dilemmas, 56, 63
self knowledge, 26
self-respect, 156
self-transposal, 84
sexuality and disability
    acting out sexually, 226
    affected by medical conditions, 234
    body image, 226
    cultural variables, 227
    effective communication
        attitudes of health professionals, 223
        Bridge and Barnum statements, 227–228
        guidelines, 227
        historical perspectives, 222
        terminology, 222
    effects of illness, 226
    examples, 226
    hospitalization, 225–226
    medication considerations, 233
    myocardial infarction, 233
    myths, 228–229
    neurophysiology, 229–231
    PLISSIT model, 223–224
    self-esteem, 229
    spinal cord injury, 231–232
shadow, definition, 6
simulations in patient education, 199

social contract, legalistic orientation, 42
social responsibility, 36
somatization, 159
Southern European societies, 154
specific suggestions level, PLISSIT model, 224
spinal cord injury, 231–232
spiritual beliefs, 155
stability, 114
stigmatization, 211–212
stress management
    burnout, 264–267
    common stressors, 262
    definition of stress, 261–262
    intervention, 268–269
    misperceptions, 263–264
    physical effects of stress, 263
    prevention, 269
    stress development model, 263
subjectivism, 39
Swisher, Laura Lee (Dolly), 67, 68
sympathy, 83–84

teenagers, interviewing, 169
Telecommunications Act of 1996, 213
teleology, 62
therapeutic communication, 83, 95–96. *See also* assertiveness skills
therapeutic effectiveness, cultural influences, 152–153
therapeutic presence, 37–38
therapeutic use of self, 4, 38–39, 82
"third ear" process, 83, 85, 86
time and space issues, 157
total body response, 232
traditionalists, 159
trans-theoretical model, 194
transactional analysis literature, 5
transcultural studies, 153–154
transtheoretical model of patient education, 195
truth, all-knowing goodness, 7

unconscious, 5
universal-ethical principle orientation, 42
US Department of Commerce, predictions on population distribution, 151

values as determinants of behavior
    defining, 35
    effect on therapeutic presence, 37–38
    ethical consciousness, 39–40
    introjected, 33–35
    moral decision-making, 40–42
    moral versus nonmoral values, 35–36
    vs needs, 35
    professional values, 36
    reinforcing healing, 38–39
    values conflicts, 36–37
veracity, 60, 67

virtue ethics, 63–64
visual (V) systems, 138
voice matching, 136

Weiss, Brian L., 252
Western medical culture, 154
Whitfield, Charles, 23
women with disabilities, 215

young-old patients, 170

Zaner, Richard, *The Context of Self*, 4

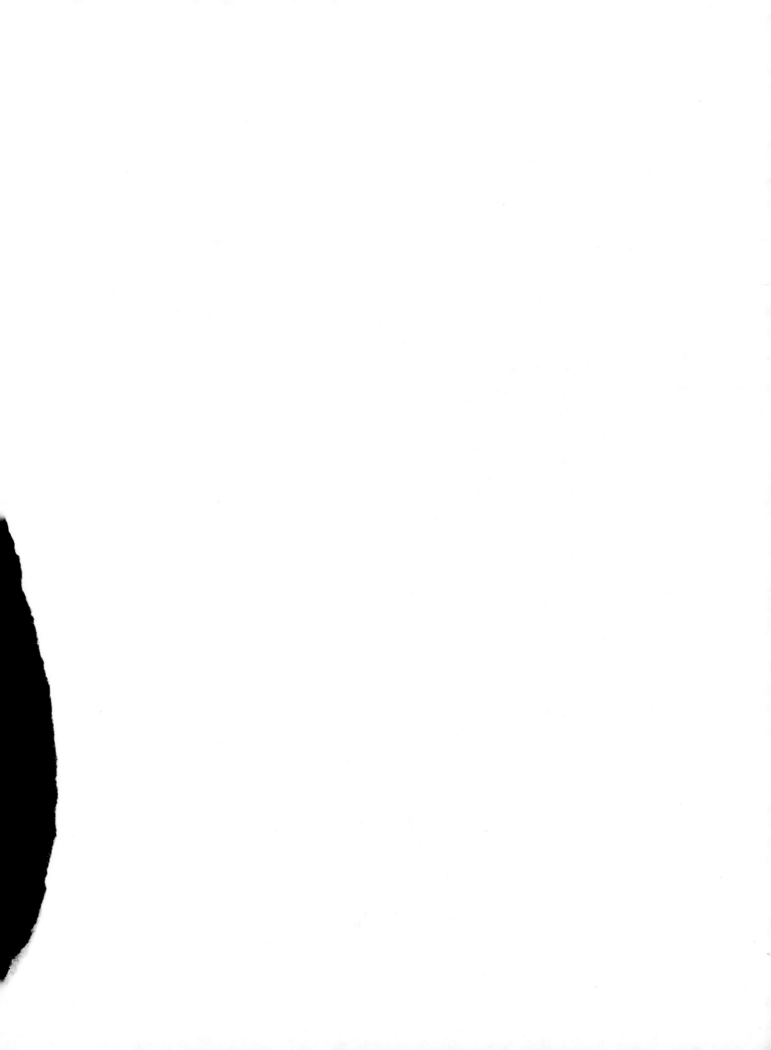

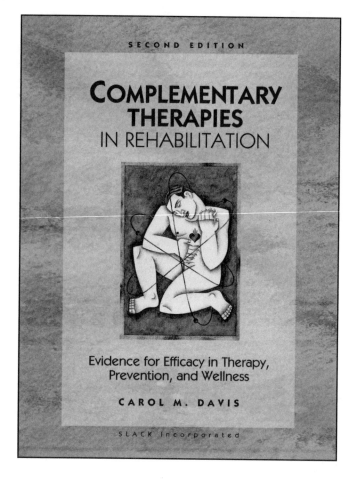
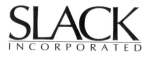